Biological Applications of Anti-Idiotypes

Volume I

Editor

Constantin A. Bona, M.D., Ph.D.
Professor of Microbiology
Mount Sinai School of Medicine
New York, New York

CRC Press, Inc.
Boca Raton, Florida

Library of Congress Cataloging-in-Publication Data

Biological applications of anti-idiotypes.

Bibliography: p.
Includes indexes.
1. Immunoglobulin idiotypes. I. Bona, Constantin A.
QR186.7.B565 1988 616.07′93 87-20833
ISBN 0-8493-6941-X (v. 1)
ISBN 0-8493-6942-8 (v. 2)
ISBN 0-8493-6940-1 (set)

Direct all inquiries to CRC Press, Inc., 2000 Corporate Blvd., N.W., Boca Raton, Florida, 33431.

International Standard Book Number 0-8493-6940-1 (Set)
International Standard Book Number 0-8493-6941-X (Volume I)
International Standard Book Number 0-8493-6942-8 (Volume II)

Library of Congress Card Number 87-20833
Printed in the United States

PREFACE

The most demanding aspect of editing a book dealing with a specialized scientific topic is covering a vast body of literature through which as much available information as possible on the subject is obtained. However, it is also undeniable that much is gained from this mandatory exercise, not only to have a deep insight into the intimate dialectic of a science and the evolution of its concepts, but also the position which a particular discipline occupies among the realm of the general sciences of nature is revealed.

Comparatively speaking, immunology is a young science. In contrast to many sciences conceived 25 centuries ago under a Hellenistic sky dominated by the postulate that the universe is governed by rules accessible to the human mind, immunology was born at the end of the last century. In spite of its youth, the rapidity at which progress in the understanding of a system was attained in immunology is rivaled in very few fields. Such an accomplishment is attributable to the application of the same principles of creativity which permitted comparable achievements in other disciplines.

The strategy of immunological research was based on analysis: namely, the dissection of the components of the immune system and synthesis of information into the formulation of concepts. Often, investigators possessed sufficient insight and understanding of their systems to allow them to cumulate concepts even before their analytical studies were completed.

Other elements have also contributed to the rapid progress in immunology. First, research tactics were continuously adapted to take advantage of recent technological advances. There is no doubt that the success of experimental work is directly related to the technological approaches employed. Second was the collective character of the research. This is probably related to the interdisciplinary character of the science. It is compulsory for an immunologist to not only keep abreast of the technology but also to be familiar with the principles of biology and medicine to understand the organization and function of the immune system and the implication of any alteration of these functions in various diseases. Of course, it is not possible to minimize the role which intuition plays in contributing to brilliant discoveries.

Intuition is an individual event which allows one to find the most suitable approach leading to a major scientific breakthrough.

I do not believe that intuition is due to chance. Rather, it represents an excellent chronological juxtaposition between the accumulation of a critical amount of analytical findings and the erudite ability of conceptual synthesis culminating in a giant strike forward. Only well-prepared persons can have such illuminating intuition.

The text of a scientific book requires a few basic elements which include the presentation of findings, concepts, and theories. The presentation of findings is an essential component of this type of publication when they are the fruit of correctly executed experiments that can be assigned to the category of "eternal truths" which are no longer susceptible to transformation or improvement. However, it should be recognized that there is a legion of findings whose presentation is just a means to achieve a more distinct goal.

Indeed, one may ask whether a histologist who spent his life peering through a microscope at slides made from a horse, in fact, knows how the horse looks or runs.

To study the lymphocyte (its structure and physiology), biosynthetic products, and genes is not a goal in itself; such studies achieve a meaningful aim only by the collective integration of all the knowledge which they provide into a coherent assembly. Newton perhaps provided the best example of this in science by understanding that the physical laws governing the fall of a stone also govern the movement of stars.

The presentation of concepts requires a keen selection process in order to retrieve from the reams of available information these seminal findings supporting the concepts as well as the exceptions. Two features should not be forgotten in this regard. First, concepts are not everlasting since they are formulated from a limited amount of available information.

It is intriguing to follow the rapid transformation of concepts and models in immunology as new findings are brought to light. The second is to place in the proper perspective the anthropocentric input in concepts which are aimed at defining objective laws to rationalize the phenomena. I feel that numerous concepts and models in immunology have too much anthropomorphic input; sometimes we must resist the temptation to formulate orderly rules for governing a system when our true mission is only to unravel them.

The third element is the presentation of theories, classifying the findings into categories in a coherent order, and integrating the concepts. Theories are also not timeless since the curiosity of the experimental investigator continuously generates new findings by challenging the established theories. Thus, the writing of a scientific book is just a beginning and each beginning is imperfect.

The goal of this book was to present findings which are supportive of the concept that the words of the idiotype dictionary and likewise self-recognition are essential for communication between lymphocyte clones while some unfaithful (''infidel'') copies of the words contained in the idiotype dictionary perhaps play a role in the functional regulation of nonlymphoid cells.

The notion of self-recognition as a regulatory force was very important for my understanding of idiotype regulation. Since immunology evolved as a discipline of microbiology, a major paradigm which dominated immunological theories was selection during phylogeny of lymphocytes to ensure the defense mechanisms. Therefore, the immune system is oriented solely towards the recognition of foreign antigens. We wanted to point out that idiotype mediated self-recognition is an important regulatory force within the immune system.

THE EDITOR

C. A. Bona, M.D., Ph.D., is Professor of Microbiology at Mount Sinai School of Medicine, New York.

Dr. Bona received his M.D. and Ph.D. degrees in Medical Science from the Faculty of Medicine, Bucharest, and his Docteur in Sciences Naturelles degree from Paris University.

Dr. Bona has published more than 150 papers in various national and international journals, 29 chapters in various monographs, 6 sections in textbooks, has edited 2 monographs, and has written 2 books on idiotypes.

His major research interest is in the idiotypy field in which he discovered the naturally occurring idiotype-specific T cells, regulatory idiotopes, epibodies, and the first demonstration that an anti-Id antibody can elicit (instead of an antigen) an immune response against a bacterial antigen. This observation stimulated the research in the utilization of idiotypes as vaccines.

CONTRIBUTORS

Volume I

Clifford J. Bellone, Ph.D.
Professor
Department of Microbiology
St. Louis University School of Medicine
St. Louis, Missouri

Kim Bottomly, Ph.D.
Associate Professor
Department of Pathology
Yale University Medical School
New Haven, Connecticut

Christian Cambillau, Dr. ès Sc.
Chargé de Recherche
Centre de Recherche sur les Mécanismes de Croissance Cristalline
Marseille, France

J.D. Capra, M.D.
Professor
Department of Microbiology
University of Texas Health Science Center at Dallas
Dallas, Texas

Dennis A. Carson, M.D.
Member
Basic and Clinical Research
Scripps Clinic and Research Foundation
La Jolla, California

Pierre-Andrè Cazenave, Ph.D.
Professor
Unité d'Immunochimie Analytique
Institut Pasteur
Paris, France

Pojen P. Chen, Ph.D.
Assistant Member
Basic and Clinical Research
Scripps Clinic and Research Foundation
La Jolla, California

Sylvie Corbet
Centre d'Immunologie
Institut National de la Santé et de la Recherche Médicale
Centre National de la Recherche Scientifique
Marseille, France

Frank W. Fitch, M.D., Ph.D.
Department of Pathology
and
The Ben May Institute
University of Chicago
Chicago, Illinois

Michel Fougereau, D.V.M., Dr Sci
Professor
Centre D'Immunologie
Institut National de la Santé et de la Recherche Médicale
Centre National de la Recherche Scientifique
Marseille, France

Sherman Fong, Ph.D.
Assistant Member
Basic and Clinical Research
Scripps Clinic and Research Foundation
La Jolla, California

Sundararajan Jayaraman, Ph.D.
Research Fellow
Department of Pathology
Harvard Medical School
Boston, Massachusetts

John F. Kearney
Professor
Department of Microbiology
University of Alabama
Birmingham, Alabama

Keith A. Knisley, Ph.D.
Postdoctoral Fellow
Department of Pathology
University of Texas Medical School
Houston, Texas

Gilbert Mazza, Dr. ès Sc.
Chargé de Recherche
Centre d'Immunologie
Institut National de la Santé et de la Recherche Médicale
Centre National de la Recherche Scientifique
Marseille, France

Kathryn Meeke, D.V.M.
Research Assistant Professor
Department of Microbiology
University of Texas Health Science Center at Dallas
Dallas, Texas

Michele Milili, Dr. Université
Technician
Centre d' Immunologie
Institut National de la Santé et de la Recherche Médicale
Centre National de la Recherche Scientifique
Marseille, France

Daniel Moinier, B.T.S.
Technician
Centre d'Immunologie
Institut National de la Santé et de la Recherche Médicale
Centre National de la Recherche Scientifique
Marseille, France

Philippe Ollier, M.D.
Centre d'Immunologie
Institut National de la Santé et de la Recherche Médicale
Centre National de la Recherche Scientifique
Marseille, France

Daniele Primi, Ph.D.
Unité d'Immunochimie Analytique
Institut Pasteur
Paris, France

José Rocca-Serra, Doctorat d'État
Maître de Conference 1 ère Classe
Centre d'Immunologie
Institut National de la Santé et de la Recherche Médicale
Centre National de la Recherche Scientifique
Marseille, France

L. Scott Rodkey, Ph.D.
Associate Professor
Department of Pathology
University of Texas Medical School
Houston, Texas

Claude Roth
Département d'Immunologie
Institut Pasteur
Paris, France

Claudine Schiff, Dr. ès Sc.
Chargé de Recherche
Centre d' Immunologie
Institut National de la Santé et de la Recherche Médicale
Centre National de la Recherche Scientifique
Marseille, France

Gerard Sommé, Dr. ès Sc.
Assistant
Département d'Immunologie
Institut Pasteur
Paris, France

J. Thèze, Dr. ès Sc.
Chef d' Unité
Département d'Immunologie
Institut Pasteur
Paris, France

Cécile Tonnelle, Dr. ès Sc.
Chargé de Recherche
Centre d'Immunologie
INSERM-CNRS
Marseille, France

Meenal Vakil, Ph.D.
Research Scientist
Department of Microbiology
University of Alabama
Birmingham, Alabama

Carol Victor-Kobrin, Ph.D.
Assistant Professor
Department of Microbiology
Mount Sinai School of Medicine
New York, New York

TABLE OF CONTENTS

Volume I

TABLE OF CONTENTS

Volume II

Chapter 1

ANTI-IDIOTYPES

C.A. Bona

TABLE OF CONTENTS

I. WHAT IS AN ANTI-IDIOTYPE?

The specificity of the antigen receptor of lymphocytic clones results from the recombination of various germline gene segments coding for the variable region of polypeptide chains of the receptor, as well as from somatic mutational events which occur within rearranged genes during the differentiation of lymphocytes.

Like enzymes, hormones, and other biologically active substances, the antigen receptor of lymphocytes has a dual property; it recognizes other chemically well-defined structures called *antigens* and can be recognized itself by virtue of its antigenic determinants called *idiotypes (Id), allotypes*, or *isotypes*.

Id are antigenic markers of the variable region of the receptor of B and T lymphocytes. Id can be divided into two major categories: individual Id (IdI) and cross-reactive Id (IdX). IdI are markers of somatic mutational events occurring in a single clone of a single individual. They reflect a discrete alteration of the genetic program of a single lymphocyte and its progeny and obviously are not inherited. IdX, on the other hand, are Id expressed on clones of various individuals of an outbred species, of all individuals of an inbred strain, and are inherited in a Mendelian manner. They are phenotypic markers of germline genes.

The Id were initially defined by serologic reagents,[1,2] which operationally were called anti-idiotypes (anti-Id). Later, it was shown that in both T- and B-cell compartments, there are clonally distributed lymphocytes which, through their combining site (also called paratope), can interact with the idiotopes borne by the antigen receptor of other clones. Indeed, the immune system of each individual contains four types of "anti-idiotypic" clones.

1. B cells producing antibodies recognizing the idiotope of the Ig receptor of other B cells. Such clones have been identified by using PFC assay in the spleens of animals immunized with antigens which elicit an oligoclonal antibody response characterized by a dominant IdX such as the antiphosphocholine or antiinulin response, respectively.[3,4] Kearney et al.[5] estimated that 18% of early B cells are anti-Id.
2. B cells which produce antibodies specific for the Id of T-cell receptor. These antibodies can recognize IdI of a single T-cell clone (also called clonotypic markers) or IdX, Id shared by various T-cell clones. Some of these antibodies then recognize IdX expressed on a large population of T cells. For example, F23.1 monoclonal antibody interacts with an Id of the Vβ chain of the T-cell receptor of about 20% of T cells from certain mouse strains.[6]
3. T-cell clones bearing an antigen receptor recognizing Id determinants of immunoglobulin receptor of B-cell clones. This type of T cell is also called an "Id-specific T cell". Such T cells were identified in various T-cell subsets such as suppressor,[7] helper,[8] or effector T cells.[9-11] It should be mentioned that Id-specific T cells can recognize Id determinants of Igs which are different from those serologically defined by anti-Id antibodies.[12]
4. T cells which recognize the Id of antigen receptor of other T cells. This kind of anti-Id T cell was described in a few experimental systems such as in animals with graft-vs.-host immunity[13] or immunity against allografts[14] (Figure 1).

We believe that the "anti-Id" B or T cells (Ab_2 lymphocytes) do not represent a particular set of clones which differ from B- or T-cell clones recognizing self, altered self, or foreign antigens (Ab_1 clones). Indeed, molecular studies showed that the usage of V gene families, the organization of gene segments encoding the variable region, and the structure of the genes are similar to those of Ab_1 antibodies.

The classification of Ab_1 and Ab_2 clones has its roots in didactics. Ab_1 clones were defined as the immunogens (i.e., Id), while the molecules obtained from immunized animals (i.e.,

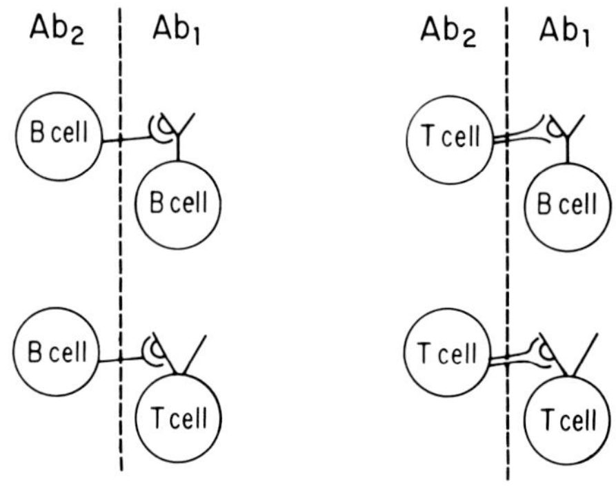

FIGURE 1. Symmetry of anti-Id (Ab_2) clones in B- and T-cell compartments.

anti-Id) were the Ab_2 clones. Actually, the interaction between clones within the immune system is based on the interaction of complementary contacting residues exposed on the surface of the antigen receptor of two different clones. These interactions can occur between the cleft or groove of one receptor and protrusion of another receptor of the lymphocyte, as well as between flat external surfaces of the receptor of two different clones. Therefore, the clones designated as Ab_1 or Ab_2 operationally define the interaction between complementary antigen receptors of two different clones.

II. PREPARATION OF ANTI-ID

The Id were discovered, studied, and characterized with anti-Id reagents. There are many ways to prepare anti-Id antibodies. While Kunkel et al.[1] prepared anti-Id antibodies in rabbits against human myeloma proteins by immunizing with soluble proteins, Oudin and Michel[2] prepared anti-Id antibodies in rabbits immunized with antigen-antibody complexes. Later, anti-Id antibodies were obtained by immunization with polymerized immunoglobulins or coupled with various protein carriers.[15] This method was particularly successful and used to prepare syngeneic anti-Id antibodies.

The specificity of anti-Id antibodies depends on on the method of immunization. Thus, Jorgensen et al.[16] have shown that there are important differences between anti-Id antibodies obtained in mice after immunization with soluble MOPC315 myeloma protein or subsequent to immunization with affinity labeled with bromoacetyl-DNP-L-lysine-MOPC315 complex. Whereas the immunization with soluble protein produced antibodies recognizing Id associated with the combining site, the immunization with affinity-labeled protein raised the productions of antibodies recognizing Id associated with framework segments.

Anti-Id antibodies against the Id of the antigen receptor of T cells were obtained subsequent to the immunization of T-cell clones or hybridoma clones[17] or mixed with adjuvants such as alum B pertussis.[18]

Based on the origin of anti-Id reagents, they can be classified into four categories:

1. Xenogeneic anti-Id obtained by the immunization of animals from different species
2. Allogeneic anti-Id obtained by the immunization across strain barriers or genetically different individuals of our outbred species
3. Syngeneic anti-Id antibodies obtained by the immunization of genetically identical individuals
4. Autologous anti-Id antibodies obtained by the immunization of the same individual from which the antibodies originated

III. WHAT RECOGNIZES AN ANTI-ID?

Anti-Id antibodies as well as Id-specific T cells define antigenic determinants of the variable region of polypeptide chains of the receptor of B and T cells. In order to localize idiotopes, it was important to establish the contribution of heavy and light chain variable regions to the expression of idiotopes borne by native molecules. In early studies, the localization of idiotopes was carried out using polyclonal anti-Id antibodies which are composed of a heterogeneous population of antibody molecules specific for various idiotopes. In the studies with anti-Id antibodies made against myeloma proteins, the bulk of antibodies required the combination of both heavy and light chains for expression of idiotopes.[19,20] The investigators rarely succeeded in obtaining anti-Id antibodies against Id of a single chain by immunization of animals with isolated heavy or light chain.

The general conclusion of these studies was that the combination of both chains is required for the expression of idiotopes. Utilization of monoclonal anti-Id antibodies and of synthetic peptides corresponding to Id determinants modified this general conclusion.

By using antibodies against synthetic peptides corresponding to the hypervariable regions of light chain (V_KIIIb) of human rheumatoid factors, Chen et al.[21] were able to determine that Wa IdX expressed on about 60% of human IgM paraproteins displaying rheumatoid factor activity is located on CDRII of variable region of light chain.

Analysis of the binding activity of a syngeneic monoclonal anti-Id antibody against PY206, an antibody specific for X31 influenza virus hemagglutinin, allowed us to determine that this antibody recognizes an idiotope located on heavy chain.[22] Indeed, this anti-Id antibody binds to PY206 native protein, as well as to heavy chain under reducing conditions, as was assessed by Western blotting analysis. By contrast, another monoclonal anti-Id antibody against VM202, an antibody specific for PR8 influenza virus hemagglutinin, binds only to native molecule and not to separate heavy or light chains[23] (Figure 2).

These data clearly show that the idiotopes recognized by anti-Id antibodies can be located on variable regions of heavy or light chain or to configurational antigenic determinants requiring the contribution of both heavy and light chains. This is also true in the case of anti-Id antibodies specific for Id of the receptor of T cells.

Recently, we prepared a syngeneic monoclonal antibody against a KLH-specific T-cell line. It also binds to a KLH-specific T-cell hybridoma called FN1-18 which recognizes the antigen with an I-E gene complementation product.[18] Study of the binding of this anti-Id antibody to variants of FN1-18 hybridoma which lost the ability to recognize KLH showed that this antibody still binds to FN1-18 variants. Molecular studies carried out on variants showed that they lost the ability to transcribe the rearranged V_β gene of the FN1-18 parental line, but synthesized the message of V_α FN1-18 and V_β of BW5147 lymphoma line used to prepare FN1-18 hybridoma.[24] These results strongly suggest that our syngeneic anti-Id antibody recognizes an idiotope located on V_α chain of FN1-18 T-cell hybridoma paired with the produce of V_β BW5147 (Table 1).

Anti-Id antibodies can recognize Id determinants associated with the combining site or with framework segments of the antigen receptor of T or B cells.

The binding of anti-Id antibodies to idiotopes associated with the combining site is inhibited by antigen. Inhibition of anti-IdX to Arsonate-binding antibodies by phenylarsonate was shown first by Brient et al.[25] and later in other antigenic systems. Similarly, in the case of T cells, an anti-Id antibody recognizing an idiotope associated with the paratope of T-cell receptor inhibits the recognition of the antigen. For example, we have shown that the binding of a syngeneic anti-Id antibody against a Lyt.1 KLH-specific helper T-cell clone inhibited the antigen-specific induced proliferation as well as the ability of this clone to help TNP-specific B cells to mount an anti-TNP-PFC response upon stimulation with TNP-KLH conjugate.[18]

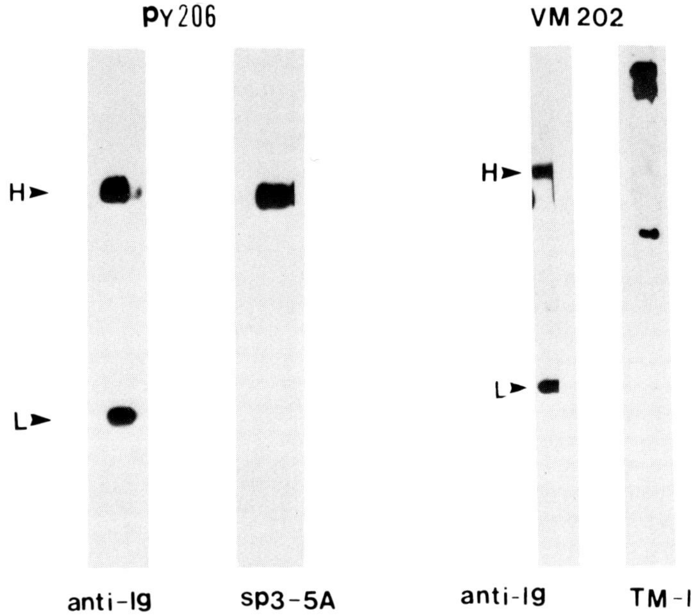

FIGURE 2. Western blots showing the binding of SP3-5A to only heavy chain of PY206 and of TM1 to only unreduced VM202 molecule.

Table 1
RELATIONSHIP BETWEEN TRANSCRIPTION OF T-CELL RECEPTOR V GENES AND THE EXPRESSION OF ID

	Rearrangement[a] of		mRNA message[b]			
T cells	V_α FN1-18	V_β FN1-18	V_α FN1-18	V_β FN1-18	V_β 86T1	FN1-18 Id[c]
FN1-18 hybridoma	+	+	+	+	+	+
BW5147	−	−	−	−	+	−
Irradiation-induced variants of FN1-18						
11	+	+	+	−	+	−
26	+	+	+	−	+	−

[a] Data obtained by Southern blotting.
[b] Data obtained by Northern blotting.
[c] Data obtained by RIA assays.

The second category of anti-Id antibodies recognizes idiotopes associated with framework segments of variable region. The reaction between anti-Id antibodies and framework-located idiotopes is not inhibited by the antigens. This category of anti-Id antibodies was clearly defined in a study carried out by Mudgett et al.[26] on rabbit anti-Id antibodies against homogenous anti-Streptococcus C antibodies. The immunodominant sugar of Streptococcus C polysaccharide is 3-0-2, *N*-acetylgalactosoaminosyl-*N*-acetylgalactosamine. The authors found in anti-Id antisera two families of antibodies: one eluted from Id immunoadsorbents with hapten and another with ammonium thiocyanate. The binding of the second population of antibodies to Id-bearing antibodies was not inhibited by hapten, since these antibodies bound to framework segments which do not contribute to the combining site of anti-Streptococcus C polysaccharide antibodies.

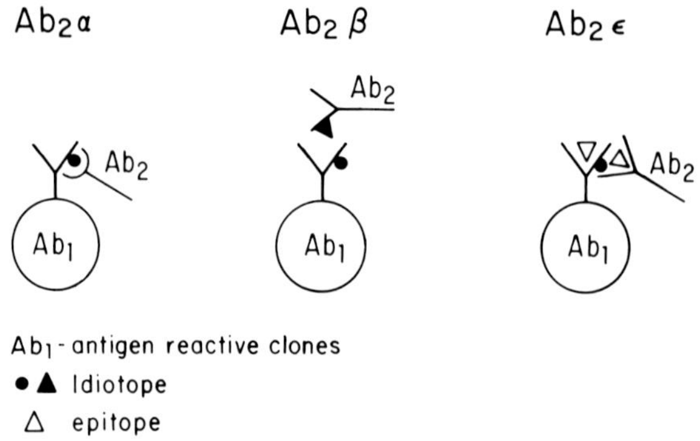

FIGURE 3. Binding particularities of $Ab_{2\alpha,\ \beta}$, and $_{\epsilon}$ to paratopes of various Ab_1.

As was mentioned above, anti-Id antibodies or T cells can distinguish between IdI and IdX. The IdX defined by anti-Id antibodies can be classified in these major categories:

1. Interspecies IdX expressed by antibodies with same antigen binding activity synthesized by various species
2. Interstrain IdX expressed by antibodies with the same specificity produced by various strains in case of a species with inbred strains
3. Intrastrain IdX expressed by antibodies produced by the individuals of a given strain.

The presence of IdX is related to the presence of DNA segments in the V gene encoding the specificity of a given antibody molecule which was conserved during phylogeny among various species or various inbred strains.

IV. FUNCTIONAL CLASSIFICATION OF ANTI-ID ANTIBODIES

Anti-Id antibodies and probably Id-specific T cells are produced by a heterogeneous population of clones which display various functions. There are numerous experimental data which demonstrated that anti-Id antibodies have a regulatory effect and are able to either stimulate or suppress the immune response (see data reviewed in Reference 27).

The enhancing and suppressive effect depends on the affinity and the amount of intentionally administered or spontaneously produced anti-Id antibodies during a given immune response against foreign or self-antigens.

It is well established that while minute amounts of anti-Id antibodies have an enhancing effect, the high concentrations cause suppression.[28,29] Jerne et al.[30] classified anti-Id antibodies into two categories, $Ab_{2\alpha}$ and $Ab_{2\beta}$. We recently added to this classification a third category, $Ab_{2\epsilon}$, standing for epibodies[31] (Figure 3).

There are no well-defined immunochemical, structural, or tridimensional properties which can distinguish these three categories of anti-Id antibodies.

$Ab_{2\alpha}s$ are produced by clones which recognize idiotopes on the receptor of B- or T-cell lymphocytes. Binding of these anti-Id antibodies to the antigen receptor of B lymphocytes can induce either activation or suppression of the corresponding clones, depending on the dose of the anti-Id antibodies. The enhancing effect is due to the direct binding of anti-Id to B cells. Rubinstein et al.[45] have shown that the $A48Id^+$ anti-levan response induced by the administration after birth of minute amounts (10 to 100 ng) of anti-A48Id antibodies can be transferred by B cells alone.

However, this does not preclude a T-cell involvement when allogeneic or xenogeneic

Table 2
EFFECT OF ANTI-ID ANTIBODY ON THE ANTIGEN RECOGNITION AND PROLIFERATION OF A T-CELL HYBRIDOMA (FN1-18)

FN1-18 incubated with	IL-2 production
Nil	−
KLH	−
$CB6F_1$ spleen cells	−
$CB6F_1$ spleen cells + KLH	+
$CB6F_1$ spleen cells + KLH + anti-Id antibody (μ)	−
$CB6F_1$ spleen cells + KLH + MOPC104 (μ)	+

Note: +, significant IL-2 production.

Table 3
ACTIVATION OF AN AUTOREACTIVE T-CELL HYBRIDOMA BY F23.1 SEPHAROSE® 4.B BEADS

QW 64 hybridoma	IL-2 production
Stimulated with nil	−
$CB6F_1$ spleen cells	+
F23.1 Sepharose® beads	+
BSA — Sepharose® beads	−

anti-Id are used. By contrast, the suppressive effect can be caused either by direct interaction of anti-Id antibodies with B cells, as was clearly documented in the inulin antigenic system,[29] or by the expansion of suppressor T cells, as was suggested in the phenylarsonate system. Indeed, in this system, Owen et al.[32] described IdX specific suppressor T cells, an observation not supported by other investigators. Thus, Rothstein et al.[33] have shown that the suppression of the IdX arsonate antibody response induced by anti-Id antibodies cannot be transferred by T cells. Similarly, anti-Id antibodies against the antigen receptor of T cells also have an enhancing or suppressor effect.

An enhancing effect was observed with anti-Id antibodies coupled with Sepharose® 4B either directed against individual[34] or largely cross-reactive Id.[6] For example, Staerz et al.[6] have shown that F23.1 monoclonal antibody specific for an antigenic determinant of the V_β chain stimulates cytolytic T-cell clones. Quartin et al.,[35] using the same antibody coupled to Sepharose® 4B, were able to stimulate the production of IL-2 of an autoreactive T-cell hybridoma (Table 2). Other anti-Id antibodies have an inhibitory effect on antigen-induced proliferation of T-cell clones or IL-2 production by T-cell hybridomas. For example, the incubation of a syngeneic anti-Id antibody raised by the immunization with a KLH-specific T-cell line inhibited the IL-2 production induced by incubation with antigen of a KLH-specific T-cell hybridoma[24] (Table 3).

I believe that we do not have a clear-cut explanation for the ability of some anti-Id antibodies to stimulate or inhibit T cells. However, it is apparent that both stimulatory or inhibitory effects of anti-Id antibodies have a direct effect on B or T cells. This concept is strongly supported by the studies involving the stimulation of T-cell clones or hybridomas by F23.1 antibody coupled to Sepharose® 4B beads. The presentation of anti-Id on beads is probably necessary, because of the low density of the antigen receptor associated with the membrane of lymphocytes.

This indicates that the effect of $Ab_{2\alpha}$ is not MHC-restricted antigen presentation and probably does not require active processing by antigen-presenting cells. In the case of B cells, $Ab_{2\alpha}$ exerts its effect in a T-independent manner, and like T-independent antigens, it stimulates the expansion of clones in small amounts and is tolerogenic in high amounts, causing suppression.

$Ab_{2\beta}s$ are anti-Id antibodies representing the internal image of the antigens. The internal image concept was introduced as a statistical necessity in the network theory.[36] If we can somehow average the three-dimensional structure of V domains of antibodies and of antigenic determinants, we should accept that the idiotopes cross react with foreign epitopes. Stated in another way, they are the internal image of the foreign antigens. There are several examples which support the concept of internal image, demonstrating that anti-Id antibodies can mimic various biologically active substances such as hormones,[37] vitamins,[38] ligand for the various receptor somatic cells,[39-41] and viral,[42-46] bacterial,[45,47] and parasitic[48,49] antigens. The receptor of various somatic cells for biologically active substances or the paratope of the antigen receptor of lymphocytic clones specific for foreign antigens sees the Id of $Ab_{2\alpha}$ like a biologically active ligand or as a foreign antigen, respectively. This interaction can be visualized as a paratope-Id binding or, in a broader view, as the interaction between two active sites. Because the chemical nature of the antigens mimicked by the $Ab_{2\beta}$ can be very different, it should be accepted that three-dimensional structures should be responsible for this molecular mimicking phenomenon. The most important consequence of this mimicking is the ability of antigen and $Ab_{2\beta}$ to compete for the same receptor. However, the binding of an $Ab_{2\beta}$ to a receptor for a foreign antigen or a receptor of a somatic cell for a biologically active substance should be of low affinity. I believe that the binding of an $Ab_{2\beta}$ mimicking a hormone will never reach the level of the affinity of the hormone for the receptor (e.g., 10^{-8} to 10^{-10} *M*).

If, indeed, the affinity of $Ab_{2\beta}$ for the receptor is low, then the $Ab_{2\beta}$ which is able to stimulate T cells instead of foreign antigens will require antigen presentation and, consequently, H-2 restriction recognition. Since it is known that helper or inducer cells require the association of foreign antigen with Class II MHC-encoded determinants and cytolytic T cells require Class I determinants, in principle, the stimulation of these T cells by $Ab_{2\beta}$ may require the presentation of anti-Id processed by accessory cells in context of Class II or I MHC-encoded antigens in order to stimulate helper or cytolytic cells, respectively.

There are several criteria which have been proposed to distinguish $Ab_{2\alpha}$ from $Ab_{2\beta}$. Until now, there has not been a universal immunochemical criterion useful to predict an anti-Id antibody exhibiting $Ab_{2\alpha}$ or $Ab_{2\beta}$ properties. Therefore, we proposed two functional criteria to distinguish these two categories of anti-Id antibodies.

A. Presentation of Anti-Id in the Context of Self-MHC-Encoded Antigens

An $Ab_{2\alpha}$, exhibiting a high affinity and interacting with the complementary Id of T- or B-lymphocytic receptor, can expand the proliferation of clones without processing anti-Id antibody and circumventing genetic restriction requirements. Indeed, anti-Id antibodies against the Id of the T-cell receptor can induce clonal proliferation in the absence of antigen processing cells by incubation of T cells with soluble anti-Id antibody or coupled to Sepharose® 4B beads.[6] Similarly, they can expand B cells in a T-independent manner.[47] By contrast, an $Ab_{2\beta}$, at least in the case of T cells, should be presented like antigen in the context of MHC-encoded antigens. If this assumption is correct, then we should conclude that the activation of B cells by $Ab_{2\beta}$ requires antigen presentation and is a T-dependent phenomenon.

This hypothesis is supported by recent data indicating that the antibodies, coupled with dendritic cells, have a stronger immunogenic effect compared to soluble antibodies.[50] Thus, whereas the stimulatory (and, perhaps, suppressive) effect of $Ab_{2\alpha}$ is pseudorestricted, the effect of $Ab_{2\beta}$ is a genetically restricted phenomenon (Figure 4).

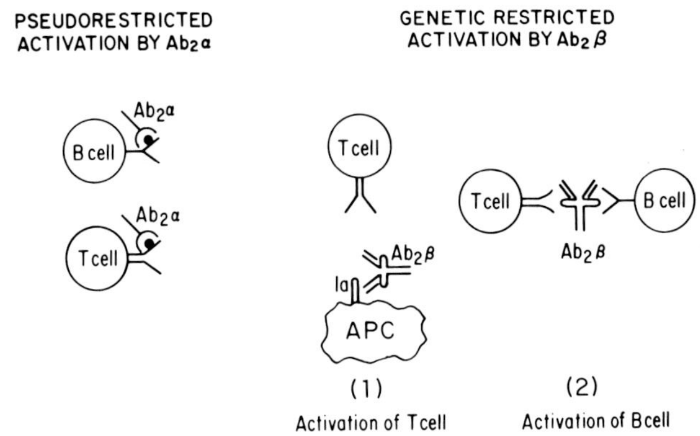

FIGURE 4. Activation pathways of B and T lymphocytes by $Ab_{2\alpha}$ and $Ab_{2\beta}$.

B. Qualitative Differences between Clones Activated by $Ab_{2\alpha}$ and $Ab_{2\beta}$

If there are qualitative differences between $Ab_{2\alpha}$ and $Ab_{2\beta}$, we may predict a different pattern of the activation of clones induced by these two categories of antibodies.

The priming effect of $Ab_{2\beta}$ is related to the binding of anti-Id antibody to a complementary Id expressed on the receptor of lymphocytic clones. From Oudin's and Cazenave's observation,[51] it was clearly established that the same idiotope can be shared by clones with various antigen specificities.

Then we predict that an $Ab_{2\alpha}$ will stimulate clones

- Id^+ $antigen^+$ (Ab_1)
- Id^+ $antigen^-$, i.e., expressing an antigen binding specificity different from that of Ab_1 (parallel set)
- Id^- $antigen^-$, i.e., anti-anti-Id clones able to bind only to the idiotope of $Ab_{2\alpha}$

$Ab_{2\beta}$ mimics the antigen.

Therefore, we can predict that an $Ab_{2\beta}$ will essentially stimulate clones reactive with antigen, i.e.,

- Id^+ $antigen^+$ (Ab_1)
- Id^- $antigen^+$ (Ab'_1)

These two criteria could represent a working hypothesis to distinguish these two major categories of Ab_2.

C. $Ab_{2\epsilon}$

Recently, we defined a third category of anti-Id antibodies which we designated as epibodies. An epibody is an anti-Id antibody that reacts with an antigen and with an idiotope of an antibody towards the same antigen.[31] The epibodies are a heterogeneous family of antibodies, since they are anti-Id antibodies which react with self-antigens, anti-Id antibodies which react with foreign antigens, and even anti-Id antibodies which can react with their own idiotopes (e.g., antibodies[43]).

The existence of epibodies is, perhaps, important in the understanding of the role of anti-Id antibodies in autoimmune diseases, since such an antibody can activate autoreactive clones instead of autoantigens. This category of anti-Id antibodies is an example of multispecific antibodies as well as an image of the Id network within a single paratope.[53]

REFERENCES

1. **Kunkel, H. G., Mannick, M., and Williams, R. C.,** Individual antigenic specificity of isolated antibodies, *Science,* 140, 1218, 1963.
2. **Oudin, J. and Michel, M.,** Une nouvelle forme d'allotype des globulines du serum de lapin apparement lie a la fouction et a la specificite anticerps, *C.R. Acad. Sci. (Paris),* 257, 805, 1963.
3. **Cosenza, H.,** Detection of antiidiotype reactive cells in the response to phosphocholine, *Eur. J. Immunol.,* 6, 114, 1976.
4. **Bona, C., Lieberman, R., Chien, C. C., Mond, J., House, S., Green, I., and Paul, W. E.,** Immune response to levan. I. Kinetics and ontogeny of anti-levan and anti-inulin antibody response and expression of crossreactive idiotype, *J. Immunol.,* 120, 1436, 1978.
5. **Kearney, J. F. and Vakil, M.,** Functional idiotype networks during B cell ontogeny, *Ann. Inst. Pasteur (Immunol.),* 137C, 77, 1986.
6. **Staerz, U. D., Rammensee, H. G., Benedetto, J. D., and Bevan, M. J.,** Characterization of a murine monoclonal antibody specific for an allotypic determinant on the T cell antigen receptor, *J. Immunol.,* 134, 3994, 1985.
7. **Bona, C. and Paul, W. E.,** Cellular basis of expression of idiotypes. I. Suppressor cells specific for MOPC460 idiotype regulate the expression of cells secreting anti-trinitrophenyl antibodies bearing 460 idiotype, *J. Exp. Med.,* 144, 592, 1979.
8. **Bottomly, K. and Mosier, D. E.,** Mice whose B cells cannot produce the T15 idiotype also lack an antigen-specific helper T cell required for T15 expression, *J. Exp. Med.,* 150, 1399, 1979.
9. **Sherr, D. H., Ju, S. T., and Dorf, M. E.,** Hapten-specific T cell responses to 4-hydroxy-3-nitrophenyl acetyl. XII. Fine specificity of antiidiotypic suppressor T cells (Ts2), *J. Exp. Med.,* 154, 1382, 1981.
10. **Jayarman, S. and Bellone, C. J.,** Hapten-specific responses to the phenyltrimethyl amino hapten. III. Mice whose delayed-type hypersensitivity responses cannot be abrogated by the presence of anti-idiotypic suppressor T cells lack a critical modulatory T cell function, *J. Exp. Med.,* 155, 1810, 1982.
11. **Binz, H. and Wigzell, H.,** Induction of specific immune unresponsiveness with purified mixed leucocyte culture-activated T-lymphoblasts as autoimmunogen. III. Proof for the existence of autoantiidiotypic killer T cells and transfer of suppression to normal syngeneic recipients by T or B lymphocytes, *J. Exp. Med.,* 147, 63, 1978.
12. **Gleason, K. and Kohler, H.,** Regulatory idiotopes. T helper cells recognize a shared VH idiotope on phosphorylcholine-specific antibodies, *J. Exp. Med.,* 156, 539, 1982.
13. **Kimura, H. and Wilson, D. B.,** Antiidiotypic cytotoxic T cells in rats with graft-versus-host disease, *Nature,* 308, 463, 1984.
14. **Lancaster, F., Chui, Y. L., and Batchelor, J. R.,** Antiidiotypic T cells suppress rejection of renal allografts in rats, *Nature,* 315, 336, 1985.
15. **Bona, C., Hooghe, R., Cazenave, P.-A., LeGuern, C., and Paul, W. E.,** Cellular basis of regulation of expression of idiotypes. II. Immunity to anti-MOPC460 idiotype antibodies increases the level of anti-trinitrophenyl antibodies bearing 460 idiotypes, *J. Exp. Med.,* 149, 815, 1979.
16. **Jorgensen, T., Gaudernack, G., and Hannestad, K.,** Immunization with the light chain and the V_L domain of the isologous myeloma protein 315 inhibits growth of mouse plasmacytoma MOPC-315, *Scand. J. Immunol.,* 11, 29, 1980.
17. **Infante, A. J., Infante, P. D., Gillis, S., and Fathman, C. G.,** Definition of T-cell idiotopes using antiidiotypic antisera produced by immunization with T cell clones, *J. Exp. Med.,* 155, 1100, 1982.
18. **Waters, S. J., Luzzatti, P. R., and Bona, C. A.,** Functional properties of T cell clones with a double specificity for alloantigens and foreign antigens, *J. Exp. Med.,* 160, 1300, 1984.
19. **Vrana, M., Rudikoff, S., and Potter, M.,** Sequence variation among heavy chains from inulin-binding myeloma proteins, *Proc. Natl. Acad. Sci. U.S.A.,* 75, 1957, 1978.
20. **Eichmann, K.,** Expression and function of idiotypes on lymphocytes, *Adv. Immunol.,* 26, 195, 1978.
21. **Chen, P. P., Fong, S., Normansell, D., Houghten, R. A., Karras, J. G., Vaughan, J. H., and Carson, D. A.,** Delineation of a cross-reactive idiotype on human autoantibodies with antibody against a synthetic peptide, *J. Exp. Med.,* 159, 1502, 1985.
22. **Moran, T. M., Monestier, M., Lai, A. C. K., Norton, G., Reale, M. A., Thompson, M. A., Schulman, J. L., Riblet, R., and Bona, C. A.,** Characterization of variable region genes and shared cross-reactive idiotypes of antibodies specific for antigens of various influenza viruses, *Virol. Immunol.,* 1, 1, 1987.
23. **Reale, M. A., Manheimer, A. J., Moran, T. M., Norton, G., Bona, C. A., and Schulman, J. L.,** Characterization of monoclonal antibodies specific for sequential influenza A/PR/8/34 virus variants, *J. Immunol.,* 137, 1352, 1986.
24. **Gascoigne, N. R. J., Waters, S., Elliott, J. F., Victor-Kobrin, C., Goodnow, C., Davis, M. M., and Bona, C. A.,** Expression of T cell receptor genes in an antigen-specific hybridoma and radiation-induced variants, *J. Exp. Med.,* 164, 113, 1986.

25. **Brient, B. W. and Nisonoff, A.,** Quantitative investigation of idiotypic antibodies. IV. Inhibition by specific haptens of the reaction of anti-hapten antibody with its idiotypic antibody, *J. Exp. Med.*, 132, 951, 1970.
26. **Mudgett, M., Coligan, J. E., and Kindt, T. J.,** Isolation and characterization of distinct antibody populations from antisera directed against idiotypes of rabbit homogenous antibodies, *J. Immunol.*, 120, 293, 1978.
27. **Bona, C. and Moran, T.,** Idiotype vaccines, *Ann. Immunol. (Inst. Pasteur)*, 136C, 299, 1985.
28. **Kohler, H.,** The response to phosphorylcholine: dissecting an immune response, *Tranplant. Rev.*, 27, 24, 1975.
29. **Bona, C., Lieberman, R., House, S., Green, I., and Paul, W. E.,** Immune response to levan. II. T-independence of suppression of cross-reactive idiotypes by antiidiotype antibodies, *J. Immunol.*, 122, 1614, 1979.
30. **Jerne, N. K., Roland, J., and Cazenave, P. A.,** Recurrent idiotopes and internal images, *EMBO J.*, 1, 243, 1982.
31. **Bona, C. A., Finley, S., Waters, S., and Kunkel, H. G.,** Antiimmunoglobulin antibodies. III. Properties of sequential antiidiotypic antibodies to heterologous anti-λ-globulins. Detection of reactivity of antiidiotype antibodies with epitopes of Fc fragments (homobodies) and with epitopes and idiotopes (epibodies), *J. Exp. Med.*, 156, 986, 1982.
32. **Owen, F. L., Ju, S.-T., and Nisonoff, A.,** Presence on idiotype-specific suppressor T cells of receptors that interact with molecules bearing the idiotypes, *J. Exp. Med.*, 145, 1559, 1977.
33. **Rothstein, T. L., Miller, R. A., Parker, D. J., Kelly, E., Vastola, P., and Marshak-Rothstein, A.,** Induction of idiotype suppression in the antiazophenyl arsonate response of T-de-leted A/J mice, *J. Exp. Med.*, 159, 1283, 1984.
34. **Haskins, K., Hannum, C., White, J., Roehm, N., Kubo, R., Kappler, J., and Marrack, P.,** The major histocompatibility complex-restricted antigen receptor on T cells. VI. An antibody to receptor allotype, *J. Exp. Med.*, 160, 452, 1984.
35. **Quartin, R. S., Monestier, M., Moran, T. M., Waters, S. J., Fredrickson, G. G., and Bona, C. A.,** Characterization of the fine specificity and antigen markers associated with the receptor of autoreactive T cell hybridomas, *J. Immunol.*, submitted.
36. **Jerne, N. K.,** Towards a network theory of the immune response, *Ann. Immunol. (Paris)*, 125C, 373, 1974.
37. **Sege, K. and Paterson, P. A.,** Use of antiidiotypic antibodies as cell-surface receptor probes, *Proc. Natl. Acad. Sci.*, 75, 2443, 1978.

37. **Sege, K. and Paterson, P. A.,** Use of antiidiotypic antibodies as cell-surface receptor probes, *Proc. Natl. Acad. Sci.*, 75, 2443, 1978.

38. **Sege, K. and Peterson, P. A.,** Antiidiotypic antibodies against antivitamin A transporting protein react with prealbumin, *Nature (London)*, 271, 167, 1978.
39. **Wassermann, N. H., Penn, A. S., Freimuth, P. I., Treptow, N., Wentzel, S., Cleveland, W. L., and Erlanger, B. F.,** Antiidiotypic route to anti-acetylcholine receptor antibodies and experimental myasthenia gravis, *Proc. Natl. Acad. Sci. U.S.A.*, 79, 4810, 1982.
40. **Schreiber, A. B., Conrand, P. O., Andre, C., Vray, B., and Strossberg, A. D.,** Anti-alprenelol anti-Id antibodies bind to β-adrenergic receptors and modulate catecholamine-sensitive adenylate cyclase, *Proc. Natl. Acad. Sci. U.S.A.*, 77, 7385, 1980.
41. **Marasco, W. A. and Becker, E. L.,** Antiidiotype as antibody against formyl peptide chemotaxis receptor of the neutrophil, *J. Immunol.*, 128, 963, 1982.
42. **Kennedy, R. C. and Dressman, C. R.,** Enhancement of the immune response to hepatitis B surface antigen: in vivo administration of antiidiotype induces anti-HBs that express a similar idiotype, *J. Exp. Med.*, 159, 655, 1984.
43. **Regan, K. J., Wunner, W. H., Wiktor, T., and Koprowski, H.,** Antiidiotypic antibodies induce neutralizing antibodies to rabies virus glycoproteins, *J. Virol.*, 48, 660, 1983.
44. **Uytdehaag, F. G. C. M. and Osterhaus, A. D. M. E.,** Induction of neutralizing antibody in mice against poliovirus type II with monoclonal antiidiotypic antibody, *J. Immunol.*, 134, 1225, 1985.
45. **Rubinstein, L. J., Goldberg, B., Hiernaux, J., Stein, K. E., and Bona, C. A.,** Idiotype-antiidiotype regulation. V. The requirement for immunization with antigen or monoclonal antiidiotypic antibodies for the activation of β2-6 and β2-1 polyfructosan reactive clones in BALB/c mice treated at birth with minute amounts of anti-A48 idiotype antibodies, *J. Exp. Med.*, 158, 1129, 1983.
46. **Stein, K. and Soderstrom, J.,** Neonatal administration of idiotype or antiidiotype primes for protection against *Escherichia coli* K13 infection in mice, *J. Exp. Med.*, 160, 1001, 1984.
47. **McNamara, M. K., Ward, R. E., and Kohler, H.,** Monoclonal idiotype vaccine against Streptococcus pneumoniae infection, *Science*, 226, 1325, 1985.

48. **Sachs, D. L.,** Induction of protective immunity using antiidiotypic antibodies: immunization against experimental trypanosomiasis, in *Idiotypy in Biology and Medicine,* Kohler, H., Urbain, J., and Cazenave, P. A., Eds., Academic Press, New York, 1984, 401.
49. **Grzyck, J. M., Capron, M., Lambert, P. H., Dissons, C., Torres, S., and Capron, A.,** An antiidiotypic vaccine against experimental schistosomiasis, *Nature,* 316, 74, 1985.
50. **Francotte, M. and Urbain, J.,** Enhancement of antibody response by mouse dendritic cells pulsed with tobacco mosaic virus or with rabbit antiidiotypic antibodies raised against a private rabbit idiotype, *Proc. Natl. Acad. Sci. U.S.A.,* 82, 8149, 1985.
51. **Oudin, J. and Cazenave, P. A.,** Similar idiotypic specificites in immunoglobulin fractions with different antibody functions or even without detectable antibody function, *Proc. Natl. Acad. Sci. U.S.A.,* 68, 2616, 1971.
52. **Bona, C. A. and Pernis, B.,** Idiotype networks, in *Fundamental Immunology,* Paul, W. E., Ed., Raven Press, New York, 1984, 577.
53. **Bona, C. A., Kang, C. Y., Kohler, H., and Monestier, M.,** Epibody: the image of the network created by a single antibody, *Immunol. Rev.,* 90, 115, 1986.

Chapter 2

STRUCTURE AND GENETICS OF AB2

K. Meek and J. D. Capra

TABLE OF CONTENTS

I. INTRODUCTION

Jerne put forth a hypothesis in 1974 that has intrigued immunologists for more than a decade.[1] He proposed that the immune response might be regulated via the unique antigenic determinants of immunoglobulin variable regions (idiotypes, Id) described earlier by Kunkel[2] and Oudin.[3] The Id determinants of each antibody molecule would be complemented by those of another, allowing protein interactions between antibody molecules, creating an Id network through which immunoglobulin expression might be controlled. A multitude of experiments followed in which manipulation of the immune response was achieved through the use of anti-idiotypic (anti-Id) reagents.[4] These studies have generally strengthened his hypothesis.

Jerne extended his ideas in 1982 by grouping Ab_2s into two functional subsets: those that recognize determinants present in the V region, and those that represent internal images of the original antigen.[5] He proposed that Ab_2s that represent internal images of the original antigen might be important in the establishment of the B-cell repertoire — with no requirement for foreign antigen. Thus, the Id network might not only be functionally important in the regulation of immune responses, but may also play a role in the establishment of the immune repertoire.

Anti-Id antibodies of both types have been described by several groups in several systems.[6,7] However, the immune repertoire is nearly complete in its capability to respond to protein antigens — immunoglobulin or not. The existence, then, of anti-Id antibodies does not necessarily infer their relevance. Thus, the physiologic significance of the Id network continues to be a source of debate.

Jerne's network theory can most simply be illustrated as follows:

$$\text{Antigen} \rightarrow Ab_1 \leftrightarrow Ab_2 \leftrightarrow Ab_3 \leftrightarrow \ \ldots \text{etc.}$$

He suggested that these interacting molecules could be generated directly from germline; not from somatic variation. Indeed, it seems logical that if anti-Id antibodies are functionally crucial, their generation should not be random. It would follow that an anti-Id response to a homogeneous antibody response should be uniform in usage of germline gene segments. Hapten systems are ideal for approaching the question of a germline-encoded network, because unlike the responses to many protein antigens, the primary responses to haptens are often homogeneous. It is not coincidental, then, that most of our knowledge of structural characteristics of anti-Id antibodies (the focus of this chapter) comes from the hapten systems.

The amount of structural information of Ab_2s available is currently somewhat limited. However, because of a heightened interest in anti-Id antibodies in therapeutics and new more efficient molecular techniques, this body of information should be greatly expanded in the next few years. At this time, we are limited to the information generated in three systems: NP, GAT, and Ars. Each system will be discussed separately, and then the parallels which can be drawn among the three will be discussed. It should be noted that with certain exceptions, the anti-Id antibodies discussed here all recognize well-characterized, recurrent murine Id. The Ab_2s studied in the NP and GAT systems are all syngeneic; both syngeneic and allogeneic Ab_2s have been studied in the arsonate system.

II. STUDIES IN THE ANTI-NP SYSTEM

Sablitzky and Rajewsky in the NP system were the first to report detailed structural information on a group of anti-Id antibodies.[8] The response of the C57BL/6 strain to the hapten (4-hydroxy-3nitro-phenyl)acetyl (NP) consists primarily of antibodies derived from one VH gene (VH186.2) and one V/(V/1) gene.[9,10] Rajewsky's group completely sequenced

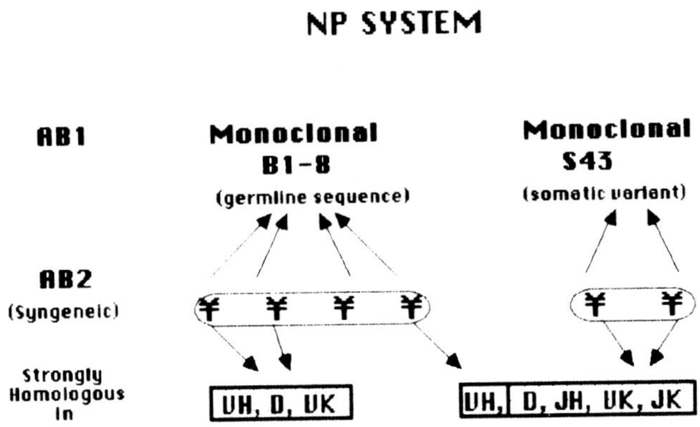

FIGURE 1. Schematic drawing of the NP anti-Id system. Circles denote serologically related groups of anti-Id antibodies. Filled squares and arrows denote structurally related molecules.

the heavy and light chain variable regions of six syngeneic monoclonal Ab_2s in this system. The antibodies were derived in two ways. Four were derived from fusions of mice immunized with an anti-NP antibody expressing the germline version of the C57BL/6 anti-NP molecule (B1-8). The other two were derived from mice immunized with a C57BL/6 anti-NP antibody (S43) which was derived from an hyperimmunized animal. This Ab_1 derives from the same germline genes as does B1-8, however, this antibody varies from the germline sequence.

Figure 1 summarizes their findings. Of the four molecules derived from immunization with the germline molecule, B1-8 recognizes B1-8, but not S43, the somatic variant. Likewise, the molecules derived from immunization with S43 recognize S43, but not B1-8.

The two Ab_2s recognizing S43 use identical germline gene segments (VH, D, JH, VK, JK) and may be clonally related. The VH gene that these molecules use is also used by one of the molecules recognizing B1-8. The other gene segments utilized by this molecule are distinct from those used by the other five Ab_2s. Two of the four recognizing B1-8 apparently are derived from the same VK, VH, and D gene segments. The fourth molecule recognizing B1-8 uses germline gene segments entirely distinct from those employed by the other five molecules.

The following conclusions can be drawn from this work. First, somatic mutation is apparent in anti-Id antibodies. This can be concluded even though the (C57BL/6) germline genes from which these molecules derive have not been isolated because of the following observations. There are sequence variations between closely related Ab_2s which, presumably, derive from the same germline elements. In addition, sequence variations are apparent in the joining and diversity segments of these molecules as compared to published germline sequences. Therefore, at least a moderate amount of somatic variation occurs.

Second, the third complementarity-determining regions (CDRs) of three of the heavy chains of these molecules are unusually long (15 amino acid residues), but are identical in *length* to each other. In part, the third CDRs are derived from known germline elements. The other three molecules have D segments of a more usual length, but are also not generated directly from known germline elements.

Finally, the authors conclude the syngeneic Ab_2s in the NP system are restricted in their use of germline gene segments. The level of the isogenic anti-Id expression is very weak in the NP system as well as in other systems.[11,12] This could be because the generation of these unusual D segments may require multiple somatic processes and, therefore, antibodies with this particular specificity would be infrequently generated and, therefore, rarely expressed. Information implying that the potential anti-Id repertoire is actually quite large

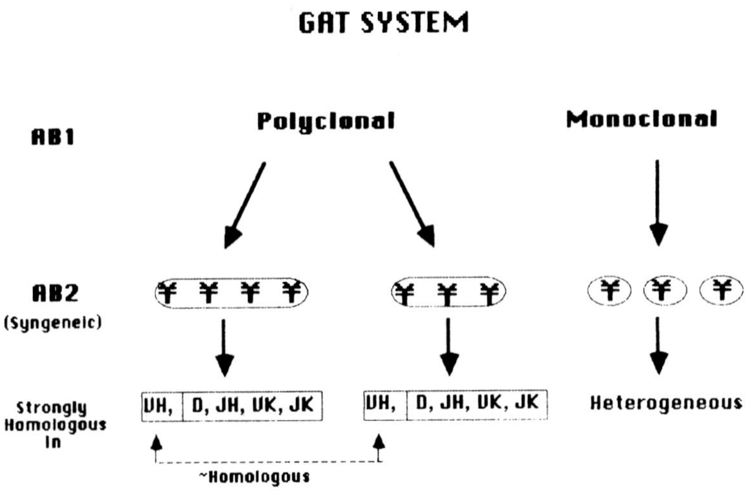

FIGURE 2. Schematic drawing of the GAT anti-Id system. Circles denote serologically related groups of anti-Id antibodies. Filled squares and arrows denote structurally related molecules.

would not support this conclusion.[11,12] Alternatively, weak syngeneic anti-Id responses could be due to some type of suppression.

III. STUDIES IN THE ANTI-GAT SYSTEM

The work of Fougereau and colleagues[7] with the BALB/c strain in the GAT system is summarized in Figure 2. Syngeneic monoclonal anti-Id antibodies were derived from mice immunized with either monoclonal or polyclonal BALB/c anti-GAT antibodies expressing the public cGAT Id.[13] When monoclonal Ab_1s served as the immunogen, Ab_2s were isolated which recognized private idiotopes only. When polyclonal anti-GAT antibodies were used as the immunogen, the Ab_2s isolated recognized public GAT idiotopes.

These molecules (recognizing public idiotopes) could then be placed into two groups serologically. One group recognized public idiotopes of the anti-GAT response in several strains of mice. The second group recognized public idiotopes present nearly exclusively on BALB/c anti-GAT antibodies.

These molecules could be grouped structurally as well. The anti-Id antibodies recognizing private GAT idiotopes were all distinct. This group was structurally completely heterogeneous, all deriving from completely different germline gene segments. This was in direct contrast to what was seen structurally in the antibodies recognizing public GAT idiotopes. The molecules within each of the two groups, although isolated from separate fusions, were nearly identical to each other, deriving from the same VH, D, JH, VK, and JK gene segments.

When comparing the VH segments of the two separate groups, it is apparent that they are also fairly closely related to each other — 94% homologous. The light chains of the two groups are quite distinct from one another. Since some variation occurs between molecules within each group, and since variations occur in the joining segments as compared to the published BALB/c germline JH and JK segments, it is apparent that some somatic mutation occurs in GAT Ab_2s, as is the case in the NP system.

Again, as in the NP system, the third CDRs of the heavy chains of these molecules are very interesting for several reasons. First, they are extremely long — 16 amino acid residues in one group of Ab_2s, 17 in the other group of AB_2s. Furthermore, none can be explained completely from any of the published germline D sequences. The D segments in one group

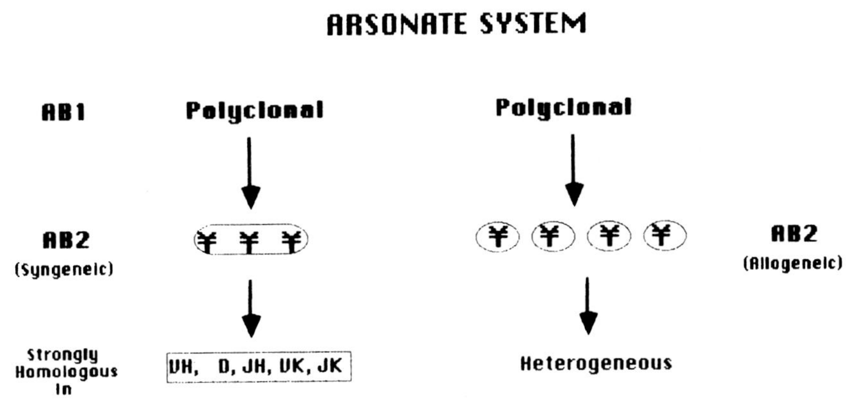

FIGURE 3. Schematic drawing of the arsonate anti-Id system. Circles denote serologically related groups of anti-Id antibodies. Filled squares and arrows denote structurally related molecules.

appear to have resulted from a double inverted fusion of two DSP2 D segments. The five prime portion appears to have derived from the noncoding strand of one DSP2 D segment; the next 17 base pairs are identical to the coding strand of another of the DSP2 D segments. A similar mechanism has been hypothesized to account for the conserved "N" segment seen in many murine antiarsonate antibodies.[14] It is quite striking that this extremely unusual D segment occurs identically in two independently derived anti-Id antibodies. The most straightforward explanation for this is that this particular D segment is selected for by antigen, in this case Ab_1s. This, therefore, implies that this structure is important for the antibodies' function.

Perhaps the most interesting aspect of the D segments of these molecules is the presence of sequences which appear to mimic the structure of the original antigen — the random terpolymer GAT (glu-ala-tyr). This proposed internal image occurs in the D segments of both groups of public anti-idiotopes as well as in the D segment of one private anti-idiotope. It has been shown that the glu-tyr residues of the GAT terpolymer are the most important for antigen binding of GAT Ab_1s. The sequence glu-glu-tyr is present in the D regions of one group of Ab_2s; whereas the sequence tyr-tyr-glu is present in the D regions of the second group of public Ab_2s.

IV. STUDIES IN THE ANTIARSONATE SYSTEM

In the Ars system, our laboratory has structurally characterized seven monoclonal anti-Id antibodies recognizing distinct public idiotopes which, in part, comprise the cross-reactive Id associated with the A/J strain's response to the hapten, para-azophenylarsonate.[15-17] In contrast to the other two studies, four of the seven Ab_2s described are allogeneic. These Ab_2s were isolated from BALB/c mice (a strain which normally does not express this Id) immunized with polyclonal Id-positive A/J antiarsonate antibodies and then boosted with a monoclonal antiarsonate antibody. The other three Ab_2s studied are syngeneic, isolated from A/J mice immunized with A/J polyclonal Id-positive antiarsonate antibodies.[18]

Figure 3 summarizes our results. The most striking feature of this study is the extreme heterogeneity of the allogeneic molecules compared to the near identity of the syngeneic molecules.[17] All four allogeneic molecules derive from different VH, D, JH, VK, and JK gene segments, whereas the three syngeneic molecules are nearly identical to one another. While clonal relatedness of the three cannot be ruled out, it is clear that the syngeneic Ab_2 response in the Ars system is extremely limited (as is the case in NP and GAT) in its level of expression and in its usage of germline gene segments.

In contrast, the allogeneic Ab_2 response is structurally heterogeneous — deriving from a large number of unrelated gene segments. This heterogeneity is also apparent serologically — each Ab_2 recognizes a different Id determinant. The amino acid residues in the A/J Ab_1s affecting expression of each of these four idiotopes had been determined through sequence information, chemical modifications, and chain recombination experiments.[19] The expression of three of the idiotopes is most dependent on amino acid residues located in the D region of the Ab_1s, whereas the expression of one idiotope is heavily influenced by the amino acid in position 59 of the heavy chain variable region. These allogeneic Ab_2s are actually, then, representative of what one would expect in an antibody response to any foreign protein — deriving from many different germline elements in response to many different antigenic determinants present on the immunogen.

The D segments of the four allogeneic Ab_2s cannot be easily explained from existing germline gene segments. It is interesting to note the high number of hydrophylic residues in the D segments of the allogeneic Ab_2s. Of particular interest is the D segment of the Ab_2 which defines the idiotope which is strongly affected by position 59 in the heavy chains of the Ab_1s. The residue which influences expression of this idiotope is the lysine in position 59 of the heavy chains of Ab_1s. The D segment of this Ab_2 begins with three aspartic acid residues. Since lysine is positively charged at physiologic pH, whereas three aspartic acids would be negatively charged, it is possible that some of the idiotope-anti-idiotope interactions in this instance may be ionic in nature.

The D segments of the three syngeneic molecules are average in length in contrast to the unusual length of the D segments of GAT and NP Ab_2s. However, as was the case in the GAT Ab_2s, they may have been generated by a novel inverted D-D fusion. Each is 14 base pairs long. The first six appear to be derived from the noncoding strand of DFL16.1; the next six appear to be from the coding strand of DSP2.6. We propose a similar mechanism, as suggested by Ollier et al. in the GAT system, to generate this unusual sequence. We hypothesize that an inverted recombination event occurs between the coding strand of one D segment and the noncoding strand of the second, using the alternative signal sequences proposed by Wood and Tonegawa.[20] Since the syngeneic molecules in this study may be clonally related, it is impossible to determine whether or not the event generating the unusual D segment seen occurs repeatedly in Ab_2s in the arsonate system, as is the case in the GAT system. Still, it is remarkable that in two of three Ab_2 systems studied, the same unique inverted D-D fusion mechanism must be invoked to explain the D segments' generation.

Since there are no germline sequences available which are more than 95% homologous to the VH or VK regions of any of the Ars Ab_2s, it is difficult to determine what effect somatic mutation has had on their generation. However, as was the case in both the NP and GAT Ab_2s, sequence variation occurs between the variable regions of closely related syngeneic molecules. Limited somatic mutation is apparent in both the JH and JK regions of both the syngeneic and allogeneic molecules. Therefore, it is clear that somatic mutation also occurs in arsonate anti-Id antibodies.

V. EXPERIMENTAL LIMITATIONS

In drawing conclusions from these studies, it is important to take several things into consideration. First and foremost, the numbers of Ab_2s studied to date are still quite small — only 23 molecules total from the three systems. Furthermore, some of these antibodies were not completely sequenced and some may represent clonal duplicates. Second, since the Ab_2s (even within a system) were generated in a variety of different ways (i.e., by immunizing with polyclonal or monoclonal reagents etc.), careful consideration must be taken in drawing generalities. Third, one must remember that the occurrence of a recurrent Id in a given immune response should be thought of as the exception and not the rule. Anti-

Id antibodies in immune responses that are not associated with a recurrent Id may not have the same characteristics as the molecules studied thus far. Still, with certain limitations, some important generalities *can* be drawn.

VI. STRUCTURAL CHARACTERISTICS OF ANTI-ID ANTIBODIES

A. Restricted Gene Usage

One of the most obvious characteristics of this group of molecules is the restriction in usage of germline elements by the molecules recognizing public Id determinants. This observation is most clearly demonstrated in the GAT system, in which molecules recognizing distinct public Id were extremely closely related structurally (more than 95% homologous), whereas molecules recognizing private idiotopes were heterogeneous. This restriction of usage of germline elements is also observed in the syngeneic Ars Ab_2s as well as in the Ab_2s recognizing the germline NP molecule. This, in part, supports Jerne's idea of coexistence of complementary sets of variable region genes in the germline. It suggests that within a single strain, a structurally distinct population induces (or is Id to) a second group of structurally distinct group of antibodies. The extreme heterogeneity of the allogeneic anti-Id antibodies would seem to support this idea. We predict that a strain which lacks a particular variable region gene segment required for a particular antibody to which a response is directed, responds as if that antibody were a foreign antigen and would not respond with a single "complementary" protein.

B. Variable Region Gene Family Usage

It is clear from these studies that there is nothing particular to the VH or VK regions of anti-Id antibodies. These molecules derive from germline heavy and kappa chain variable genes which can easily be placed within variable region families already described. While the gene segment usage is restricted in a given anti-Id response, the gene usage, in general, by these antibodies is not biased to any heavy chain variable region or kappa variable region family. The J558 family is employed most by far, but this, of course, is undoubtedly due to its large size. None of the molecules derives from a heavy chain variable region gene of the 7183 family, so anti-Id antibodies which are in a sense antiself antibodies do not follow the bias which has been reported in other antiself antibodies in usage of that gene family.

C. Somatic Variation

It is quite clear that somatic variation does occur in anti-Id antibodies. There are multiple examples of somatic mutation in the joining segments of the anti-Id antibodies from all three systems, and, indeed, it does not seem surprising that anti-Id antibodies should be affected by the same diversifying mechanisms that affect Ab_1s. However, since there are no germline sequences available for any of these molecules, it is nearly impossible to judge to what *degree* somatic mutation has affected the variable regions of these molecules. Since there are no examples of germline Ab_2s available, it is impossible to judge whether or not somatic mutation alters their anti-Id characteristics. There are many examples of antibodies that have undergone somatic mutation in which the specificity is unaltered. It is, therefore, unclear if somatic mutation is significant in the generation of Ab_2s, and it remains uncertain whether or not the Id network is germline encoded.

D. Heavy Chain Diversity Segments

The D segments of a majority of the Ab_2s studied thus far seem to share several characteristics. In more than half the NP and GAT Ab_2s, the third CDRs are extremely long — 15 to 17 amino acid residues. The third CDRs in murine heavy chains can vary in length from 7 to 19 amino acids. Although the third CDRs of the Ars Ab_3s are of a more usual length (ten amino acid residues) than those in the GAT and NP systems, they do share another structural characteristic. In all three systems studied to date, a high proportion of the Ab_2s appears to have generated their D segments by novel mechanisms. None appear to have been generated directly from germline. It is very striking that in two GAT Ab_2s (independently derived) and three Ars Ab_2s (possibly clonally related), the D segments appear to derive from an unusual inverted D-D fusion. Although a similar mechanism has been proposed to generate the D segments in antibodies that are not anti-Id in specificity,[14] the proportion of the sequence generated from the inverted fusion was small compared to the proportion generated from germline elements in the normal orientation (only one amino acid residue). In contrast, nearly half of the D segments in these Ab_2s are generated from the inversion.

There are examples of antibodies that are not anti-Id in nature that have extremely long D segments. There are also many examples of D segments in Ab_1s that cannot be easily explained by existing germline gene segments. In order to determine whether or not the observation that Ab_2s consistently seem to generate their D segments through novel mechanisms, a detailed statistical analysis will have to be conducted comparing all known antibody D segment structures with their specificities taking into account the selection pressures put on the system by our sampling method. Still, it is tempting to speculate on the importance of these novel D segments to anti-Id antibodies.

Several possibilities exist. First, the syngeneic anti-Id responses studied to date are all restricted in their level of expression. If these novel D segments are necessary for the Ab_2s' specificities, and the event that generates these structures represents a relatively rare rearrangement, then molecules with the appropriate specificity would be rare in the B-cell repertoire and their expression would be only at a low level. But rearrangements of this type have been observed in antibodies which are not anti-idiotopes even though the portion of the third CDR generated through the mechanism was rather small.[14] It may well be, then, that this unusual rearrangement mechanism is not as rare as it may have first appeared. In addition, well before any structural studies of Ab_2s had been concluded, several investigators made the observation in several systems that even though isogenic anti-Id responses are weak, the potential repertoire of B cells expressing anti-Id determinants is relatively large.[11,12] If this is generally the case, one is left only with Id suppression as the explanation for the low frequency of these molecules.

One final hypothesis from these studies is the following. The observation that Ab_2s are restricted in their level of expression offers an explanation for the "overexpression" of their "complementary" antibodies and, thus, the expression of recurrent Id, in general, by Ab_1s in these systems.

An enormous amount of insight into the mechanisms which control the immune system can be derived from these studies. The benefits that may possibly derive in beginning to understand how the immune system may be more effectively manipulated by perturbing the Id network are just beginning to be realized and are obviously important in their own right. Structural studies of anti-Id antibodies will undoubtedly be important in learning how to accomplish this most effectively and efficiently. Still the most intriguing aspect of further structural and serologic studies like these is that they may provide the opportunity to make clear the real significance of the Id network.

REFERENCES

1. **Jerne, N. K.,** Towards a network theory of the immune system, *Ann. Immunol. (Paris),* 125, 373, 1974.
2. **Kunkel, H. B., Mannik, M., and Williams, R. C.,** Individual antigenic specificity of isolated antibodies, *Science,* 140, 1218, 1963.
3. **Oudin, J. and Michel, M.,** Une nouvelle form d'allotypie des globulines gamma du serum lapin apparemet liée à la fonction et à la specificité anticorps, *C.R. Hebd. Seances Acad. Sci. Ser. D Sci. Nat.,* 257, 805, 1963.
4. **Moser, M., Leo, O., Kiernaux, J., and Urbain, J.,** Idiotypic manipulation in mice: Balb/c mice can express the cross-reactive idiotype of A/J mice, *Proc. Natl. Acad. Sci.,* 80, 4474, 1983.
5. **Jerne, N. K., Roland, J., and Cazenave, P. A.,** Recurrent idiotopes and internal images, *EMBO J.,* 1, 243, 1982.
6. **Dildrop, R., Bovens, J., Siekevitz, M., Beyreuther, K., and Rajewsky, K.,** A V region determinant (idiotope) expressed at high frequency in B lymphocytes is encoded by a large set of antibody structural genes, *EMBO J.,* 3, 517, 1984.
7. **Legrain, P., Rocca-Serra, J., Moulin, A., Fougereau, M., and Buttin, G.,** A single VH gene associated with a variety of D- and J-segments encodes for a large family of ABPC48 related antibodies induced by anti-idiotypic immunization, *Mol. Immunol.,* 22 (4), 437, 1985.
8. **Sablitzky, F. and Rajewsky, K.,** Molecular basis of an isogenic anti-idiotypic response, *EMBO J.,* 3, 3005, 1984.
9. **Rajewsky, K. and Takemori, T.,** Genetics, expression, and function of idiotypes, *Annu. Rev. Immunol.,* 1, 569, 1983.
10. **Reth, M., Hammerling, G. J., and Rajewsky, K.,** Analysis of the repertoire of anti-NP antibodies in C57B46 mice by cell fusion. I. Characterization of antibody families in the primary and hyperimmune response, *Eur. J. Immunol.,* 8, 393, 1978.
11. **Seppalla, J. T. and Eichmann, K.,** Induction and characterization of isogeneic anti-idiotypic antibodies to Balb/c myeloma S117: lack of reactivity with major idiotypic determinants, *Eur. J. Immunol.,* 9, 243, 1979.
12. **Schuler, W., Weiler, E., and Kolb, M.,** Characterization of syngeneic anti-idiotypic antibody against the idiotype of Balb/c myeloma protein J558, *Eur. J. Immunol.,* 7, 649, 1977.
13. **Ollier, P., Rocca-Serra, J., Somme, G., Theze, J., and Fougereau, M.,** The idiotypic network and the internal image: possible regulation of a germline network by paucigene encoded Ab2 (anti-idiotypic) antibodies in the GAT system, *EMBO J.,* 4, 3681, 1985.
14. **Milner, E. C. B., Meek, K., Rathbun, G., Tucker, P. T., and Capra, J. D.,** Are anti-arsonate antibody N-segments selected at both the protein and the DNA level, *Immunol. Today,* 7, 36, 1986.
15. **Milner, E. C. B. and Capra, J. D.,** VH families in the antibody response to p-azophenylarsonate: correlation between serology and amino acid sequence, *J. Immunol.,* 129, 193, 1982.
16. **Capra, J. D., Slaughter, C. A., Milner, E. C. B., Estess, P., and Tucker, P. T.,** The cross-reactive idiotype of A strain mice. Serological and structural analysis, *Immunol. Today,* 3, 332, 1982.
17. **Meek, K., Jeske, D., Alkan, S., Urbain, J., and Capra, J. D.,** Structural characterization of syngeneic and allogenic anti-idiotypic antibodies in the anti-arsonate system, *Monogr. Allergy,* in press.
18. **Alkan, S.,** Structural and serological analysis of cross-reactive idiotypes: comparison of heavy and light chain families of anti-arsonate antibodies, *Ann. Immunol. (Inst. Pasteur),* 135c, 31, 1984.
19. **Jeske, D., Milner, E. C. B., Leo, O., Moser, M., Marvel, J., Urbain, J., and Capra, J. D.,** Molecular mapping of idiotopes of anti-arsonate antibodies, *J. Immunol.,* 136, 2568, 1986.
20. **Wood, C. and Tonegawa, S.,** Diversity and joining segments of mouse immunoglobulin heavy chain genes are closely linked and in the same orientation: implications for the joining mechanism, *Proc. Natl. Acad. Sci. U.S.A.,* 80, 3030, 1983.

Chapter 3

MOLECULAR BASIS OF ANTI-ID ANTIBODIES CARRYING INTERNAL IMAGE OF ANTIGENS ($Ab_{2\beta}$)

M. Fougereau, C. Cambillau, S. Corbet, G. Mazza, M. Milili, D. Moinier, P. Ollier, J. Rocca-Serra, C. Roth, C. Schiff, G. Sommé, J. Thèze, and C. Tonnelle

TABLE OF CONTENTS

I. INTRODUCTION

The idiotypic (Id) network, as proposed by Jerne[1] and first approached by serial immunizations performed in different animals,[2-4] may be written, in an oversimplified way, as the cascade:

$$Ag \rightarrow Ab_1 \rightarrow Ab_2 \rightarrow Ab_3$$

in which Ag is the original (''external'' or ''foreign'') antigen, Ab_1 the responding antibody (Id) which, in turn, may elicit the synthesis of Ab_2 or anti-Id antibodies. More recently, Jerne et al.[5] proposed that within the Ab_2 populations, two types of molecules could be distinguished: the so-called $Ab_{2\alpha}$, recognizing the Ab_1 idiotopes (true anti-idiotypic [anti-Id] set), and the $Ab_{2\beta}$, complementary to the Ab_1 paratope and, thus, appearing as an internal image of the antigen. The concept of internal image stems from the possibility of raising Ab_3 antibodies that would recognize the original antigen.[5] This has been demonstrated in a number of systems and opens a potential approach to Id vaccines. If one takes into account both the antigenic characteristics of Ab_1 molecules, four discrete types of Ab_3 molecules may be anticipated:[6] $Id^- Ag^-$, $Id^+ Ag^-$, $Id^- Ag^+$, $Id^+ Ag^+$, the latter being very similar to Ab_1 and termed $Ab_{1'}$. An *a priori* disjunction of the internal image from the Id set in $Ab_{2\beta}$ molecules may lead to the production of Ab_3 of the $Id^- Ag^+$ type, as described by Jerne et al.[5] In addition to this classification, $Ab_{2\epsilon}$, or epibodies,[7] have also been described as recognizing both the original antigen and the Ab_1 idiotopes.

A major issue which is still largely controversial[8] concerns the physiological role of the Id network. Besides the possibility to regulate specifically the immune response (a view which is supported by manipulation of the Id cascade, see Reference 9 for a review), more profound would be the idea, originally centered on the internal image concept,[1] that the Id network may find its major physiological significance in playing a key role for the emergence of the antibody repertoire[10,11] by providing a built-in selective pressure. Three requirements are needed for the network to play such a role: (1) the cascade should spontaneously occur within one single animal (this was first shown in the mouse for the phosphorylcholine [PC] system[12]); (2) a germline network should be operational; (3) a structural basis for an internal image should be identified.

II. THE ''GAT'' MODEL

A. General Features

We have been studying the characteristics of the Id cascade both at the expression and germline levels using the GAT, a random synthetic terpolymer (Glu^{60} Ala^{30} Tyr^{10}) as the original antigen. It induces, in a number of inbred strains of mice, anti-GAT (Ab_1) antibodies, most of which express public Id specificities, termed C-GAT[13] or pGAT[14]. The presence of these Id specificities strongly correlates with a preferential recognition of Glu-Tyr-containing epitopes.[15] The expression of pGAT idiotopes requires the presence of both the H and the L Ab_1 chains.[16] Hybridomas have been derived in syngeneic situation in the BALB/c strain, at each of the three levels of the cascade.[17-19] A summary of many characteristics of the selected materials is given in Table 1. Most polyclonal Ab_1 antibodies express the pGAT Id specificities and four $pGAT^+$ hybridomas were selected for detailed analysis.

Ab_2 hybridomas have been prepared either by immunization with $pGAT^+$ mAb_1s or with polyclonal Ab_1s. Immunization with individual mAb_1s only led to production of mAb_2s that were directed against private Ab_1 idiotopes. Raising Ab_2s that would recognize Ab_1 public epitopes required that polyclonal mAb_1s were used for immunization.[18] Eleven hybridomas were selected, from which seven recognized public idiotopes on the Ab_1 molecules. These

Table 1
MAIN FEATURES OF THE "GAT" ID CASCADE

	mAb_1	mAb_2			mAb_3		
Strain	BALB/c	BALB/c			BALB/c		
Fusion partner	X63.Ag8.653	SP2.0 Ag			SP2.0 Ag		
Idiotopes	pGAT$^+$ (20 and 22 specificities associated to pGAT)	"Internal image" (+ not identified Id)			pGAT$^+$	pGAT$^+$	pGAT$^-$
Anti-idiotopes		α-Id20	α-Id22	α "private"			α "private"
GAT recognition	+	–	–	–	+	–	–
Number of V regions sequenced (mRNA)							
H	4 (γ1)	3 (γ1)	2 (γ1)	3 (γ1)	2 (μ) 2(γ1)	2 (μ) 1 (γ1)	1 (γ2a)
κ	4	4	3	2	4	3	1

Table 2
MAIN CHARACTERISTICS OF Ab_1 AND $Ab_{1'}$ HYBRIDOMAS[a]

Hybridomas	Isotypes	Anti-GAT activity	pGAT expression
Ab_1			
G8 Ca 1.7	γ1κ	+	+
G5 Bb 2.2	γ1κ	+	+
G7 Ab 2.9	γ1κ	+	+
G8 Ad 3.8	γ1κ	+	+
$Ab_{1'}$			
22.8	μκ	+/−	+
22.176	μκ	−	+
20.11	γ1κ	+	+
22.186	μκ	+	+
20.33	μκ	+	+
20.8	γ1κ	+	+

[a] Data are taken from References 22, 23 (G series), and 25 (20 and 22 series).

Ab_2s could be classified into two groups: group 20 (four members) identified an idiotope common to all three strains tested (BALB/c, DBA/2, C57BL/6), whereas group 22 (three members) allowed recognition of an idiotope frequently restricted to the BALB/c strain. The pGAT specificities expressed on Ab_1 were shown to be associated to these two discrete idiotopes.

One member of each group $Ab_{2\text{-}20}$ and $Ab_{2\text{-}22}$ was selected to produce Ab_3 antibodies. Production of Ab_3 was quite easy and a rather large collection of hybridomas was obtained and characterized.[19] The most striking feature was that most mAb_3s expressed the pGAT specificities, as Ab_1 did. Among those, a large majority was also GAT specific as shown either by direct binding or inhibition experiments, whereas a minority was not. So three groups could be distinguished between the Ab_3, from the four potential ones:[6] Id^+ Ag^+ ($Ab_{1'}$), Id^+ Ag^-, and Id^- Ag^-. Ab_3 was of the IgM or IgG1 class. Ab_1 and Ab_2 were IgG, mostly of the γ1 type. At all three levels, the light chain was of the κ type.

B. Stimulation by Ab_2 Antibodies Elicits Ab_3, Most of Which Use the Same V_H Germline Gene as Ab_1

Using various genomic libraries and a V_H cDNA probe that was GAT specific (Ab_1), three genes were isolated, termed H10, H4a-3, and H2b-3, that all pertained to the V_HII family,[20] within which they constitute a sub-sub group, expressing 95% homologies, including the first intron and the 3′ noncoding region.[21] These germline gene sequences were compared with Ab_1 and $Ab_{1'}$ heavy chains expressed in hybridomas, for which main characteristics appear in Table 2.

The first line of evidence that mAb_1s might be encoded by the same V_H germline gene was derived from mRNA sequencing performed in the four analyzed Ab_1 ($pGAT^+$) hybridomas[22] and also by sequencing of a cDNA-specific clone[23] which was further used to isolate the above-mentioned germline genes.[21] It turned out that two hybridomas use one of these germline genes, termed H10, straightforward, without any substitution — with the exception of the 3′ terminal nucleotide involved in the V-D junction (Figure 1). It was shown by Southern blotting experiments and by comparing with the sequences of 19 isolated and sequenced V_H genes[21,24] that the two remaining hybridomas derive by a few somatic mutations from the H10 germline.

```
            1                                   10                                      20
H 10        GAG GTT CAG CTG CAG CAG TCT GGG GCA GAG CTT GTG AAG CCA GGG GCC TCA GTC AAG TTG TCC TGC ACA GCT TCT
H 4a-3      --- --- --- --- --- --- --- --- --T --- --- --- -G- --- --- --- -T- --- --- --- --- --- -A- --- ---
H 2b-3      --- --- --- --- --- --- --- --- --- --- --- --- -G- T-- --- --- --- --- --- --- --- --- --- --- ---

G8 Ca1.7    --- --- --- --- --- --- --- --- --- --- --- --- --- --- --- --- --- --- --- --- --- --- --- --- ---
G5 Bb2.2                            --- --- --- --- --- --- --- --- --- --- --- --- --- --- --- --- --- --- ---
G7 Ab2.9                                        --- --- --- --- --- --- --- --- --- --- --- --- --- --T --- ---
G8 Ad3.8                                        --- --- --- --- --- --- --- --- --- --- --- --- --- --- --- ---

                            30                                      40                                      50
H 10        GGC TTC AAC ATT AAA GAC ACC TAT ATG CAC TGG GTG AAG CAG AGG CCT GAA CAG GGC CTG GAG TGG ATT GGA AGG
H 4a-3      --- --- --- --- --- --- TA- --- --- --- --- --- --- --- --- --- --- --- --- --- --- --- --- --- T--
H 2b-3      --- --- --- --- --- --- TA- --- --- --- --- --- --- --- --- --- --- --- --- --- --- --- --- --- T--

G8 Ca1.7    --- --- --- --- --- --- --- --- --- --- --- --- --- --- --- --- --- --- --- --- --- --- --- --- ---
G5 Bb2.2    --- --- --- --- --- --- --- --- --- --- --- --- --- --- --- --- --- --- --- --- --- --- --- --- ---
G7 Ab2.9    --- --- --- --- --- --- --- --- --- --- --- --- --A --- --- --- --- --- --- --- --- --- --- --- ---
G8 Ad3.8    --- --- --T --- --- --- --- --- --- --- --- --- --- --- --- --- --- --- --- --- --- --- --- --- ---

22.8                    --- --- --- --- --- --- --- --- --- --- --- --- --- --- --- --- --- --- --- --- --- ---
22.176                  --- --- --- --- --- --- --- --- --- --- --- --- --- --- --- --- --- --- --- --- --- ---
20.11                   --- --- --- --- --- --- --- --- --- --- --- --- --- --- --- --- -X- --- --- --- --- ---
22.186                                                                          --- --- --- --- --- --- --- ---

                    a                                   60                                      70
H 10        ATT GAT CCT GCG AAT GGT AAT ACT AAA TAT GAC CCG AAG TTC CAG GGC AAG GCC ACT ATA ACA GCA GAC ACA TCC
H 4a-3      --- --- --- -A- --- --- --- --- -T- --- --- --- --- --- --- --- --- --- -G- --- --- --- --- --- ---
H 2b-3      --- --- --- -A- --- --- G-- --- G-- --- -C- --- --- --- --- --- --- --- --- --G --T --- --- --- ---

G8 Ca1.7    --- --- --- --- --- --- --- --- --- --- --- --- --- --- --- --- --- --- --- --- --- --- --- --- ---
G5 Bb2.2    --- --- --- --- --- --- --- --- --- --- --- --- --- --- --- --- --- --- --- --- --- --- --- --- ---
G7 Ab2.9    --- --- --- --- --- XA- --- -G- --- --- -G- --- --- --- --- --X X-- --A --- --- --- --- --- --- ---
G8 Ad3.8    --- --- --- --- --A --- --- --- --- --- --- --- --- --- --- --- --- --A --- --- --- A-- --- --- ---

22.8        --- --- --- --- --- --- --- --- --- --- --- --- --- --- --- --- --- --- --- --- --- --- --- --- ---
22.176      --- --- --- --- --- --- --- --- --- --- --- --- --- --- --- --- --- --- --- --- --- --- --- --- ---
20.11       --- --- --- --- --- -T- --- --- -G- --- --- --- --- --- --- --- -G- -GX --- --- --- --- --- --- ---
22.186      --- --- --- -X- --- --- --- --- --- --- --- --- --- --- --- --- --- --- --- --- --- --- --- --- ---
20.33       --- --- --- --- --- --- --- --- --- --- --- --- --- --- --- --- --- --- --- --- --- --- --- --- ---
20.8                        --- --- --- --- --- --- --- --- --- --- --- --- --- --- --- --- --- --- --- --- ---

                                80              a   b   c                           90
H 10        TCC AAC ACA GCC TAC CTG CAG CTC AGC AGC CTG ACA TCT GAG GAC ACT GCC GTC TAT TAC TGT GCT AGA
H 4a-3      --- --- --- --- --- --- --- --- --- --- --- --- --- --- --- --- --- --- --- --- --- --- ---
H 2b-3      --- --- --- --- --- --- --- --- --- --- --- --- --- --- --- --- --- --- --- --- --- AA- GC-

G8 Ca1.7    --- --- --- --- --- --- --- --- --- --- --- --- --- --- --- --- --- --- --- --- --- --- --G
G5 Bb2.2    --- --- --- --- --- --- --- --- --- --- --- --- --- --- --- --- --- --- --- --- --- --- --G
G7 Ab2.9    --- -G- G-- --- --- --- --- --- --- --- --- --- --- -G- --- --- --A --- --- --- --- A-- --G
G8 Ad3.8    --- --- --- --- --- --- --- T-- --- --- --- --- --- --- --- --- --A --- --C --- --- --- ---

22.8        --- --- --- --- --- --- --- --- --- --- --- --- --- --- --- --- -X- --- --- --- --- --- ---
22.176      --- --- --- --- --- --- --- --- --- --- --- --- --- --- --- --- --- --- --- --- --- --- ---
20.11       --- --- --- --- --- --- --- --- --- --- --- --- --- --- --- --- --- --- --- --- --- --- ---
22.186      --- --- --- --- --- --- --- --- --- --- --- --- --- --- --- --- --- --- --- --- --- --- ---
20.33       --- --- --- --- --- --- --- --- --- --- --- --- --- --- --- --- --- --- --- --- --- ---
20.8        --- --- --- --- --- --- --- --- --- --- --- --- --- --- --- --- --- --- --- --- --- --- ---
```

FIGURE 1. The H-10 germline gene encodes V_H-GAT-specific Ab_1 and $Ab_{1'}$ sequences. Germline genes of the H series[21] are compared with Ab_1 (G series[22,23]) and $Ab_{1'}$ (20 and 22 series)[25] nucleotide sequences. (Reproduced from *J. Exp. Med.*, 1986, 163, 573, by copyright permission of The Rockefeller University Press.)

In Figure 1 is also given the comparison of the H10 sequence with six $mAb_{1'}$ V_H regions. All of these $Ab_{1'}$ had been produced by immunization with monoclonal Ab_2.[18,19] All express the pGAT specificities and all but two (22.8 and 22.176) were GAT specific as determined either by direct fixation or inhibition tests.[25] Five of these (22.8, 22.176, 22.186, 20.33, 20.8) had sequences that were completely identical over the region analyzed, which begins from codon 29 to 54.[25] As it was previously shown that, in the GAT system, mutations accumulated preferentially in the COOH-terminal half of the V_H region,[22] it seems likely that the entire V_H of these hybridomas express the H10 germline gene without modification. Hybridoma 20.11 had four differences from the germline sequence.

The absence of the low level of somatic mutations observed in $Ab_{1'}$ antibodies may be the result of several factors: (1) fusions were made with lymphocytes derived from one single immunization. This is consistent with the existence of a majority of μ chains, although it should be recalled that fusion was performed 1 month after immunization. The absence of mutation might, thus, be simply related to a low rate of division of IgM expressing B cells; (2) alternatively, the system may tend not to accumulate mutations, because in Ig-Ig interactions of the Id network, the optimal fit might be already insured by germline gene-encoded antibodies.

We also have evidence that, in the GAT system, V_κ germline genes are used preferentially.[47] As the expression of the pGAT Id specificities relies on the presence of both the H and L chains, this clearly suggests a very strict role of a given member of the Id cascade for the restricted expression of an Id, which is largely dependent on the utilization of germline gene sequences.

The J regions were all J_H4 and $J_\kappa 2$, in both cases essentially in their germline form.

The Ab_3 that was not related to the GAT system neither for Id ($pGAT^-$) nor for GAT binding — thus, pertaining to the Id^- Ag^- set[6] — used unrelated V_H and V_κ sequences.[23]

Analysis of the Ab_1/Ab_3 D regions revealed very interesting features that will be discussed separately later. It may already be stressed, however, that among the Ab_3 expressing the $pGAT^+$ specificities, only those which have an Ab_1-like D region bound GAT, suggesting, therefore, in this system a key role to the D region for antigen recognition, whereas the public pGAT idiotopes should rather be considered a germline marker of a very restricted V_H-V_κ pairing.

C. Amino Acid Sequences of Ab_2 H and L Variable Regions and the Localization of a Possible Internal-Image-Like Structure within the D Region

1. Hybridomas

Preparation of the Ab_2 hybridomas has been described in detail by Sommé et al.[18] In brief, two types of fusions were prepared. One used spleen cells from BALB/c mice that had been immunized with monoclonal GAT-specific G5 Bb 2.2 Ab_1, coupled to KLH. The fusion partner was the SP 2.0 Ag nonsecreting cell line. This type of fusion led to hybridomas 9, 12, and 13 which all produced Ab_2 antibodies directed against private specificities of the immunizing Ab_1 Id.

For the second type of fusions, lymphocytes originated from BALB/c, mice immunized with polyclonal GAT-specific polyclonal Ab_1 coupled to KLH and using the same fusion partner. All hybridomas were derived from the same fusion, with the exception of HP27. The monoclonal Ab_2s produced by these hybridomas allowed definition of two groups: group 20 (HP20, 21, 24, 25) and group 22 (HP22, 27, 29), on the basis of the recognition of discrete public idiotopes pertaining to the pGAT mosaic.

2. Analysis of the Sequences

Amino acid sequences were derived from mRNA data both for the heavy and the light chains of the various Ab_2 molecules.[26] These data appear in Figures 2 and 3. Distinction between groups 20 and 22 antibodies predominantly relies on deep differences in the light chain sequences, which are clearly group specific, and, also, on the structure of the D regions which differ both in length (11 amino acids for group 22 and 10 for group 20) and in sequences. This would point to the crucial participation of the light chain (probably including the J_κ-encoded section) and the D region of Ab_2 for *idiotope recognition* on the Ab_1 molecules. The nucleotide sequences of Ab_2 which recognize private specificities were very different from those of groups 20 and 22, with the exception of HP 12 heavy chain, which contains a V_H amino acid sequence 94% homologous to that of HP 20, but which possesses a completely different D region, both in size (six amino acids instead of ten) and in sequence, and a different V_κ domain.

3. A Possible Sequential Internal Image

An intriguing feature is the presence of the sequence *Tyr-Tyr-Glu,* and *Glu-Glu-Tyr* in the D regions of group 22 and 20, respectively (Figure 3). Since anti-GAT (Ab_1), $pGAT^+$ antibodies recognize primarily Glu-Tyr determinants,[17] it is tempting to propose that these sequences may reflect the internal images of the original antigen. The possibility that group 20 or group 22 Ab_2 may contain an internal image was implicit from the possibility of raising

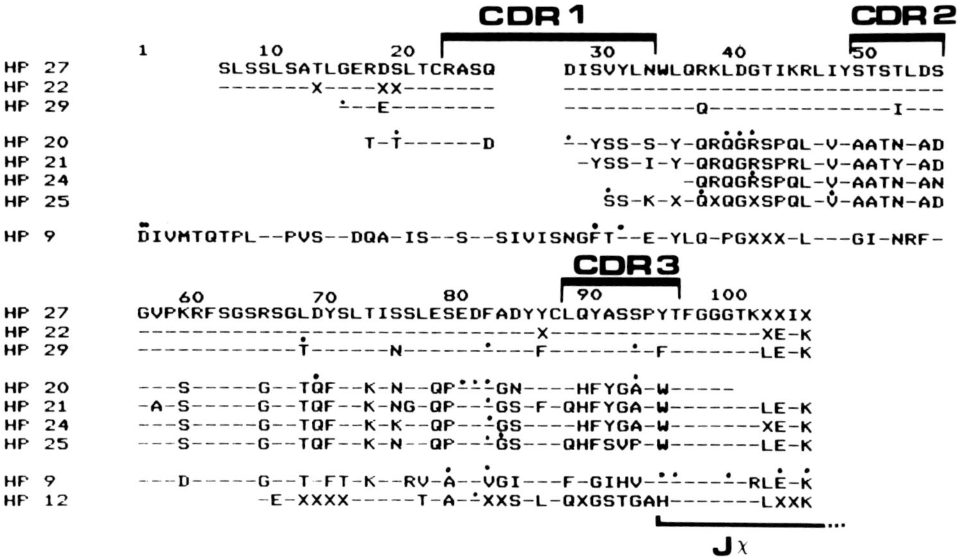

FIGURE 2. Ab_2-V_κ amino acid sequences derived from mRNA analysis. HP27, 22, 29 define group 22; HP20, 21, 24, 25 define group 20. Others are antiprivate specific. (Taken from Ollier, P., Rocca-Serra, J., Sommé, G., Thèze, J., and Fougereau, M., *EMBO J.*, 4, 3681, 1985. With permission.)

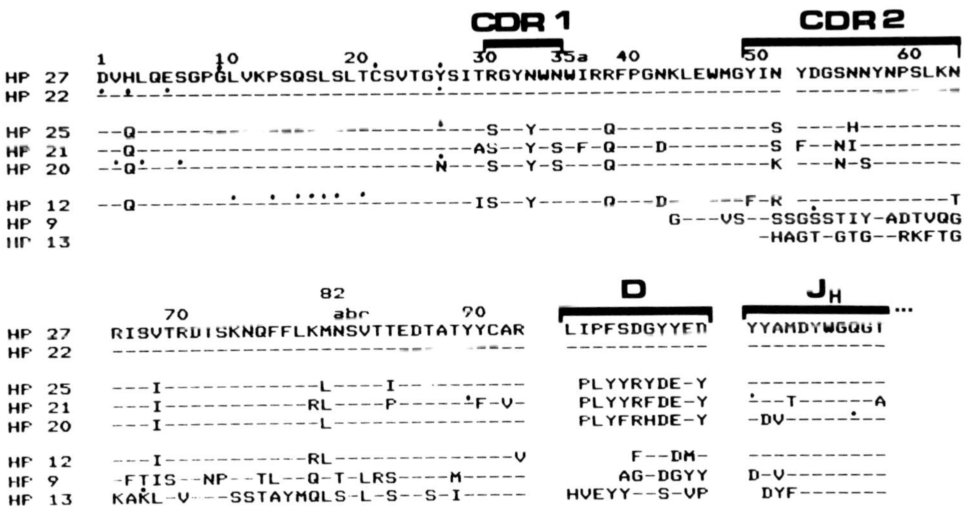

FIGURE 3. Ab_2-V_H amino acid sequences derived from mRNA analysis. (Taken from Ollier, P., Rocca-Serra, J., Sommé, G., Thèze, J., and Fougereau, M., *EMBO J.*, 4, 3681, 1985. With permission.)

Ab_3 of the $Ab_{1'}$ type, possessing both the pGAT idiotopes and the GAT specificity.[25] According to the nomenclature proposed by Jerne et al.,[5] the "GAT" Ab_2 would, thus, appear of the $Ab_{2\beta}$ type. Ab_1-Ab_2 or Ab_2-$Ab_{1'}$ interactions might, thus, involve, among several possible CDR-CDR interactions, D regions of the Ab_2 antibodies. If one considers the possibility that the Ab_1 D region is implicated in the GAT binding,[22] an Id-anti-Id recognition in the GAT system might involve a D-D interaction between Ab_1 and Ab_2, seen as a paratope-internal image recognition. In Table 3 are computed all CDR sequences of H and L chains of all three levels (Ab_1, Ab_2, Ab_3/$Ab_{1'}$) of the GAT Id system. It is remarkable that, taking into account the percentage of aromatic residues and the overall net charge of

Table 3
HYPERVARIABLE REGIONS OF THE GAT SYSTEM

			Aromatic residues on the considered region (%)	Net charge
$Ab_1/Ab_{1'}$				
Heavy chains		31		
	CDR1	DTYMH	16	−1
		50		
	CDR2	RIDPANGNTKYDPKFQ	6	+1
	D	GWLRRD (Ab_1)	16	+1
Light chains		24		
	CDR1	RSSQSIVHSNGNTYLY	12	+1
		50		
	CDR2	RVSNRFS	12	+2
		89		
	CDR3	FQGTHVPHT	11	0
		S		
Ab_2				
Heavy chains		31		
	CDR1	RGYNWN (HP22)	40	+1
		SGYYWS (HP20)	50	0
		50		
	CDR2	YINYDGSNNYNPSLKN (HP22)	19	0
	D	LIPFSDG*YYED* (HP22)	27	−3
		PLYFRHD*EEY* (HP20)	30	−2
		Internal image-like sequences		
Light chains		24		
	CDR1	RASQDISVYLN (HP22)	9	0
		RASDDIYSSLS (HP20)	9	−1
		50		
	CDR2	STSTLDS (HP22)	0	−1
		AATNLAD (HP20)	0	−1
		89		
	CDR3	LQYASSPYT (HP22)	22	0
		LHFYGAPWT (HP20)	33	0

each CDR, some complementarities are clearly apparent. For instance, most CDRs of Ab_2 are negatively charged, whereas most CDRs of the $Ab_1/Ab_{1'}$ set are positively charged. Taking, also, into consideration the percentage of aromatic residues, it may be possible that some interactions are of crucial importance, such as Ab_1 D-Ab_2 D (already discussed), but also Ab_1(L-CDR2)-Ab_2(L-CDR2) or, alternatively, the cross combination. Elucidation of these interactions will obviously rely on 3-D analysis, but recent data obtained by Chen et al.,[27] who succeeded in raising anti-Id antibodies against rheumatoid factor by injecting synthetic CDRs, certainly are compatible with the importance of CDR-CDR interactions in the Id network. As the geometry of the CDRs obeys a clear order, despite individual differences that dictate the antibody specificity, one is faced with the necessity that some interactions are possible, whereas others are not. In the GAT system, the key role played by the D region in the recognition of antigen and in the internal image construction may lead to propose that D-D regions represent one anchor of the Ab_1-Ab_2 or Ab_2-Ab_3 interactions. In this system, other interactions, implicating other CDRs, should account for at least a fraction of the "true" idiotopes-anti-idiotopes binding. This is represented in a very naive way in Figure 4 and may be largely refined by model building of the 3-D structure, using

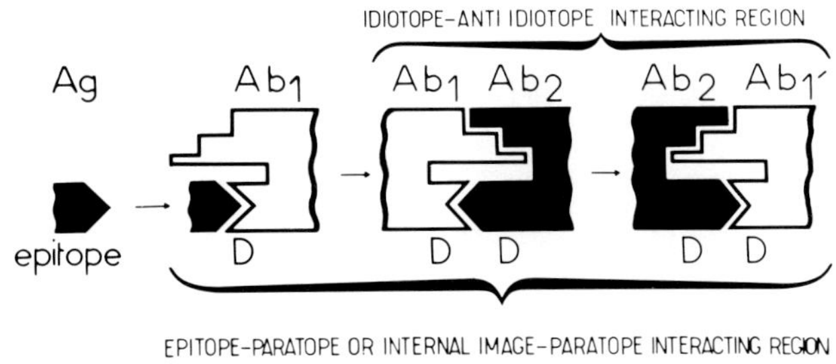

FIGURE 4. A simplified "clutch" model for CDR interactions in the GAT Id cascade.

as a reference crystallographic data obtained for different myeloma proteins with binding activity. Such an approach, centered on the search for ionic interactions between the D regions of Ab_1 and Ab_2 partners, will be discussed in a later section.

D. Elicitation of Anti-GAT Antibodies by Synthetic Peptides Containing the Ab_2-D Region Sequences

In order to test whether the Ab_2-D regions might indirectly act as mimicking the GAT antigen, peptides containing one or the other of the characteristic 20 and 22 major D sequences were synthesized according to the solid-phase procedure.[28] Due to technical and/or solubility problems, a slight modification of the original sequences was brought in, so that synthetic peptides had the following structures (stretches corresponding to the D region are italicized):

20: Lys-Lys-Ala-Arg-*Pro-Leu-Tyr-Phe-Arg-His-Asp-Glu-Glu-Tyr*-Tyr
22: Cys-Ala-Arg-*Leu-Ile-Pro-Phe-Ser-Asp*-Ala-*Tyr-Tyr-Glu-Asp*-Tyr

These peptides were then separately coupled to BSA and injected into BALB/c mice. Antibodies produced were specific of each peptide (Figure 5). As can be observed in Figure 6, a noticeable fraction of these antibodies was able to recognize the GAT terpolymer, thus, bringing direct evidence that an Ab_2-D-region-like structure was able to act as the original antigen of the Id cascade according to the prediction of the internal image hypothesis. Antibodies that were produced as a response to the synthetic peptides did not bear the commonly expressed pGAT public specificities identified on Ab_1[17] and $Ab_{1'}$[25] of the GAT Id cascade. This observation, therefore, suggests that portions of the Ab_2 molecules which are responsible for inducing the pGAT idiotopes are distinct from the internal image, implying a duality of structures that can act separately on the regulation of the Id network. This is consistent with the observation, in several systems, that Ab_3 may express Ab_1 idiotopes without recognizing the original antigen[25,29] and, more evidently, that discrete antibodies recognizing the same antigenic determinant may bear very distinct idiotopes.

The general organization of the internal image in the context of the germline expression of the GAT Id cascade is summarized in Table 4.

E. A Three-Dimensional Model for Ab_1/Ab_2 Interactions

A number of 3-D structures of immunoglobulin (Ig) Fab fragments has been determined.[31-33] It has been shown from 3-D comparisons that the domain organization is quite similar within a given Ig, but also between different ones. From sequence alignments, modeling, or partial crystallographic data, it is now believed that this domain is the building block of the super family of molecules of the immune system (Ig, MHC, T-cell receptors), which could all have derived from a common ancestor.[34] This domain is made of seven β-strands forming a barrel and contains a disulfide bridge surrounded by a core of hydrophobic

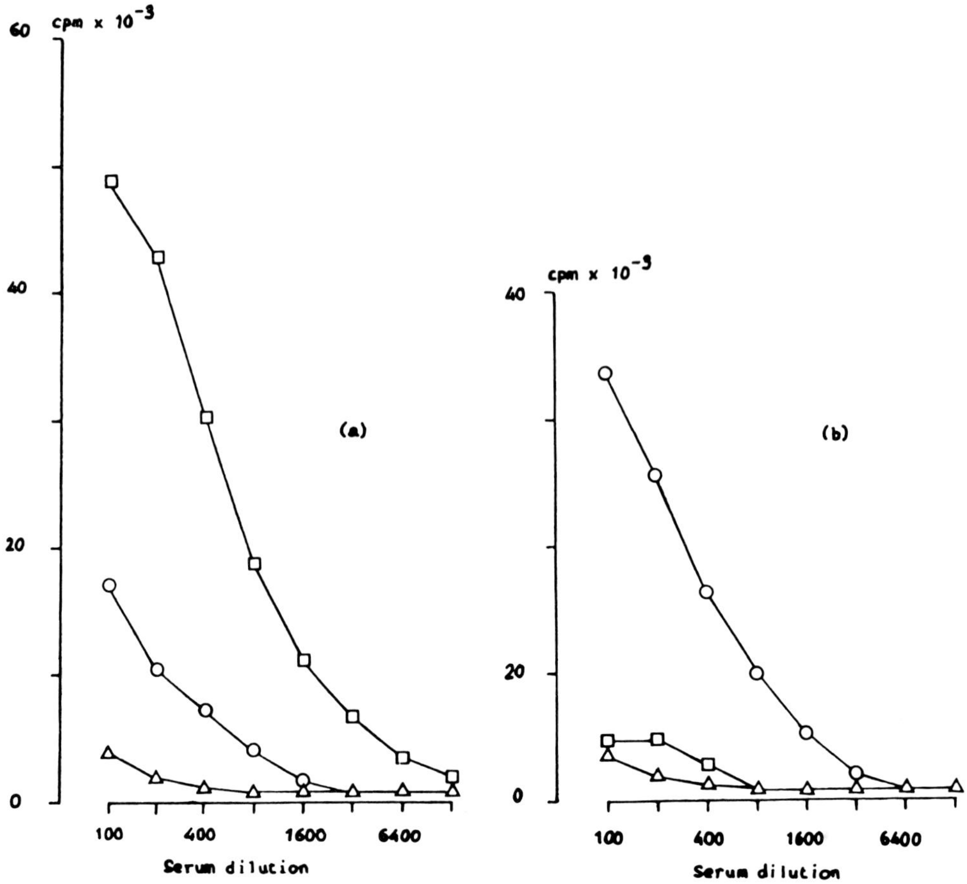

FIGURE 5. Binding to synthetic peptides 20 and 22. Binding profiles of sera from mice immunized with synthetic peptide 20 (○) or 22 (□) to synthetic peptides 20 (b) and 22 (a); △ = sera from nonimmunized mice. The binding profiles shown in Figures 5 and 6 correspond to sera obtained from the last bleeding. (Taken from Mazza, G., Ollier, P., Sommé, G., Moinier, D., Rocca-Serra, J., van Rietschoten, J., Thèze, J., and Fougereau, M., *Ann. Inst. Pasteur/Immunol.*, 136D, 259, 1985. With permission.)

residues.[35-37] The main conformational differences are found in loops, especially the ones bearing the hypervariable residues.

With such a knowledge on the structure of Fab fragments and on the GAT Id cascade, it seemed interesting to build models of the Ab_1 and Ab_2 partners and their complex.

1. Sequences Alignment and Models Building

Figure 7 presents the sequences alignment between three crystallographically determined Fabs, human Kol[31] and New[33] and mouse McPC 603,[32] together with the sequences of Ab_1 G5 and Ab_2 HP22 from GAT. This alignment is straightforward in most of the sequences, except in some hypervariable areas where it is ambiguous, i.e., L1, H2, and especially H3. In this latter case, we deliberately aligned the R-R 101-102 of Ab_1 with the E-D 108-109 in Ab_2 to emphasize the fact that they might be related in terms of internal image.

The models of Ab_1 G5 and Ab_2 HP22 were derived from the McPC Fab crystallographic structure present in the Protein Data Bank.[38] T.A. Jones FRODO system of programs was used all along in this work.[39] With this program, residues can be replaced according to the amino acids sequences alignment and atoms deleted or introduced with proper stereochemistry from a dictionary. Main chain atoms are thereby kept, and side-chain atoms are po-

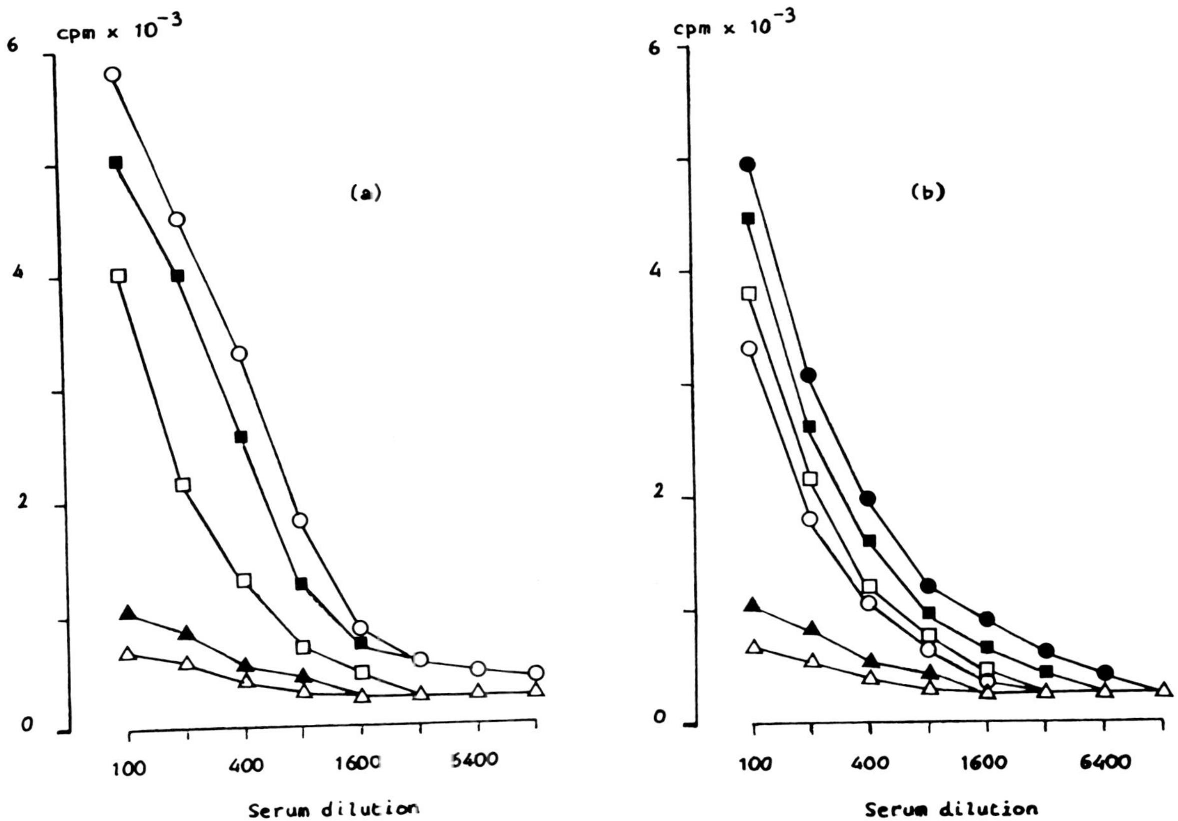

FIGURE 6. Binding to GAT. Binding profiles to GAT of sera from individual mice (○, ■, □) immunized with BSA-synthetic peptide 20 conjugate (a) and from individual mice (●, ■, □, ○) immunized with BSA-synthetic peptide 22 conjugate (b). △ = sera from nonimmunized mice; ▲ = sera from mice immunized with BSA alone. The GAT binding assay was performed on PVC plates coated with GAT as already described. (Taken from Mazza, G., Ollier, P., Sommé, G., Moinier, D., Rocca-Serra, J., van Rietschoten, J., Thèze, J., and Fougereau, M., *Ann. Inst. Pasteur/Immunol.*, 136D, 259, 1985. With permission.)

```
Light chain                                                           L1
Kol D S V L T Q - P P S A S G T P G Q R V T I S C S G|T S S N I - - - - G S D|
New                                           S C T G|S S S N I - - - G A G N|
Mcp D I V M T Q S P S S L S V S A G D R V T M S C K S|S Q S L L N S G N Q K N|

AB1 D V V M T Q T P L S L P V S L G D Q A S I S C R S|S Q S I V H S N - G N T|
                                                    |^ 26               36 ^|
AB2             S L S S L S A T L G E R D S L T C R A|S Q D I - - - - - - - S V|
                                                    |^ 20               25 ^|
                                               L2
Kol S V V W Y Q Q L P G M A P K L L I Y|R D A M R P S|G V P D R F S G S K S G
New H V K W Y Q Q L P G T A P K L L I F|- - - - - - -|H N N A R F S V S K S G
Mcp F L A W Y Q Q K P G Q P P K L L I Y|G A S T R E S|G V P D R F T G S G S G

AB1 Y L Y W Y L Q K P G Q S P K L L I Y|R V S N R F S|G V P D R F S G S G S G
                                      |^ 55    61 ^|
AB2 Y L N W L Q R K L D G T I K R L I Y|S T S T L D S|G V P K R F S G S G S G
                                      |^ 44    50 ^|
                                                    L3
Kol T S A S L A I S G L E A E D E S D Y Y C A S|W N N S D N|A Y V F G T G T K
New S S A T L A I T G L Q A E D E A D Y Y C Q S|Y D R S - -|L R V F G G G T K
Mcp T D F T L T I S S V Q A E D L A V Y Y C Q N|D H S Y P L|- - T F G A G T K

AB1 T D F T L K I S R V E A E D M G V Y Y C F Q|G T N V P H|- - T F G G G T K
                                            |^ 96  101 ^|
AB2 L D Y S L T I S S L E S E D F A D Y Y C L Q|Y A S S P Y|- - T F G G G T K
                                            |^ 85   90 ^|
```

```
Heavy chain
                                                            H1
Kol  E V Q L V Q S G G G V V Q P G R S L R L S C S S S G F I F|S S Y|A M Y W Y
New    V Q L E Q S G P G L V R P S Q T L S L T C T V S G T S F|D D Y|Y S T W V
Mcp  E V K L V E S G G G L V Q P G G S L R L S C A T S G F T F|S D F|Y M E W V

AB1  E V Q L A Q S G A E L V K P G A S V K L S C T A S G F N I|K D T|Y M H W V
                                                              |^ 29|
AB2  D V H L Q E S G P G L V K P S Q S L S L T C S V T G Y S I|T R Y|N W N W I
                                                           30|^  G|
                               H2
Kol  R Q A P G K G L E W V A|I I W D D G S|- - D Q H Y A D S V K G R F T I S R
New  R Q P P G R G L E W I G|Y V F Y H G -|- - T S D T D T P L R S R V T M L V
Mcp  R Q P P G K R L E W I A|A S R N K G N|K Y T T E Y S A S V K G R F I V S R

AB1  K Q R P E Q G L E W I G|R I D P A N G|- - N T K Y D P K F Q G K A T I T A
                            |^ 49    55 ^|
AB2  R R F P G N K L E W M G|Y I N Y D G -|- - S N N Y N P S L K N R I S V T R
                            |^ 51   56 ^ |

Kol      N D S K N T L F L Q M D S L R P E D T G V Y F C A R
New      N T S K N Q F S L R L S S V T A A D T A V Y Y C A R
Mcp      D T S Q S I L Y L Q M N A L R A E D T A I Y Y C A R

AB1      D T S S N T A Y L Q L S S L T S E D T A V Y Y C A R

AB2      D T S K N Q F F L K M N S V T T E D T A T Y Y C A R

Kol     |D G G H G F C S S A S C F|G P D Y W G Q Q T P V
New     |D L I A G - - - - - - - -|C I D V W G Q G S L V
Mcp     |N Y Y G S T W - - - - - -|Y F D V W G A G T T V

AB1     |- - - - - - G W L R E D -|A M D Y W G Q G T S V
        |            ^ 98  103 ^  |
AB2     |L I P F S D G Y Y E D Y Y|A M D Y W G Q G T
        |^ 99              111 ^  |
                  H3
```

FIGURE 7. Sequence alignment between three crystallographically determined Fabs, human Kol[31] and New[33] and mouse McPC 603[32] (PMC), with the sequences of Ab_1 G5 and Ab_2 HP22 from GAT. The hypervariable loops are within boxes and are called L 1-3 for the light chain, H 1-3 for the heavy one.

Table 4
THE INTERNAL IMAGE AND THE GERMLINE ORGANIZATION OF THE GAT ID CASCADE

GAT	Ab_1	Ab_2	Ab_3	
			Id^+	Id^-
Public idiotopes (pGAT = Id^+)	Id^+	anti-Id	Id^+	Id^-
V_H germline genes	1 V_H: "H10" (common to V_H NP[a])	1 V_H ?	1 V_H = "H10"	Unrelated genes
V_H expressed genes	Germline and variants	Germline and variants	Mostly germline	—
V_κ germline genes	1 V_κ = "κ1.A5"	2 V_κ ?	1 V_κ = "K5.1"	—
V_κ expressed genes[a]	Somatic variants		Somatic variants	
D regions	Five amino acids positive net charges	LIPFSDGYYED (germline?) or PLYFRHDEEY	Anti-GAT$^+$ ↓ Ab_1-D-like; Anti-GAT$^-$ ↓ Different from D Ab_1	
Synthetic peptides		Ab_2-D-region-like peptides (negative net charge) coupled to KLH or BSA	Anti-peptides	↗ anti-GAT$^+$ (Ag^+ Id^-) ↘ anti-GAT$^-$ (Ag^- Id^-)

[a] V_κ germline genes sequences are from Reference 47.

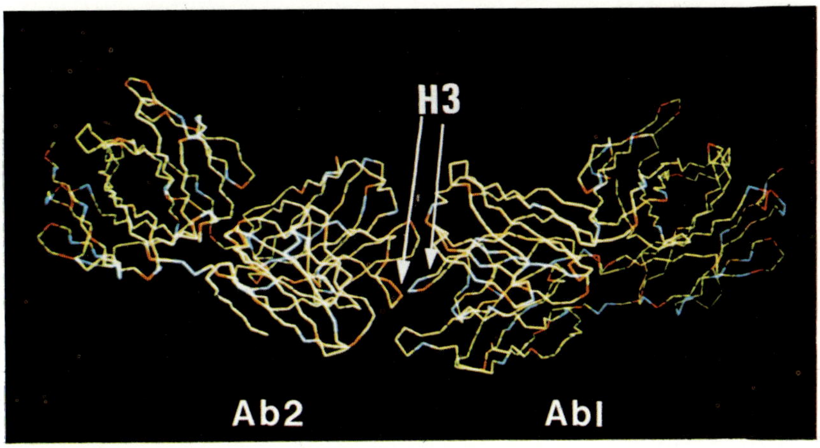

PLATE 1 View of Ab_1-Ab_2 Fabs "best" complex. C atoms are displayed and link together. Acidic residues, red; basic, blue; others, yellow. Note H3-H3 interaction at center.

PLATE 2: See overleaf.

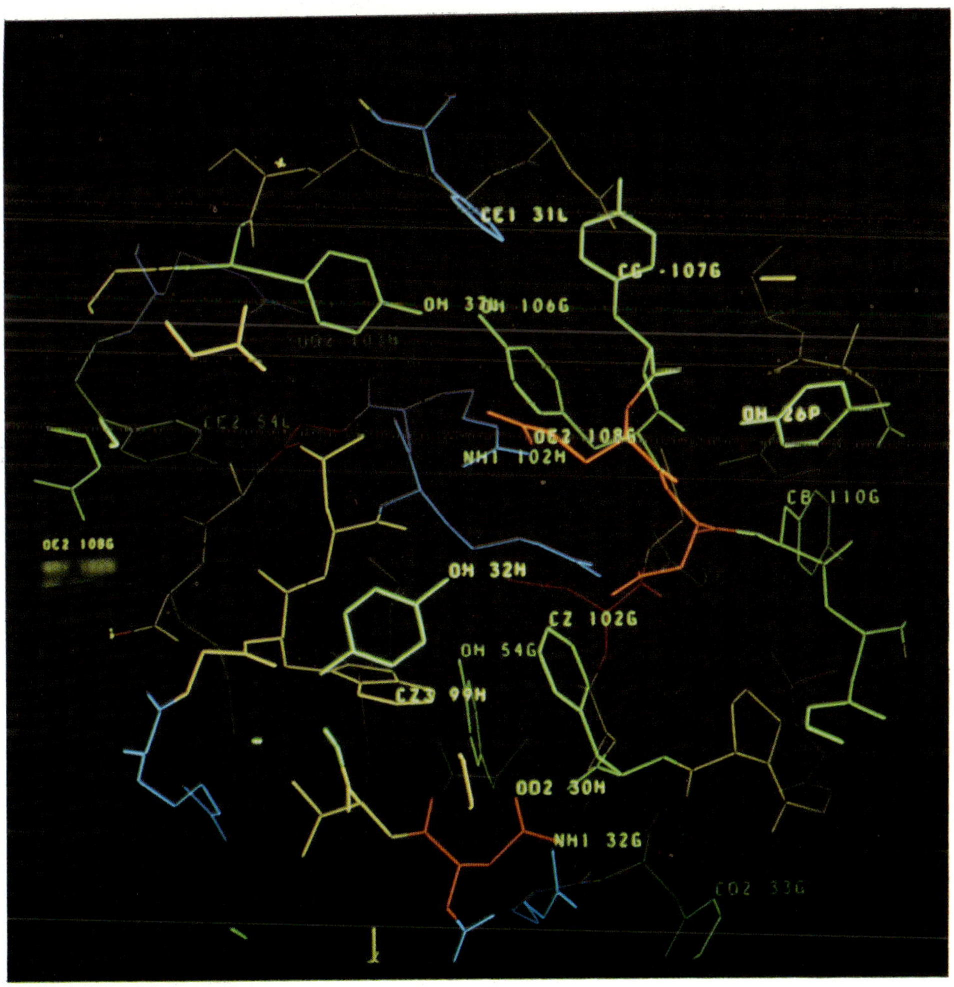

PLATE 3 Close-up view of central contact area between Ab_1 and Ab_2 in the model of their complex. Acidic residues, red; basic, blue; aromatic, green; other types, yellow.

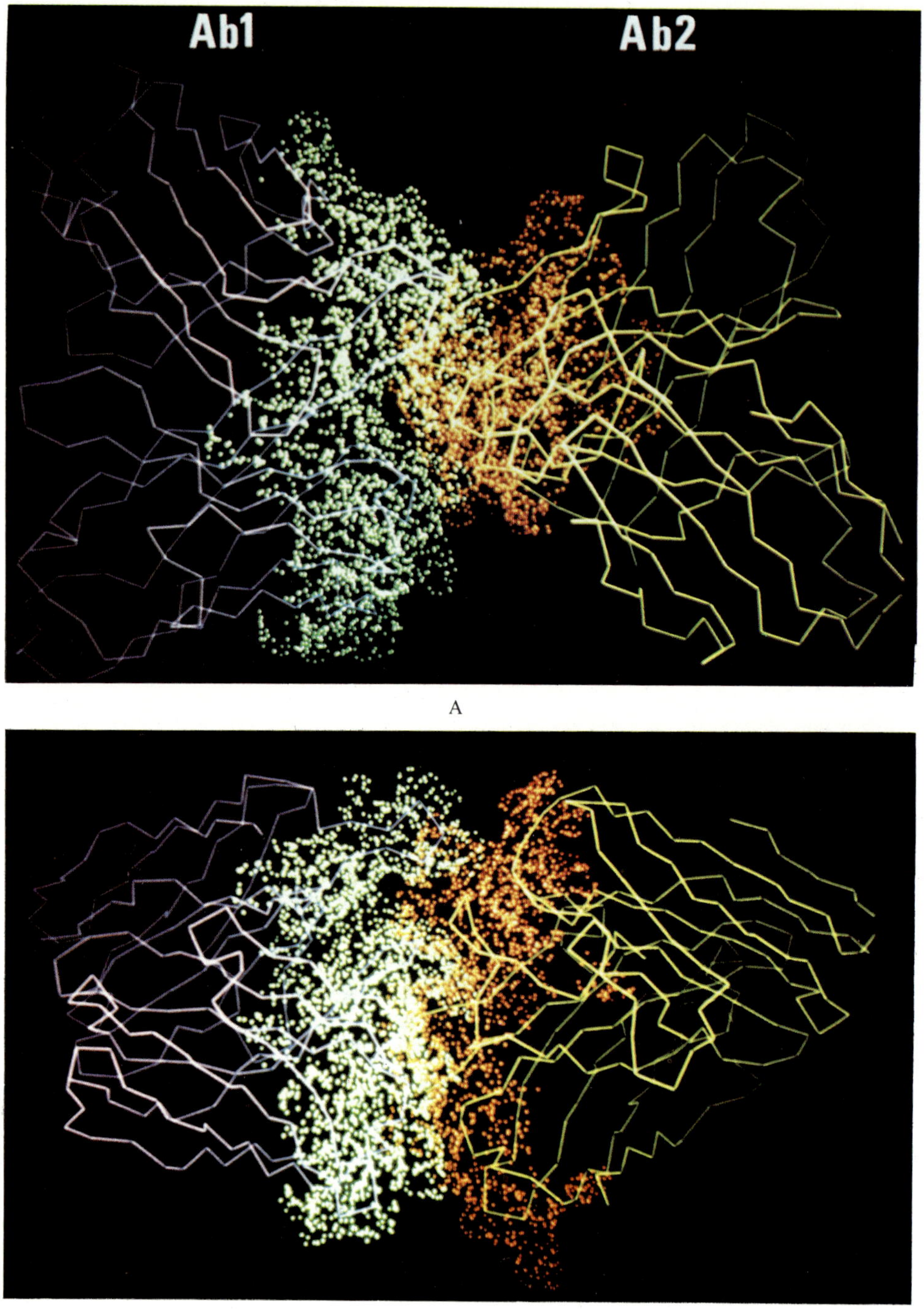

A

B

PLATE 2 View of the variable domains of the Ab_1-Ab_2 complex, displayed with their water-accessible surface.[46] Ab_1 is on the left side. Views (A) and (B) are 90° from each other.

sitioned as close to the original side chain as possible. Residues can also be deleted and new ones can be inserted, taken from the dictionary. Inserted residues are modeled manually on the graphics display to the most plausible conformation. At the end, the models are energy minimized using EREF[40] to give a chemically relevant structure. This method is widely used in 3-D modeling[41,42] (and references therein).

The model of Ab_1 was the easiest to build, since it requires only a few deletions in L1(1), H2(2), and H3(1) and no insertion. The model of Ab_2 requires more drastic changes: a large number of deletions in L1(6) and H2(3). Moreover, in the H3 area, six insertions should be made. In order to avoid an *ab initio* building of this loop, we picked up the H3 loop from the Kol Fab structure where it has the same length, without prejudice of the exact structure of this loop.

2. Complex Modeling

In the absence of any physical data, the modelization of the complex from the Ab_1 and Ab_2 Fab models was based on two arguments:

1. The importance of the H3 hypervariable loop in the GAT system has been extensively discussed above, in line with other systems.[43,44] These observations can be related to the structural observation in Fabs that H3 is located in the middle of the "front" area of the fragment, surrounded by the five other hypervariable loops (Figure 8). In the GAT system especially, a H3-H3 (D-D) contact has been postulated, based on charged residues complementarities. In the case of the G5-HP22 complex, this would involve residues 101-102 vs. 108-109 (see Figure 7).
2. The contact area between a Fab and its antigen has been shown to be large, *circa* 20 × 20 Å.[45] We postulated such a large interaction in the Ab_1-Ab_2 complex.

Therefore, we docked Ab_1 and Ab_2, keeping in mind these two points, so to check if they were compatible together and could lead to a relevant 3-D model. Practically, the models were docked "manually" using the FRODO screen option FBRT (rigid body translation-rotation) to produce a small number of complex models. The contact faces of the Fabs were then surfaced using Connolly's MS program (water-accessible surface[46]). The "best" model was selected on the criterion of the largest contact area. Both H3 regions were then modeled manually to establish the two ion pairs, respectively, R 101-E 108 and R 102-D 109.

3. Model Examination

Plate 1 (following page 36) represents the "best" model of the Ab_1-Ab_2 Fabs complex. In Plates 2A and B (facing page), the two variable domains of each Fab are displayed with their contact surfaces. The two views are 90° from each other. The contact area is about 12 × 20 Å. Plate 3 (following page 36) is a close up of the central contact area. The two ion pairs are surrounded by a large number of aromatic residues, predominantly tyrosines. This hydrophobic core probably exalts the importance of having balanced charges in this area. The description of other contacts between hypervariable loops is far beyond the limit that one should give to the model, since a slight tilt around the complex axis could bring different residues into contact.

In conclusion, the construction of this model confirmed the hypothesis that Ab_1 and Ab_2 may interact through a large contact area. In the center of this area, a highly specific interaction (two ion pairs), exalted by the presence of an hydrophobic surrounding, can probably be associated with the "internal image" concept.

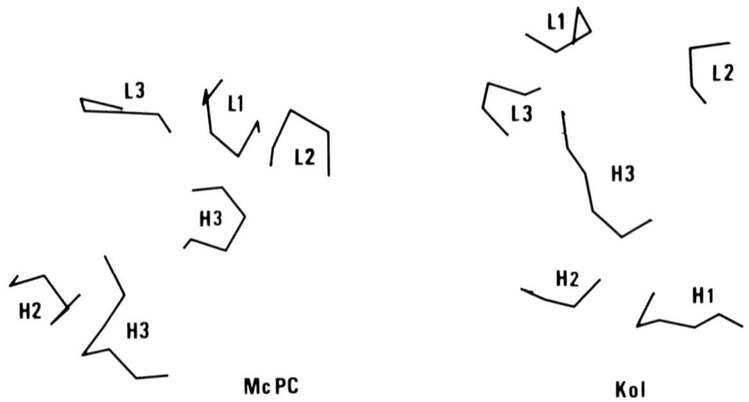

FIGURE 8. Front view of the McPC and Kol Fab hypervariable loops.

REFERENCES

1. **Jerne, N. K.,** Towards a network theory of the immune system, *Ann. Immunol. (Inst. Pasteur),* 125C, 373, 1974.
2. **Oudin, J. and Michel, M.,** Une nouvelle forme d'allotypie des globulines γ du sérum de lapin apparemment liée à la spécificité des anticorps, *C.R. Acad. Sci. (Paris),* 257, 805, 1963.
3. **Urbain, J., Wikler, M., Franssen, J. D., and Collignon, C.,** Idiotypic regulation of the immune system by the induction of antibodies against anti-idiotypic antibodies, *Proc. Natl. Acad. Sci. U.S.A.,* 74, 5126, 1977.
4. **Cazenave, P. A.,** Idiotypic-anti-idiotypic regulation of antibody synthesis in rabbits, *Proc. Natl. Acad. Sci. U.S.A.,* 74, 5122, 1977.
5. **Jerne, N. K., Roland, J., and Cazenave, P. A.,** Recurrent idiotopes and internal images, *EMBO J.,* 1, 243, 1982.
6. **Schnurr, I.,** Idiotypes, Antigens on the Inside, workshop at the Basel Institute for Immunology, Hoffman La Roche, Basel, 1981, 122.
7. **Bona, C. S., Finley, S., Waters, S., and Kunkel, H. G.,** Anti-Ig antibodies. III. Properties of sequential anti-idiotypic antibodies to heterologous anti-γ-globulins. Detection of reactivity of anti-idiotype antibodies with epitopes of Fc fragments (homobodies) and with epitopes and idiotopes (epibodies), *J. Exp. Med.,* 156, 986, 1982.
8. **Urbain, J., Brait, M., Bruyns, C., Demeur, C., Dubois, P., Francotte, M., Franssen, J.-D., Hiernaux, J., Leo, O., Marvel, J., Meyers, P., Moser, M., Slaoui, M., Tassignon, J., Urbain-Vansanten, G., Van-Acker, A., Wickler, M., Willems, F., and Wuilmart, C.,** The idiotypic network: order from the beginning or order out of chaos, *Curr. Top. Microbiol. Immunol.,* 119, 127, 1985.
9. **Rajewsky, K. and Takemori, K.,** Genetics, expression and function of idiotypes, *Annu. Rev. Immunol.,* 1, 569, 1983.
10. **Urbain, J., Wuilmart, C., and Cazenave, P. A.,** Idiotypic regulation in immune networks, *Contemp. Top. Mol. Immunol.,* 8, 113, 1981.
11. **Jerne, N. K.,** Idiotypic network and other preconceived ideas, *Immunol. Rev.,* 79, 1, 1984.
12. **Cosenza, H. and Kohler, H.,** Specific inhibition of plaque formation to phosphorylcholine by antibody against antibody, *Science,* 176, 1027, 1972.
13. **Ju, S. T., Kipps, T. J., Thèze, J., Benacerraf, B., and Dorf, M. E.,** Idiotypic analysis of anti-GAT antibodies. I. Presence of common idiotypic specificities in both responder and non-responder mice, *J. Immunol.,* 121, 1034, 1978.
14. **Thèze, J. and Moreau, J. L.,** Genetic control of the immune response to the GAT terpolymer. I. Interstrain and interspecies cross-reactive idiotype, *Ann. Immunol. (Inst. Pasteur),* 129C, 721, 1978.
15. **Thèze, J. and Sommé, G.,** Genetic control of the immune response to the terpolymer GAT. Characterization of a cross-reactive idiotype associated with anti-GAT antibodies from responder and nonresponder mice, *Eur. J. Immunol.,* 9, 294, 1979.

16. **Sommé, G., Rocca-Serra, J., Leclercq, L., Moreau, J. L., Mazie, J. C., Moinier, D., Fougereau, M., and Thèze, J.,** Contribution of the H and L chains of the combining site to the idiotypic specificities of mouse anti-GAT antibodies, *Mol. Immunol.*, 19, 1011, 1982.
17. **Leclercq, L., Mazie, J. C., Sommé, G., and Thèze, J.,** Monoclonal anti-GAT antibodies with different fine specificities express the same public idiotype, *Mol. Immunol.*, 19, 1001, 1982.
18. **Sommé, G., Roth, C., Mazie, J. C., Salem, P., and Thèze, J.,** Public and individual idiotopes in the anti-GAT response: analysis by monoclonal antibodies, *Eur. J. Immunol.*, 13, 1023, 1983.
19. **Roth, C., Sommé, G., Schiff, C., and Thèze, J.,** Immune response against GAT: immunization with monoclonal anti-idiotypic antibodies leads to the predominant stimulation of idiotypically similar Ig with an anti-GAT activity, *Eur. J. Immunol.*, 15, 576, 1985.
20. **Kabat, E. A., Wu, T. T., Bilofsky, H., Reid-Miller, M., and Perry, M.,** Sequences of Proteins of Immunological Interest, U.S. Department of Health and Human Services, National Institutes of Health, Bethesda, Md.,1983.
21. **Schiff, C., Milili, M., Hue, I., Rudikoff, S., and Fougereau, M.,** Genetic basis for expression of the idiotypic network. One unique IgV_H germline gene accounts for the major family of Ab1 and Ab3 ($Ab_{1'}$) antibodies of the GAT system, *J. Exp. Med.*, 163, 573, 1986.
22. **Rocca-Serra, J., Matthes, H. W., Kaartinen, M., Milstein, C., Thèze, J., and Fougereau, M.,** Analysis of antibody diversity: V-D-J mRNA nucleotide sequence of 4 anti-GAT monoclonal antibodies, *EMBO J.*, 2, 867, 1983.
23. **Schiff, C., Milili, M., and Fougereau, M.,** Immunoglobulin diversity: analysis of the germ-line V_H gene repertoire of the murine anti-GAT response, *Nucl. Acids Res.*, 11, 1007, 1983.
24. **Schiff, C., Milili, M., and Fougereau, M.,** Functional and pseudogenes are similarly organized and may equally contribute to the extensive antibody diversity of the Ig V_H II family, *EMBO J.*, 4, 1225, 1985.
25. **Roth, C., Rocca-Serra, J., Sommé, G., Fougereau, M., and Thèze, J.,** The gene repertoire of the GAT immune response: comparison of the V_H V_κ and D regions used by anti-GAT antibodies and monoclonal antibodies produced after anti-idiotypic immunization, *Proc. Natl. Acad. Sci. U.S.A.*, 82, 4788, 1985.
26. **Ollier, P., Rocca-Serra, J., Sommé, G., Thèze, J., and Fougereau, M.,** The idiotypic network and the internal image: possible regulation of a germ-line network by paucigene encoded Ab2 (anti-idiotypic) antibodies in the GAT system, *EMBO J.*, 4, 3681, 1985.
27. **Chen, P. P., Fong, S., Normansell, D., Houghton, R. A., Karras, J. G., Vaughan, J. H., and Carson, D. A.,** Delineation of a cross-reactive idiotype on human autoantibodies with antibody against a synthetic peptide, *J. Exp. Med.*, 159, 1502, 1984.
28. **Merrifield, R. B.,** Solid phase synthesis. I. The synthesis of a tetrapeptide, *J. Am. Chem. Soc.*, 85, 2149, 1963.
29. **Urbain, J., Wuilmart, C., and Cazenave, P. A.,** *Contemp. Top. Mol. Immunol.*, 8, 113, 1981.
30. **Mazza, G., Ollier, P., Sommé, G., Moinier, D., Rocca-Serra, J., van Rietschoten, J., Thèze, J., and Fougereau, M.,** A structural basis for the internal image in the idiotypic network: antibodies against synthetic Ab2-D regions cross-react with the original antigen, *Ann. Inst. Pasteur/Immunol.*, 136D, 259, 1985.
31. **Marquart, M., Deisenhofer, J., Huber, R., and Palm, W.,** Crystallographic refinement and atomic models of the intact immunoglobulin molecules Kol and its antigen-binding fragment at 3.0 A and 1.9 A resolution, *J. Mol. Biol.*, 141, 369, 1980.
32. **Segal, D. M., Padlan, E. A., Cohen, G. H., Rudikoff, S., Potter, M., and Davies, D. R.,** The three-dimensional structure of a phosphorylcholine-binding mouse immunoglobulin Fab and the nature of the antigen binding site, *Proc. Natl. Acad. Sci. U.S.A.*, 71, 4298, 1974.
33. **Poljak, R. J., Amzel, L. M., Chen, B. L., Phizackerley, R. P., and Saul, F.,** The three-dimensional structure of the Fab′ fragment of a human myeloma immunoglobulin at 2.0 A resolution, *Proc. Natl. Acad. Sci. U.S.A.*, 71, 3440, 1974.
34. **Williams, A. F.,** Immunoglobulin-related domains for cell surface recognition, *Nature (News Views)*, 314, 579, 1985.
35. **Amzel, L. M. and Poljak, R. J.,** Three-dimensional structure of immunoglobulins, *Annu. Rev. Biochem.*, 48, 579, 1985.
36. **Davies, D. R. and Metzger, H.,** Structural basis of antibody function, *Annu. Rev. Immunol.*, 1, 87, 1983.
37. **Lesk, A. M. and Chothia, C.,** Evolution of proteins formed by beta-sheets. II. The core of the immunoglobulin domains, *J. Mol. Biol.*, 160, 325, 1982.
38. Protein Data Bank, Chemistry Department, Brookhaven National Laboratory, Upton, N.Y., 1973.
39. **Jones, T. A.,** *Computational Crystallography*, Sayre, D., Ed., Clarendon Press, Oxford, 1982.
40. **Jack, A. and Levitt, M.,** Refinement of large structures by simultaneous minimization of energy and R factor, *Acta Crystallogr.*, A34, 931, 1978.
41. **Travers, P., Blundell, T. L., Sternberg, M. J. E., and Bodmer, W. F.,** Structural and evolutionary analysis of HLA-D region products, *Nature*, 310, 235, 1984.
42. **Eklund, H., Horjales, E., Jornvall, H., Branden, C. I., and Jeffery, J.,** Molecular aspects of functional differences between alcohol and sorbitol dehydrogenases, *Biochemistry*, 24, 8005, 1985.

43. **Radbruch, A., Zaiss, S., Kappen, C., Bruggemann, M., Beyreuther, K., and Rajewsky, K.,** Drastic change in idiotypic but not antigen-binding specificity of an antibody by a single amino-acid substitution, *Nature*, 315, 506, 1985.
44. **Krawinkel, U., Zoebelein, G., Bruggemann, M., Radbruch, A., and Rajewsky, K.,** Recombination between antibody heavy chain variable-region genes: evidence for gene conversion, *Proc. Natl. Acad. Sci. U.S.A.*, 80, 4997, 1983.
45. **Amit, A. G., Mariuzza, R. A., Phillips, S. E. V., and Poljak, R. J.,** Three-dimensional structure of an antigen-antibody complex at 6 A resolution, *Nature*, 313, 1, 1985.
46. **Connolly, M. L.,** Analytical molecular surface calculation, *J. Appl. Crystallogr.*, 16, 548, 1983.
47. **Corbet, S., Corbet, S., Milili, M., Fougereau, M., Schiff, C.,** Two V_κ germline genes related to the GAT idiotypic network account for the major subfamilies of the mouse V_κ I variability subgroup, *J. Immunol.*, 138, 932, 1987.

Chapter 4

MOLECULAR BASIS OF EPIBODY REACTIVITY*

P. P. Chen, S. Fong, and D. A. Carson

TABLE OF CONTENTS

* This is the publication number 4349BCR from the Research Institute of Scripps Clinic, La Jolla. P.P. Chen is an Investigator of the Arthritis Foundation. S. Fong is a recipient of a Research Career Development Award (AG00279) from the National Institute of Aging. Funding for this research supported in part by grants AM35218, AG04100, and AM25443 from the National Institutes of Health.

I. INTRODUCTION

Idiotypes (Id) are unique antigenic determinants of Ig molecules, defined serologically by anti-idiotypic (anti-Id) antibodies.[1,2] Conceptually, this implies that an anti-Id antibody (Ab_2) recognizes and binds to a determinant (i.e., idiotope) on the immunizing Ig (Ab_1). However, recent studies demonstrate that some antibodies against "cross-reactive Id" (CRI) mimic the antigen of the respective Ab_1, and, thus, Ab_2 is recognized and bound by the Ab_1.[3] The latter type of anti-Id antibodies are called homobodies, internal images, or $Ab_{2\beta}$,[4-10] while the first type of anti-Id is called $Ab_{2\alpha}$.[7]

In addition to these two types of anti-Id antibodies, Bona et al.[12] recently described yet amother anti-Id antibody. The antibody binds to both the Id of Ab_1 (a human monoclonal IgM anti-IgG antibody, a rheumatoid factor/RF) and the antigen (human IgG) recognized by Ab_1. This anti-Id is called an epibody or $Ab_{2\epsilon}$.[11,12]

Among human monoclonal IgM RF from unrelated individuals with cryoglobulinemia, Kunkel and colleagues described two major CRI, termed Wa and Po.[13-16] They include 60 and 20% of monoclonal IgM-RF, respectively. Moreover, all Wa-CRI-positive IgM RF contain light chains of the kIIIb sub-subgroup, which constitutes only about 13% of Ig κ chains;[17,18] and amino acid sequence analyses of two Wa-positive RF revealed that their light chain variable regions are extremely homologous, while their heavy chain variable regions are heterogeneous.[19] These data strongly indicate that the Wa-CRI is associated mainly with the light chains of RF. This conclusion has recently been verified. The accumulated data indicate that the Wa-CRI is localized to the second complementarity-determining region (CDR) on RF κ light chains.[20-22]

During the last few years, we have studied the Id of human RFs. First, we made "conventional" polyclonal anti-Id ($Ab_{2\alpha}$ type) against the serum RF from a patient with rheumatoid arthritis and used this reagent to show that the RF Id were inherited among the related members of a family.[23] Second, we prepared a "conventional" murine monoclonal anti-Id 17.109 ($Ab_{2\alpha}$ type) against the human monoclonal IgM-RF Sie.[24-26] Third, we generated a polyclonal anti-CRI that mimicked human IgG (i.e., the antigen of human RF) and demonstrated that this reagent suppressed in vitro RF production by pokeweed mitogen-stimulated human peripheral blood lymphocytes.[28,29] Fourth, to study the structural and genetic basis of RFs in outbred human populations, we used synthetic peptides (corresponding to the CDR of some human monoclonal IgM RFs) to induce anti-Id.[20-22,25,30-33] Among these synthetic CDR peptide-induced antibodies, we found one that reacted with both a CRI of human RF and the antigen of human RF.[31] Very recently, we also generated a monoclonal anti-Id that reacts with both human RF and human IgG.[34] In this communication, we shall review the reported observations concerning epibodies and discuss the possible molecular basis for these peculiar anti-Id.

II. INDUCTION OF MURINE POLYCLONAL EPIBODIES WITH A MONOCLONAL ANTIBODY[11]

To characterize the Id of the Wa-CRI-positive human IgM-RF Glo, Bona et al.[11] immunized 11 different strains of mice four times intraperitoneally with the intact Glo protein emulsified in complete Freund's adjuvant (CFA). The immune sera were absorbed with an irrelevant IgM(kIII) protein, Ch, coupled to Sepharose®4B.[11] All strains of mice produced anti-Id that reacted with the RF Glo. However, the A/J anti-Glo antiserum displayed a peculiar binding activity. When analyzed by radioimmunoassay (RIA), the absorbed A/J anti-Glo antiserum bound to microtiter wells precoated with 50 μg/mℓ of various IgM(kIII) paraproteins, including Glo, Pg, Dau, Sa, and Ga, but not to wells precoated with the IgM Ch (Table 1, Experiment I). Glo and Pg have anti-IgG activity, while the rest have no known

Table 1
THE BINDING PROPERTIES OF A/J ANTI-GLO ANTIBODIES[10]

		Antigens						
		RIA binding assay (cpm)[a]						HA assay[b]
Experiment	**Sample**	**Glo**	**Pg**	**Dau**	**Ch**	**IgG**	**Fc**	**Glo**
I	BALB/c anti-Glo	1,643	1,174	143	42	—[c]	—	>12
	A/J anti-Glo	2,942	2,734	2,114	209	—	—	—
II	BALB/c anti-Glo	—	—	—	—	290	—	—
	A/J anti-Glo	—	—	—	—	13,804	—	—
III	A/J anti-Glo absorbed with							
	None	—	—	—	—	—	8,897	7
	Glo	—	—	—	—	—	6,380	3
	IgG	—	—	—	—	—	4,467	3
	Glo Fab	—	—	—	—	—	6,667	2
	IgG Fc	—	—	—	—	—	5,669	4
	Dau	—		—		—	6,117	5
	Ch	—	—	—	—	—	8,767	7

[a] Microtiter wells were coated with antigens at 50 μg/mℓ, except IgG-Fc (at 30 μg/mℓ). cpm expressed are the mean of triplicates, after subtracting the nonspecific binding to wells precoated with fetal calf serum proteins.

[b] Hemagglutination/HA titers of the anti-Glo antiserum were measured using sheep erythrocytes coated with the protein Glo. The results are $1/\log_2$ (highest dilution of antiserum that caused agglutination).

[c] Not done.

specificity. The results showed that A/J anti-Glo antibodies recognized a CRI shared by a very high proportion of human IgM(kIII) proteins, and that the CRI were likely to be associated with their light chains.

Subsequently, these authors found that the anti-CRI bound to wells precoated with 50 μg/mℓ of human IgG (Table 1, Experiment II). Moreover, the binding activity to both RF Glo and human IgG were simultaneously decreased upon absorption with either the RF Glo or human IgG (Table 1, Experiment III). Together, the data suggested that the anti-Glo antibodies reacted with both a CRI marker and the antigen of the human IgM RF Glo. This novel anti-Id was called "epibody/$Ab_{2\epsilon}$".

It should be noted that not all antihuman IgG antibodies in the A/J anti-Glo antiserum are epibodies. A careful examination of the data in the third experiment of Table 1 suggests that there are two components in the anti-Glo antiserum (Table 2). The first component has epibody properties and reacts with the RF Glo, non-RF Dau, and human IgG, but not with the non-RF Ch paraprotein. This antibody can be removed by absorption with Glo-coupled Sepharose®4B. The second component of the antiserum consists of antihuman IgG antibodies which are induced nonspecifically or indirectly and are not absorbed by the Glo-coupled Sepharose®4B.

Table 2
TWO COMPONENTS IN A/J ANTI-GLO ANTISERUM[a]

	Reactivity with				
Antibody	**Glo**	**Dau**	**Ch**	**IgG**	**Comments**
Epibody	+	+	−	+	Antibodies which can be removed by the Glo-column
Anti-IgG	−	−	−	+	Glo-absorbed anti-Glo antiserum

[a] These two putative components are deduced from the binding activities of various antiserum samples toward IgG-Fc and RF-Glo in the third experiment of Table 1: (1) subtract 4467 (IgG-absorbed) from 8897 (not absorbed); the result 4430 is the total specific anti-Ig activity in the anti-Glo antiserum; (2) subtract 3 (Glo-absorbed) from 7 (not absorbed); the result 4 is the total specific anti-Glo in the anti-Glo antiserum; (3) subtract 6380 (Glo-absorbed) from 8897; the result 2517 is the IgG-binding activity of the "epibody". Comparing with the total IgG-binding activity 4430, the additional Ig-binding (in excess of 2517) is due to the "anti-IgG" component.

III. INDUCTION OF RABBIT POLYCLONAL EPIBODIES WITH A SYNTHETIC PEPTIDE[31]

The structural correlates of Id have been pursued in several well-defined antibody systems.[35-40] The results suggest that the CDR of both the heavy and light chains are the structural correlates of Id determinants. Recently, synthetic peptides have been used to induce antibodies specific for preselected determinants in intact proteins.[41-45] This finding prompted us, as well as others, to use synthetic peptides (corresponding to the selected CDR sequences) to generate anti-Id of predefined specificity in an effort to delineate the structural basis of Id.[20-22,25,30-33,46] In a large series of experiments, these peptide-induced anti-Id, together with amino acid sequence data, have allowed us to study the genetic basis of CRI in outbred human populations.[18-22,25,30-33,47-49]

During the generation and characterization of a panel of such peptide-induced anti-Id, we unexpectedly encountered a peculiar anti-Id induced by a peptide, designated PGL1. It was composed of Cys-Arg-Ala-Ser-Gln-Ser-Val-Ser-Ser-Ser-Tyr-Leu-Ala, corresponding to amino acid residues 23-34 (first CDR and the adjacent first framework region) of the RF Glo light chain.[18,49] Rabbits were immunized three times with PGL1, conjugated to keyhole limpet hemocyanin, in CFA. Thereafter sera were collected and analyzed for both anti-PGL1 and anti-Glo activity by enzyme-linked immunosorbent assay (ELISA).[31]

All three immunized rabbits produced high titer anti-PGL1 antibodies, while only two produced anti-Glo antibodies. The results of one representative antiserum are shown in Table 3. As can be seen, anti-PGL1 antibodies reacted specifically with the PGL1 peptide, and significantly with the RF Glo, as compared with pooled human IgM which was coated at a 25-fold higher concentration. The control peptide (PSH3, corresponding to the third CDR of the heavy chain of the IgM-RF Sie and composed of Glu-Trp-Lys-Gly-Gln-Val-Asn-Val-Asn-Pro-Phe-Asp-Tyr-Gly-Gly-Cys) has been shown to induce antibodies specific for a private Id on the RF Sie heavy chains.[30,32]

Since RF Glo reacts with rabbit IgG, an immunoblot assay was used to demonstrate conclusively the anti-Id activity of the anti-PGL1 antibodies.[30,31] In a typical experiment, RF Glo and the control, pooled human IgG (Cohn fraction II) were separated into heavy and light chains by electrophoresis under reducing conditions in a 10% polyacrylamide gel

Table 3
INDUCTION OF ANTI-ID WITH PGL1 PEPTIDES

		Binding A_{405} × 1000 to antigens[b]							
Line	**Samples**[a]	**PSH3**	**PGL1**	**BSA**	**Glo**	**IgM**	**IgG**	**(Fab')$_2$**	**Fc**
1	Buffer only	1	1	1	15	55	88	11	17
2	Preimmunize	38	37	24	189	139	285	91	78
3	Immune serum	57	1527	17	*367*	173	*531*	*610*	268
4	Anti-Hu Ig	ND	ND	9	1796	1835	1863	1821	1301

[a] Sera were diluted 1:100 in borate-buffered saline with 0.5% bovine serum albumin (BSA). The immune serum was collected on day 14 after the third immunization. The IgG fraction of polyspecific antihuman Ig was used at 1 μg/mℓ.

[b] Antigens were used at the following concentrations: PSH3, PGL1, and Glo at 2μg/mℓ; BSA at 1 mg/mℓ; IgM, IgG, (Fab')$_2$, and Fc at 50 μg/mℓ. Absorbance at 405 nm was amplified 1000-fold and expressed.

containing sodium dodecyl sulfate (SDS), and then the polypeptides were electroblotted onto nitrocellulose paper. Subsequently, the paper was treated sequentially with: (1) phosphate-buffered saline (PBS) containing 5% BSA to block nonspecific protein binding sites; (2) anti-PGL1 antiserum (diluted 1:10 with borate-buffered saline [BBS] containing 5% BSA); (3) BBS wash; (4) radiolabeled protein A (0.1 μCi/mℓ in PBS/2.5% BSA); and (5) BBS wash.

Figure 1 shows that the anti-PGL1 antibodies reacted specifically with the Glo light chains, but not with the heavy chain of Glo nor with the light chains of pooled human IgG. Moreover, the binding to the Glo light chains was completely inhibited by the PGL1 peptide (Figure 1), but not by the PSH3 peptide (data not shown). Subsequently, the specificity of the anti-PGL1 antibodies was analyzed against a panel of human monoclonal IgM-RF paraproteins. The antibodies reacted with the separated κ light chains of the monoclonal IgM RF paraproteins Gar, Glo, Got, Neu, Pal, and Pay, but not with the κ light chains of the RF Lay (Figure 2 in Reference 31). The anti-PGL1 antibodies did not bind to the heavy chains of any IgM RF. Thus, the synthetic PGL1 peptide induced an anti-Id against a CRI associated with the κ light chains of several human IgM RF autoantibodies. The structural basis of this CRI is defined by the PGL1 amino acid sequence.

However, the PGL1-induced anti-Id also reacted surprisingly with the separated γ chains of pooled human IgG, but not with the separated light chains of the same pooled human IgG. To probe the possible structural basis for this peculiar observation, three experiments were performed. As shown in Figure 1, the binding of the anti-PGL1 antiserum to γ chains was inhibited partially by the PGL1 peptide. Under the same conditions, the control PSH3 peptide did not inhibit binding (data not shown). However, it should be noted that the peptide inhibition of binding to γ chains was not as complete as to Glo light chains. Based on the intensity of the autoradiographs, we estimated that a maximum of 70% of the binding was inhibitable. This result suggests that there are at least two sets of anti-γ components in the "polyclonal" anti-PGL1 antiserum, and that only one set recognizes the PGL1-associated epitopes on the IgG γ chains.

Second, to verify that the same antibody molecules bound to both Glo light chains and IgG γ chains, the anti-PGL1 antiserum was passed through a human IgG-coupled Sepharose®4B column, and the eluate was analyzed by the immunoblot method. Figure 2 shows

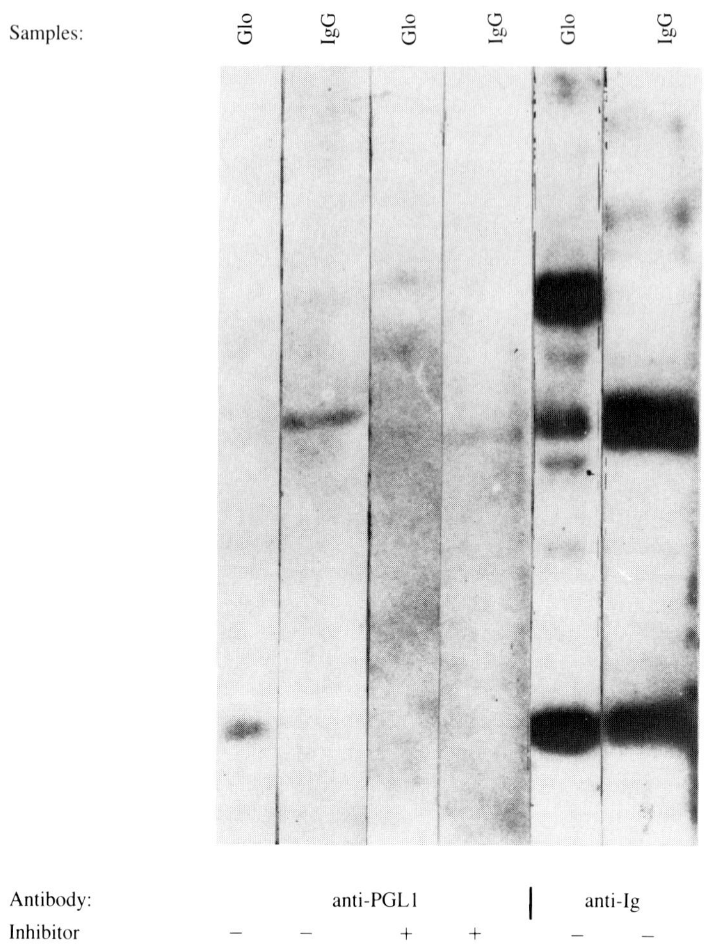

FIGURE 1. The epibody activity of the anti-PGL1 antiserum. 10 μg of each sample was loaded into each slot. After electrophoresis and blotting, the samples on the paper were incubated with the indicated antibodies with or without the PGL1 peptide. (Reproduced from *The Journal of Experimental Medicine*, 1985, 161, 323, by copyright permission of The Rockfeller University Press.)

that the eluate reacted with both Glo light chains and IgG γ chains, but not with IgG light chains. Again, the binding to Glo light chains, but not to IgG γ chains, was completely inhibited by the PGL1 peptide. On the other hand, the IgG-absorbed anti-PGL1 antiserum still bound to the Glo light chain. The binding was inhibited entirely by the PGL1 peptide (data not shown). When analyzed against a panel of monoclonal IgM-RF paraproteins by immunoblotting, the eluate bound to the light chains of Gar, Glo, Got, and Neu, but not to Lay light chains. In each case, binding was completely inhibited by the PGL1 peptide, but not by the PSH3 peptide (data not shown).

Third, to characterize more precisely the γ determinants recognized by the anti-PGL1 antiserum, microtiter wells were precoated with either human IgG, IgM, $(Fab')_2$ fragments of IgG, or the Fc fragments of IgG. As can be seen in Table 3, the anti-PGL1 antiserum bound better to the $(Fab')_2$ than to the Fc.

Taken together, these results confirm the existence of epibodies. The experiments also indicate that there are three components in the anti-PGL1 antiserum (Table 4): (1) conventional anti-Id that react with Glo light chains only, and whose antibody reactivity is completely inhibited by PGL1; (2) epibodies that react with both Glo light chain and IgG, and whose

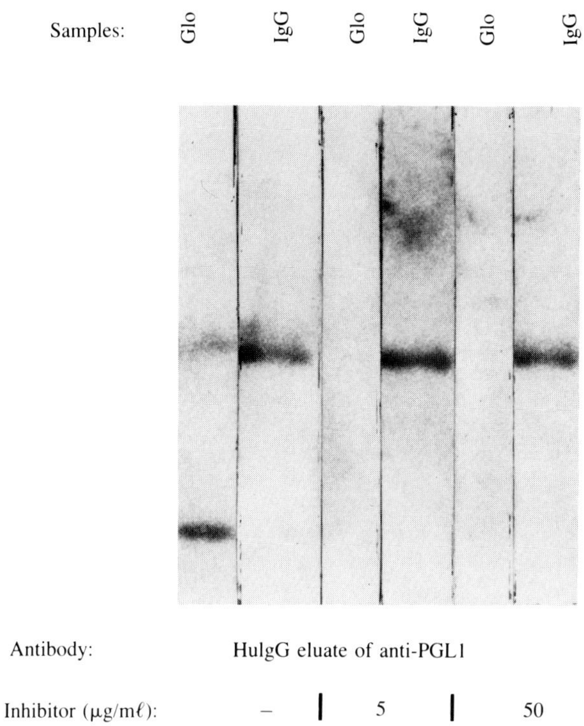

FIGURE 2. Human IgG affinity-isolated, anti-PGL1 antibodies consisted of two sets: epibodies and anti-IgG antibodies. Nitrocellulose paper with the indicated samples were incubated with antibodies (0.5 μg/mℓ) with or without the inhibitor PGL1. (Reproduced from *The Journal of Experimental Medicine*, 1985, 161, 323, by copyright permission of The Rockefeller University Press.)

Table 4
THREE COMPONENTS IN THE ANTI-PGL1 ANTISERUM

	Reactivity with				
Antibody	**Glo**	**Glo light**	**IgG**	**IgG heavy**	**PGL1**
Anti-Glo, conventional	+	+	–	–	+
Epibody	+	+	+	+	+
Anti-IgG	–	–	+	+	–
	Inhibition of Binding by PGL1[a]				
Anti-Glo, conventional	±[b]	+	NA[c]	NA	+
Epibody	±	+	–	+	+
Anti-IgG	NA	NA	–	–	NA

[a] Inhibition of binding to intact protein was done by ELISA (data not shown).
[b] PGL1 at 500 μg/mℓ gave about 10% inhibition.
[c] Not applicable.

Reproduced from *The Journal of Experimental Medicine,* 1985, 161, 323, by copyright permission of the Rockfeller University Press.

antibody reactivity is inhibitable by PGL1; and (3) anti-IgG antibodies that react with IgG only, and whose binding is not inhibited by PGL1. The epibodies react with both separated IgG γ chains and intact IgG, and probably recognize some determinant(s) in the first domain of the γ chain constant region.

It should be pointed out that the epibody component constitutes only a very small portion of overall anti-PGL1 antibodies, and that its binding to the separated Glo light chain and IgG γ chain is of low affinity. Moreover, the peptide inhibition of the anti-PGL1 binding to both intact Glo and intact IgG is not as efficient as that to the Glo light chains and γ chains, suggesting that the binding to intact Glo and intact IgG is of even lower affinity. Similar to the A/J anti-Glo antiserum, the anti-PGL1 serum contains some antihuman IgG antibodies which are induced indirectly, possibly through the immune network or other unknown mechanisms.

IV. INDUCTION OF A MURINE MONOCLONAL EPIBODY WITH POLYCLONAL ANTIBODIES[34]

Homobodies (internal image anti-Id) potentially represent ideal reagents for the manipulation of RF production by human peripheral blood lymphocytes from unrelated individuals. Previously, we reported that homobodies/$Ab_{2\beta}$ could be specifically enriched from a rabbit polyclonal anti-CRI antiserum using an affinity column conjugated with rabbit antibodies to the Fc fragment of human IgG.[27] Subsequently, we showed that such enriched homobodies could suppress the in vitro production of IgM-RF by pokeweed mitogen-stimulated human peripheral blood lymphocytes.[28] These results prompted us to generate monoclonal homobodies to human RF.

BALB/c mice were immunized with a mixture of human monoclonal IgM-RF, emulsified in CFA. The paraproteins included Glo (kIIIb, Wa-CRI positive), Pal, Lay (kI, Po-CRI positive), Pom (kIIIa, Po-CRI positive), and Koh (lambda). Three days after boosting with the pooled RF in saline, the splenic lymphocytes were fused with x63-Ag.8 myeloma cells. The hybridoma supernatants were screened by ELISA for anti-Id capable of inhibiting the binding of the same pooled RF to human IgG. During these experiments, we unexpectedly obtained one clone (c147) that reacted with both a CRI marker on RF as well as the antigen (IgG) recognized by human RF.

Supernatants from c147 inhibited 85 to 100% of the binding of various immunizing RF to human IgG (Table 5). Moreover, the c147 supernatants inhibited the binding of polyclonal RF Mei (from a patient with rheumatoid arthritis) to human IgG. In contrast, the c147 supernatants did not inhibit significantly the binding of human polyclonal IgM antithyroglobulin to thyroglobulin. These results show that the monoclonal antibody c147 is an anti-Id that recognizes a CRI expressed by a majority of human IgM-RF, but not by IgM antithyroglobulin antibodies.

To characterize the inhibitory activity of this anti-CRI antibody, we assessed its ability to bind directly to the RF (Ab_1) and to human IgG (the antigen of RF). Table 6 shows that the antibody c147 bound specifically to polyclonal RF, but not to non-RF IgM. Furthermore, the antibody c147 also reacted with human IgG, but not at all with rabbit IgG (Table 6). In contrast, the control monoclonal IgG1 antibody Scl did not bind to either human IgG or rabbit IgG. Table 6 also shows that the c147 bound better to the $(Fab')_2$ than the Fc fragments of IgG, albeit not as well as to the intact IgG molecule.

A series of control experiments were performed to ensure that the hybridoma antibody c147 represented a monoclonal antibody. First, the hybridoma c147 was subcloned twice at one cell per well. Second, the c147 antibodies were shown to bear only one type of light chain marker (κ) and only one subclass marker of heavy chain (γ 1).[34] Third and most important, the binding activities of c147 to both RF and human IgG were simultaneously absorbed by, and eluted from, a human IgG-Sepharose®4B column.[34]

Table 5
ANTIBODY c147 INHIBITS RF BINDING TO IgG

Antibody/antigen	Inhibition (%)
RF Ley/IgG	100
RF Pom/IgG	100
RF Koh/IgG	85
Pooled RF/IgG	82
RF Mei/IgG	90
Anti-Tg/Tg	20

Note: Mitrotiter wells were precoated with either human IgG (1 μg/mℓ) or human thyroglobulin/Tg (20 μg/mℓ). To test inhibition activity, c147 supernant or culture medium was first mixed with various antibody samples (i.e., RF or IgM anti-Tg). After 1 hr incubation at room temperature, the mixture was distributed to the wells and the bound RF or anti-Tg was detected with enzyme-linked antihuman μ antibodies.
RF Mei is a polyclonal IgM-RF.

Table 6
ANTIBODY c147 BINDS TO HUMAN RF AND HUMAN IgG

	Antibody binding (A_{405} × 1000) to antigens						
	Experiment 1[a]				Experiment 2[b]		
Samples[c]	RF	IgM	IgG	R.IgG	IgG	$(Fab')_2$	Fc
Med	175	2	24	11	—	—	—
Scl 1:2	202	4	34	23	—	—	—
c147 1:2	519	23	853	150	—	—	—
c147 1:160	—	—	—	—	1288	386	108

Note: —, not done.

[a] The microtiter wells were precoated with the following antigens: RF (Mei, polyclonal) IgM at 5 μg/mℓ; human IgG and rabbit IgG at 60 μg/mℓ.

[b] The wells were precoated with: the $(Fab')_2$ and Fc fragments of human IgG, and intact IgG at 0.1 μmol.

[c] The supernants containing antibodies were used at 1:2 or 1:160 dilution. The control monoclonal antibody, Scl, is an IgG1, antihuman T cell.

Table 7
MAJOR CHARACTERISTICS OF THREE EPIBODIES

Epibody	Ab_1	Ag	Main epitopes recognized: Ab_1	Main epitopes recognized: Epibody
Glo-induced murine polyclonal	RF Glo	Human IgG	Fc (r2,r3)	Fc (r2,r3)
Peptide-induced rabbit polyclonal	RF Glo	Human IgG	Fc (r2,r3)	$(Fab')_2$ (r1)
RF-induced murine monoclonal	RF, including Glo	Human IgG	Fc (r2,r3)	$(Fab')_2$ (r1)

Together, these results strongly suggest that the antibody c147 is a monoclonal epibody that binds both to a CRI on human RF and to the antigen of human RF (i.e., human IgG). In addition, similar to the synthetic peptide-induced epibodies, c147 binds preferentially to the $(Fab')_2$ fragment of human IgG.

V. DISCUSSION

An epibody/Ab2ε is defined as an anti-Id that reacts with both the Id of a particular antibody and the respective antigen of this antibody. The existence of epibodies was first described by Bona et al. in 1982.[11] These authors pointed out that the antigenic determinants recognized by epibodies may not be the same determinants that induce the production of the antibody Ab_1, and may just be "bystander" epitopes on the antigen that by chance mimic the Id on the Ab_1. Since the first report of epibodies, there have been only two other examples of such anti-Id, as described in the previous sections.[31] The major characteristics of these three epibodies are summarized in Table 7.

Importantly, all three known epibodies are specific for Id on anti-IgG antibodies. This represents a striking difference from the homobodies ($Ab_{2\beta}$) that have been previously described, not to mention conventional anti-Id ($Ab_{2\alpha}$). To date, homobodies have been shown to be induced by antibodies to various antigens, including insulin, the adrenergic antagonist alprenolol, the major histocompatibility complex (MHC), and many infectious agents (such as hepatitis B virus and Streptococcus pneumoniae) (reviewed in References 8 to 10). Is the restriction of epibodies to RF just a coincidence? To approach this question, one needs to consider the possible structural basis of epibody reactivity.

The structural basis of Id recognized by "conventional" anti-Id ($Ab_{2\alpha}$) has been studied in several well-defined antibody systems.[35-40] The results suggest that CDR of heavy and light chains are the structural correlates of Id determinants. Noticeably, in the murine antidextran system, one private Id and one CRI have been assigned, respectively, to the third and the second CDR of the heavy chain.[37] However, in most other cases, it has been extremely difficult to associate a particular Id determinant with a specific amino acid sequence.[50] Rather, anti-Id induced by intact Ig, like antibodies induced by other intact proteins, typically recognize determinants dependent upon tertiary and/or quaternary conformation.[40,50,51]

Recently, synthetic peptides have been used to induce antibodies specific for preselected determinants in intact proteins.[41-45] These findings prompted us, as well as others, to examine in an analogous fashion the structural basis of Id, through the generation of antibodies against synthetic peptides corresponding to CDR of particular antibody molecules.[20,30,46] Using this novel approach, we successfully associated the Wa-CRI with the second CDR of the CRI-positive light chains.[20-22]

Since homobodies were first predicted,[4,5] anti-Id have been demonstrated that mimic diverse antigens, ranging from polypeptides and polysaccharides to a simple organic compound such as alprenolol.[8-10] In most cases, it has been impossible to find amino acid sequence homologies between the homobodies and their respective antigens/ligands. Most likely, "conformational likeness" is responsible for the mimicry. However, in the cases where antigens/ligands are polypeptides, it is possible that a short stretch of homologous amino acid sequence can account for the mimicry. In this regard, Wilson et al. discovered 2469 stretches of 6-amino acids that were identical in apparently unrelated proteins from the 24 different protein superfamilies.[52]

This information provides a clue toward understanding the molecular basis of epibody phenomena. Among the three epibodies described, two were induced by the RF Glo light chain or its peptide fragment, while the third one (c147) was induced by a mixture of five different IgM RF. The latter proteins included Glo(κIII), as well as Pal (κIII), Pom (κIII), Lay(κI), and Koh(lambda). Since Pal is strongly positive for all three RF-associated light chain CRIs (i.e., PGL1, PSL2, and PSL3),[21,22,31] it is very likely that the Pal light chain variable region is identical or almost identical to the Glo light chain variable region sequence, as is the case for the monoclonal RF Cur, Flo, Gar, and Glo.[21,22,32] Thus, Glo and Glo-like light chains may be the major antigen component that induced c147.

Figures 3A and 3B show a sequence comparison between the Glo light chain variable region[22] and the human Ig γ 1 constant region (NBRF:ghhu.brf), using the computer programs "compare" and "dotplot" developed by The University of Wisconsin Genetic Computer Group. The top panel identifies the regions in both sequences that share 4 out of 13 amino acids, while the bottom panel identifies the regions that share 4 out of 7 amino acids. The human IgM μ chain constant region (NBRF:mhhu.brf) is used as a control. As can be seen, there are 15 short stretches that share four amino acids in a window of seven amino acids (Figure 3B). Among these 15 homologous stretches, 8 are in the first domain. This may explain why two of the three epibodies bind preferentially to the $(Fab')_2$ fragment of human IgG.

Among eight homologous stretches in the first γ domain, one corresponds to positions 28 to 34 in the Glo sequence, and to positions 70 to 77 in the first constant region domain of the γ chain, i.e., positions 192 to 199 according to Kabat et al.[53] The sequences are SVSSSYLA in Glo and TVPSSSLG in the γ chain, respectively. This finding is consistent with our suggestion that the SSS sequence is the molecular basis of the anti-PGL1 epibody.[31]

Numerous investigations using dextran and homopolymers of amino acids have concluded that the antibody binding site can accommodate a hexasaccharide or tetrapeptide.[54] In addition, analyses of the antigenic determinant size of protein antigens revealed that a determinant consisted of a pentapeptide or tetrapeptide (reviewed in Reference 55). Moreover, in the case of the C-terminal pentapeptide of tobacco mosaic virus (TMV), Leu-Asp-Ala-Thr-Arg, the Leu-Asp could be replaced by *N*-octanoyl.[55] This suggested that the anti-TMV antibodies recognized specifically the tripeptide Ala-Thr-Arg, while the Leu-Asp enhanced the antibody binding by providing hydrophobicity. Thus, SSS may be the core determinant recognized by the anti-PGL1 antibodies, while adjacent Val-Pro and Leu in Ig γ may enhance the antibody binding.

Among the remaining seven homologous stretches in the second and the third γ domains, there are two interesting areas. The first one is *TLTISR*LE*PE* (residues 72 to 81 in Glo) vs. *TLMISR*T*PE* (residues 133 to 141 in the second γ chain domain). The second one is LSLSPG, residues 11 to 16 in Glo and residues 324 to 329 in the third γ chain domain. Either one or both of these homologous stretches may form the determinant recognized by the A/J anti-Glo epibodies.

Thus, it is likely that a short stretch of homologous amino acid sequences shared by many human RF antibody variable regions and the constant region of human IgG γ chain is the structural basis for the epibodies induced by Glo and the Glo peptide fragment (PGL1). However, since c147 reacts with various RFs that have quite different light chain variable regions, "conformational mimicry" may also contribute to its epibody activity.

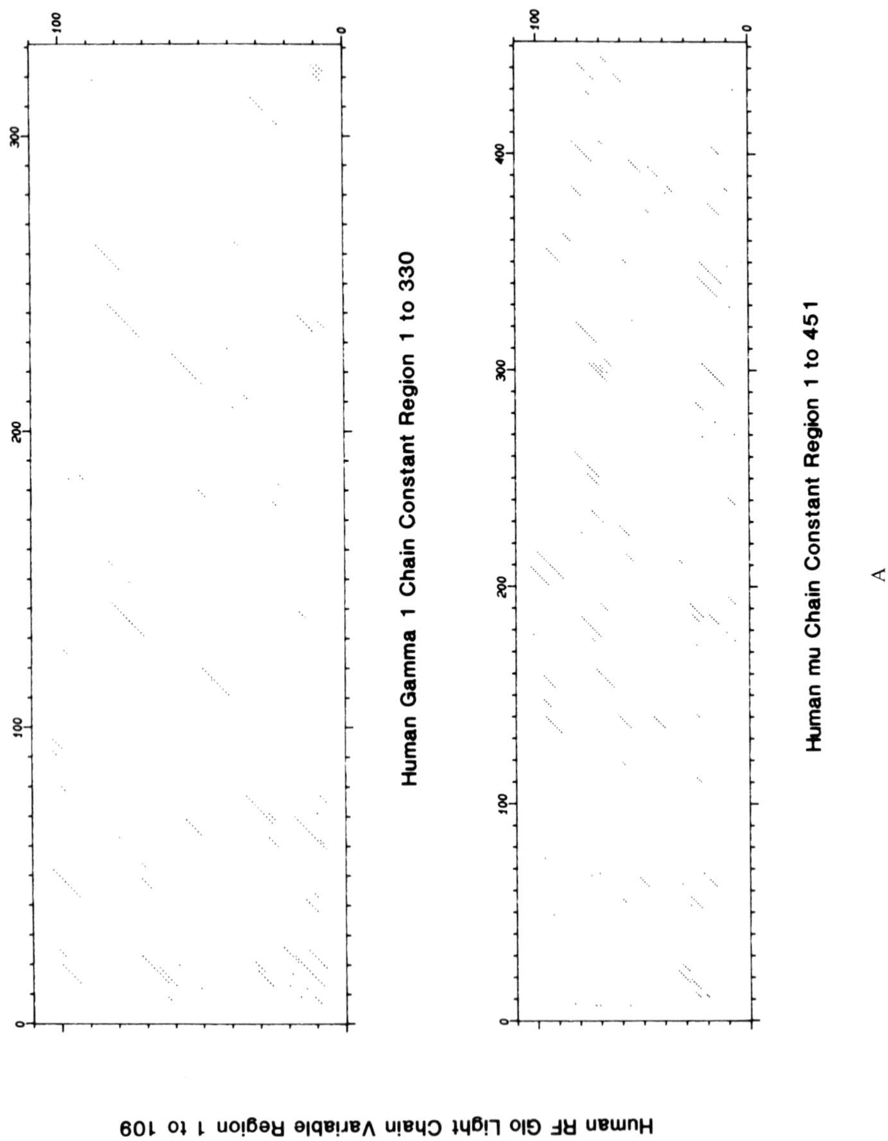
Human Gamma 1 Chain Constant Region 1 to 330
Human mu Chain Constant Region 1 to 451
Human RF Glo Light Chain Variable Region 1 to 109
A

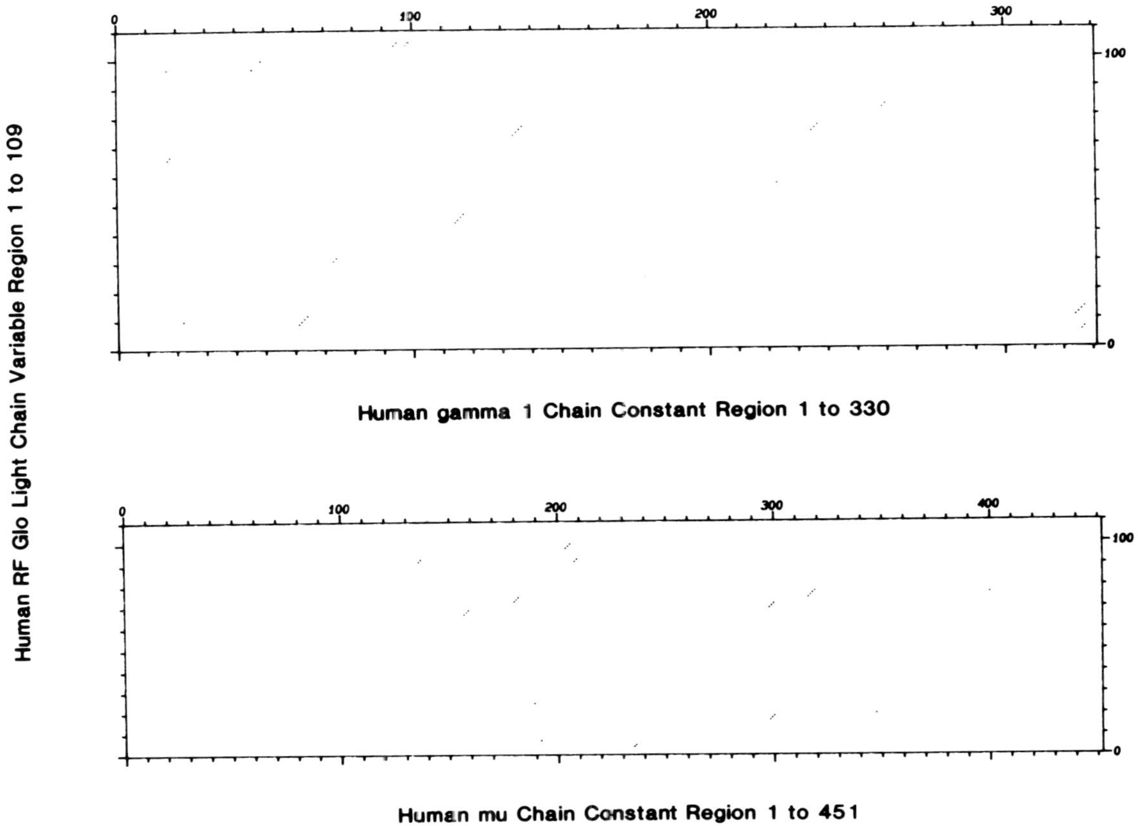

B

FIGURE 3. Amino acid sequence comparison of the Glo light chain variable region and the human IgG 1 gamma chain. The computer programs of The University of Wisconsin Genetic Computer Group and protein sequence database from the National Biomedical Research Foundation (NBRF) are used. Figure A identifies regions in both sequences that share 4 of 13 amino acids, while Figure B identifies regions that share 4 of 7 amino acids. The human IgM μ chain is used as a control.

All domains of Ig molecules probably derived from a single primordial domain during evolution. Hence, it is not surprising that RF variable regions and the γ chain constant regions share many short stretches of identical or homologous amino acid sequences, and/or share some similar conformational determinants. Among these homologies, some apparently cause cross reactivities between RF and IgG. Accordingly, epibodies are likely to be common among anti-Id for RF. Along the same line, epibodies may be observed among anti-Id induced by other anti-Ig antibodies (such as anti-allotype antibodies), and, to a lesser extent, by antibodies against antigens belonging to the Ig-superfamily (such as MHC antigens, T-cell receptors, Fc receptors,..., etc.).[56,57]

ABBREVIATIONS

Ab_1, anti-epitope antibody
Ab_2, anti-idiotypic antibody
BBS, borate-buffered saline
BSA, bovine serum albumin
CDR, complementarity-determining region
CFA, complete Freund's adjuvant
CRI, cross-reactive idiotype
ELISA, enzyme-linked immunosorbent assay
HA, hemagglutination
Id, idiotype
PBS, phosphate-buffered saline
PGL1, synthetic peptide corresponding to the light chain-CDR 1 of the RF Glo
PSH3, synthetic peptide corresponding to the heavy chain-CDR 3 of the RF Sie
RF, rheumatoid factor
RIA, radioimmunoassay

REFERENCES

1. **Kunkel, H. G., Mannik, M., and Williams, R. C.,** Individual antigenic specificity of isolated antibodies, *Science,* 140, 1218, 1963.
2. **Oudin, J. and Michel, M.,** Une nouvelle forme d'allotypie des globulines gamma du serum de lapin, apparemment liee a la fonction et la specificite anticorps, *C. R. Acad. Sci.,* 257, 805, 1963.
3. **Sege, K. and Peterson, P. A.,** Use of anti-idiotypic antibodies as cell surface receptor probes, *Proc. Natl. Acad. Sci. U.S.A.,* 75, 2443, 1978.
4. **Lindenmann, J.,** Speculation on idiotypes and homobodies, *Ann. Immunol. (Inst. Pasteur),* 124C, 171, 1973.
5. **Jerne, N. K.,** Towards a network theory of the immune system, *Ann. Immunol. (Paris),* 125c, 373, 1974.
6. **Nisonoff, A. and Lamoyi, E.,** Implications of the presence of an internal image of the antigen in anti-idiotypic antibodies: possible application to vaccine production, *Clin. Immunol. Immunopathol.,* 21, 397, 1981.
7. **Jerne, N. K., Roland, J., and Cazenave, P.-A.,** Recurrent idiotypes and internal images, *EMBO J.,* 1, 243, 1982.
8. **Strosberg, A. D.,** Anti-idiotype and anti-hormone receptor antibodies, *Biol. Semin. Immunopathol.,* 6, 67, 1983.
9. **Kohler, H., Muller, S., and Bona, C.,** Internal antigen and immune network, *Proc. Soc. Exp. Biol. Med.,* 178, 189, 1985.
10. **Bona, C. A. and Moran, T.,** Idiotype vaccines, *Ann. Immunol. (Inst. Pasteur),* 136C, 299, 1985.
11. **Bona, C. A., Finley, S., Waters, S., and Kunkel, H. G.,** Anti-immunoglobulin antibodies. III. Properties of sequential anti-idiotypic antibodies to heterologous anti-gamma globulins. Detection of reactivity of anti-idiotype antibodies with epitopes of Fc fragments (homobodies) and with epitopes and idiotopes (epibodies), *J. Exp. Med.,* 156, 986, 1982.

12. **Bona, C. A.,** Epibodies: a particular set of anti-idiotypes specific for autoantibodies, *Clin. Immunol. (Newsl.),* 6, 87, 1985.
13. **Kunkel, H. G., Agnello, V., Joslin, F. G., Winchester, R. J., and Capra, J. D.,** Cross-idiotypic specificity among monoclonal IgM proteins with anti-gammaglobulin activity, *J. Exp. Med.,* 137, 331, 1973.
14. **Bonagura, V. R., Kunkel, H. G., and Pernis, B.,** Cellular localization of rheumatoid factor idiotypes, *J. Clin. Invest.,* 69, 1356, 1982.
15. **Powell, R. and Agnello, V.,** Characterization of complement-fixing activity and cross-idiotypes of rheumatoid factors in idiopathic mixed cryoglobulinemia, *Clin. Immunol. Immunopathol.,* 29, 146, 1983.
16. **Kunkel, H., Posnett, D., and Pernis, B.,** Anti-immunoglobulins and their idiotypes: are they part of the immune network, *Ann. N.Y. Acad. Sci.,* 418, 324, 1983.
17. **Kunkel, H. G., Winchester, R. J., Joslin, F. G., and Capra, J. D.,** Similarities in the light chains of anti-gamma-globulins sharing cross-idiotypic specificities, *J. Exp. Med.,* 139, 128, 1974.
18. **Ledford, D. K., Goni, F., Pizzolato, M., Franklin, E. C., Solomon, A., and Frangione, B.,** Preferential association of kappa-IIIb light chains with monoclonal human IgM-kappa autoantibodies, *J. Immunol.,* 131, 1322, 1983.
19. **Andrews, D. W. and Capra, J. D.,** Complete amino acid sequence of variable domains from two monoclonal human anti-gamma globulins of the Wa cross-idiotypic group: suggestion that the J segments are involved in the structural correlate of the idiotype, *Proc. Natl. Acad. Sci. U.S.A.,* 78, 3799, 1981.
20. **Chen, P. P., Fong, S., Normansell, D., Houghten, R. A., Karras, J. G., Vaughan, J. H., and Carson, D. A.,** Delineation of a cross-reactive idiotype on human autoantibodies with antibody against a synthetic peptide, *J. Exp. Med.,* 159, 1502, 1984.
21. **Chen, P. P., Goni, F., Fong, S., Jirik, F., Vaughan, J. H., Frangione, B., and Carson, D. A.,** The majority of human monoclonal IgM rheumatoid factors express a primary structure-dependent cross-reactive idiotype, *J. Immunol.,* 134, 3281, 1985.
22. **Goni, F., Chen, P. P., Pons-Estel, B., Carson, D. A., and Frangione, B.,** Sequence similarities and cross-idiotypic specificity of L chains among human monoclonal IgM-K with anti-gammaglobulin activity, *J. Immunol.,* 135, 4073, 1985.
23. **Pasquali, J.-L., Fong, S., Tsoukas, C. D., Vaughan, J. H., and Carson, D. A.,** Inheritance of IgM rheumatoid factor idiotypes, *J. Clin. Invest.,* 66, 863, 1980.
24. **Carson, D. A. and Fong, S.,** A common idiotype on human rheumatoid factors identified by a hybridoma antibody, *Mol. Immunol.,* 20, 1081, 1983.
25. **Fong, S., Chen, P. P., Gilbertson, T. A., Fox, R. I., Vaughan, J. H., and Carson, D. A.,** Structural similarities in the kappa light chains of human rheumatoid factor paraproteins and serum immunoglobulins bearing a cross-reactive idiotype, *J. Immunol.,* 135, 1955, 1985.
26. **Fox, R. I., Chen, P. P., Carson, D. A., and Fong, S.,** Expression of a cross-reactive idiotype on rheumatoid factor in patients with Sjogren's syndrome, *J. Immunol.,* 136, 477, 1986.
27. **Fong, S., Gilbertson, T. A., and Carson, D. A.,** The internal image of IgG in cross-reactive anti-idiotypic antibodies against human rheumatoid factors, *J. Immunol.,* 131, 719, 1983.
28. **Fong, S., Gilbertson, T. A., Chen, P. P., Vaughan, J. H., and Carson, D. A.,** Modulation of human rheumatoid factor-specific lymphocyte responses with a cross-reactive anti-idiotype bearing the internal image of antigen, *J. Immunol.,* 132, 1183, 1984.
29. **Fong, S., Gilbertson, T. A., Chen, P. P., Karras, J. G., Vaughan, J. H., and Carson, D. A.,** The common occurrence of internal image type anti-idiotypic antibodies in rabbits immunized with monoclonal and polyclonal human IgM rheumatoid factors, *Clin. Exp. Immunol.,* 64, 570, 1986.
30. **Chen, P. P., Houghten, R. A., Fong, S., Rhodes, G. H., Gilbertson, T. A., Vaughan, J. H., Lerner, R. A., and Carson, D. A.,** Anti-hypervariable region antibody induced by a defined peptide. A new approach for studying the structural correlates of idiotypes, *Proc. Natl. Acad. Sci. U.S.A.,* 81, 1784, 1984.
31. **Chen, P. P., Fong, S., Houghten, R. A., and Carson, D. A.,** Characterization of an epibody: an anti-idiotype which reacts with both the idiotype of rheumatoid factors (RF) and the antigen recognized by RFs, *J. Exp. Med.,* 161, 323, 1985.
32. **Chen, P. P., Goni, F., Houghten, R. A., Fong, S., Goldfien, R. D., Vaughan, J. H., Frangione, B., and Carson, D. A.,** Characterization of human rheumatoid factors with seven anti-idiotypes induced by synthetic hypervariable-region peptides, *J. Exp. Med.,* 162, 487, 1985.
33. **Goldfien, R. D., Chen, P. P., Fong, S., and Carson, D. A.,** Synthetic peptides corresponding to third hypervariable region of human monoclonal IgM rheumatoid factor heavy chains define an immunodominant idiotype, *J. Exp. Med.,* 162, 756, 1985.
34. **Fong, S., Chen, P. P., and Carson, D. A.,** Anti-idiotypic antibodies to human rheumatoid factor. Isolation and characterization of monoclonal anti-idiotypic antibodies with "internal image" and "epibody" properties, in preparation.
35. **Weigert, M., Raschke, W. C., Carson, D., and Cohn, M.,** Immunochemical analysis of the idiotypes of mouse myeloma proteins with specificity for levan or dextran, *J. Exp. Med.,* 139, 137, 1974.

36. **Capra, J. D. and Kehoe, J. M.,** Structure of antibodies with shared idiotype: the complete sequence of the heavy chain variable regions of two immunoglobulin M anti-gamma globulins, *Proc. Natl. Acad. Sci. U.S.A.*, 71, 4032, 1974.
37. **Schilling, J., Clevinger, B., Davie, J. M., and Hood, L.,** Amino acid sequence of homogeneous antibodies to dextran and DNA rearrangements in heavy chain V-region gene segments, *Nature*, 283, 35, 1980.
38. **Pawlita, M., Mushinski, E., Feldmann, R. J., and Potter, M.,** A monoclonal antibody that defines an idiotype with two subsites in galactan-binding myeloma proteins, *J. Exp. Med.*, 154, 1946, 1981.
39. **Rajewsky, K. and Takemori, T.,** Genetics, expression, and function of idiotypes, *Annu. Rev. Immunol.*, 1, 569, 1983.
40. **Rudikoff, S.,** Immunoglobulin structure-function correlates: antigen binding and idiotypes, *Contemp. Top. Mol. Immunol.*, 9, 169, 1983.
41. **Sutcliffe, J. G., Shinnick, T. M., Green, N., Liu, F., Niman, H. L., and Lerner, R. A.,** Chemical synthesis of a polypeptide predicted from nucleotide sequence allows detection of a new retroviral gene product, *Nature*, 287, 801, 1980.
42. **Walter, G., Scheidtmann, K., Carbone, A., Laudano, A. P., and Doolittle, R. F.,** Antibodies specific for the carboxy- and amino-terminal regions of simian virus 40 large tumor antigen, *Proc. Natl. Acad. Sci. U.S.A.*, 77, 5197, 1980.
43. **Lerner, R. A.,** Tapping the immunological repertoire to produce antibodies of predetermined specificity, *Nature*, 299, 592, 1982.
44. **Sutcliffe, J. G., Shinnick, T. M., Green, N., and Lerner, R. A.,** Antibodies that react with predetermined sites on proteins, *Science*, 219, 660, 1983.
45. **Young, C. R., Schmitz, H. E., and Atassi, M. Z.,** Antibodies with specificities to preselected protein regions evoked by free synthetic peptides representing protein antigenic sites or other surface locations: demonstration with myoglobulin, *Mol. Immunol.*, 20, 567, 1983.
46. **McMillan, S., Seiden, M. V., Houghten, R. A., Clevinger, B., Davie, J. M., and Lerner, R. A.,** Synthetic idiotypes: the third hypervariable region of murine anti-dextran antibodies, *Cell*, 35, 859, 1983.
47. **Klapper, D. G. and Capra, J. D.,** The amino acid sequence of the variable regions of the light chains from two idiotypically cross reactive IgM anti-gamma globulins, *Ann. Immunol. (Inst. Pasteur)*, 127C, 261, 1976.
48. **Pons-Estel, B., Goni, F., Solomon, A., and Frangione, B.,** Sequence similarities among kIIIb chains of monoclonal human IgMk autoantibodies, *J. Exp. Med.*, 160, 893, 1984.
49. **Capra, J. D. and Kehoe, J. M.,** Hypervariable regions, idiotype and the antibody-combining site, *Adv. Immunol.*, 20, 1, 1975.
50. **Capra, J. D. and Fougereau, M.,** Structural correlates of idiotypes. One from column A, one from column B, *Immunol. Today*, 4, 177, 1983.
51. **Benjamin, D. C., Berzofsky, J. A., East, I. J., Curd, F. R. N., Hannum, C., Leach, S. J., Margoliash, E., Michael, J. G., Miller, A., Prager, E. M., Richlen, M., Sercarz, E. E., Smith-Gill, S. J., Todd, P. E., and Wilson, A. C.,** The antigenic structure of proteins: a reappraisal, *Annu. Rev. Immunol.*, 2, 67, 1984.
52. **Wilson, I. A., Haft, D. H., Getzoff, E. D., Tainer, J. A., Lerner, R. A., and Brenner, S.,** Identical short peptide sequences in unrelated proteins can have different conformations: a testing ground for theories of immune recognition, *Proc. Natl. Acad. Sci. U.S.A.*, 82, 5255, 1985.
53. **Kabat, E. A., Wu, T. T., Bilofsky, H., Reid-Miller, M., and Perry, H.,** Sequences of Proteins of Immunological Interest, National Institute of Health, U.S. Department of Health and Human Services, Bethesda, Md., 1983.
54. **Goodman, J. W.,** Immunogenicity and antigenic specificity, in *Basic and Clinical Immunology*, Stites, D. P., Stobo, J. D., Fudenberg, H. H., and Wells, J. V., Eds., Lange Medical, Los Altos, Calif., 1982, 21.
55. **Benjamini, E., Michaeli, D., and Young, J. D.,** Antigenic determinants of proteins of defined sequences, *Curr. Top. Microbiol. Immunol.*, 58, 85, 1972.
56. **Williams, A. F.,** Molecules in the immunoglobulin superfamily, *Immunol. Today*, 5, 219, 1984.
57. **Matsunaga, T.,** Evolution of the immunoglobulin superfamily by duplication of complementarity, *Immunol. Today*, 6, 260, 1985.

Chapter 5

MONOCLONAL ANTIBODIES SPECIFIC FOR V_H AND V_K ISOTYPES AS PROBES FOR THE ANALYSIS OF THE V GENE REPERTOIRE

D. Primi and P.-A. Cazenave

TABLE OF CONTENTS

I. INTRODUCTION

One of the most fascinating aspects of the immune system is that its components are enormously diversified and capable of interacting with an almost infinite number of antigens. Following the dogma "one gene one protein", it has been, in fact, difficult to understand how an organism which contains in its genome no more than 2 to 3 $\times$ 10^5 genes could produce millions of different immunoglobulin molecules. The answer to this paradox came from molecular biology studies that conclusively demonstrated that the variable (V) regions of immunoglobulin chains are encoded by multiple germline DNA segments which are joined into functional variable regions during B-cell ontogeny.[1,4]

The V_H and V_k loci of the mouse are currently estimated to consist of a few hundred genes.[5,6] These genes fall into families defined by the homology of their nucleic acid sequences and the size of these families varies widely from one to another.[5] The antibody repertoire is then determined by the number of V_H and V_L genes as well as by multiple joining gene segments (J_k, J_λ, J_H, and D_H). The combinatorial product of these segments, however, gives only a minimal estimate of the potential repertoire, since other mechanisms, i.e., somatic mutations[7] and imprecision in the joining of the DNA segments,[8] can, in fact, increase the potential antibody diversity of several orders of magnitude. Thus it can be calculated that the potential immunoglobulin repertoire of a mouse can, in fact, consist of as many as 10^9 specificities. The complete solution of the genetic mechanisms responsible for immunoglobulin diversity, however, has also posed some important questions that have not been completely resolved as yet. The most important one concerns the finality of such an enormous potential repertoire. These considerations become evident if one considers that the number of B cells present at any moment in the life of a mouse is at least one order of magnitude inferior to the number of potentially available specificities. In addition, numerous reports in the literature demonstrate that certain immune responses are of very limited heterogeneity and often encoded by only one germline V_H gene.[9-12] It is also important to underline that this clonal dominance phenomenon cannot be explained by the choice of the animal to utilize the best-fitted gene to cope with immunogen. The immune response of BALB/c mice to phosphorylcholine antigens, for instance, is dominated by the utilization of the V_HT15 gene product.[13-15] If, however, these mice are tolerized neonatally with anti-idiotypic (anti-Id) antibodies directed against the V_HT15 gene product, their PC immune response during the recovery time is no longer encoded by the T15V_H, but the affinity of the antibody produced is comparable to that of untreated animals.[16,17] Thus, even though these animals possess several V_H genes which can be utilized in their anti-PC response, they repeatedly utilize only the V_HT15 one. The general concept that the enormously diversified potential antibody repertoire is a necessity for the immune system to cope with the antigenic universe can be seriously further questioned on the basis of two general observations. The first one is based on the work of de Pasquier et al.[18] who demonstrated that, although the immunoglobulin repertoire of Xenopus is extremely restricted, this animal can virtually produce immunoglobulins against any antigenic determinant. The second line of evidence which clouds the concept of direct relationship between diversity and polyspecificity rests on the work of Weiss et al.[19] These authors demonstrated that mice suppressed for k chains and that, therefore, can only utilize the two V_λ light chains can, after repeated antigenic challenges, respond to a variety of antigens including those to which the specific antibodies normally produced are encoded by Vk genes. These evidences synergize in suggesting that, firstly, even inbred animals utilize only a fraction of their potential repertoire, and, secondly, that polyspecificity does not necessarily require the combinatorial expression of the immunoglobulin gene segments available in many mammalians.

These observations, therefore, demand serious reconsiderations of the evolutionary pressure which tends to maintain such a diversified potential repertoire.

During the last few years, our laboratory has been particularly interested in this problem and here we will review some of the experiments that we designed to gain some clues to this puzzle.

II. THE EXPERIMENTAL SYSTEM

Immunoglobulin repertoire studies imply the possibility of studying the expression and the regulation of given V_H or V_k genes. In the past years, repertoires have been studied by analyzing antibodies specific for certain antigenic determinants or positive for given idiotypes (Id). Although both these methodologies have provided an impressive amount of information, the interpretations of some of the results obtained have been difficult. The main limitation with this approach is that Id are conformational antigens and, consequently, can be expressed on immunoglobulins encoded by different V_H-V_L pairs. Recently, for instance, Meek et al.[20] demonstrated that, under particular circumstances, BALB/c mice can produce antiarsonate antibodies idiotypically undistinguishable from those produced by A/J animals. Nucleotide sequences, however, revealed that the antibodies produced by the two mouse strains utilize completely different V_H genes. These studies, therefore, demonstrate that anti-Id antibodies cannot be unequivocally utilized as V_H gene probes.

An alternative approach to the study of immunoglobulin gene expression has been recently made possible by the availability of DNA probes specific for V_H gene families. The utilization of these probes, however, requires considerable amounts of homogeneous material and, consequently, it cannot be utilized to analyze the products of normal, nontransformed B lymphocytes. In addition to this, some V gene families contain large numbers of genes which are not distinguished by the relevant probe.[5]

In view of these considerations, we looked for alternative approaches which would allow us to study the expression of one or few V genes in normal B cells. The solution to this problem came from observations by Devaux et al.[21-23] and Desaymard et al.[24] who described two monoclonal antibodies which, respectively, recognize the V_HT15 and V_k21D E gene products. The interactions of these molecules with the relevant Ig segment are highly specific and completely independent from the light chain (in the case of the anti-V_HT15) or the heavy chain (in the case of the anti-V_k21D-E) to which these segments are associated. Another interesting feature of these reagents is that they recognize all the allelic forms of the relevant gene product in all the laboratory mouse strains tested. All these characteristics distinguish them from classical anti-Id antibodies and we suggest they be defined as anti-V_H or anti-V_k isotypes.

These probes meet all our requirements since they provided us with the means to analyze the expression of a given V_H and V_k gene both in the serum and in normal nontransformed B cells. Most importantly, as these reagents recognize all the allelic forms of the V_k21D-E and V_HT15 segments, these monoclonal antibodies could also be used to analyze the effect of V gene polymorphism on the expression of the B-cell repertoire.

A. The Levels of V_HT15 and V_k21D-E in the Normal Sera of Inbred Mice

The availabilty of monoclonal antibodies specific for V_H and V_k gene products offered us a unique opportunity to study the levels of the expression of these two gene segments independently from the antibody specificity of the immunoglobulins to which they are utilized. This analysis was also interesting to assess whether any of the known immunologically relevant loci influence the serum expression of given V gene products. Rudikoff and Potter described a PC-binding myeloma protein of C57BL/6 origin with a V_H region 96% homologous to the T15 one.[25] The substitutions found at position 14 and 16 were present in all the induced C57BL/6 anti-PC antibodies and, therefore, it is likely that these alternatives are encoded in the C57BL/6 germline and, consequently, that this gene represents the C57BL/

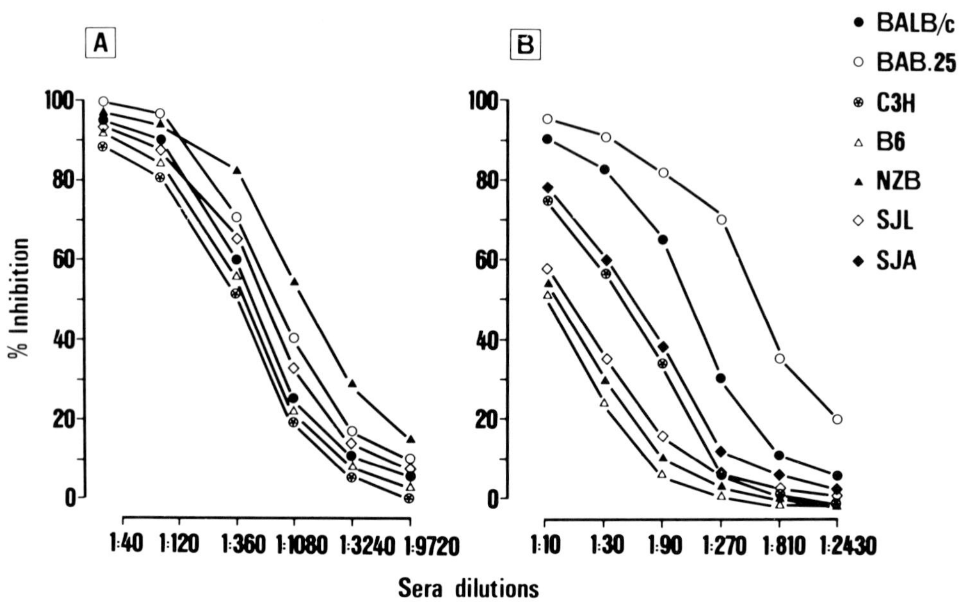

FIGURE 1. Analysis of the property of the sera of the indicated mice to inhibit the M511-TC54 (B) and the 14.4.4. (V_k21E)-H106-131 (A) interactions.

6 allelic form of the T15V_H. This allele is also shared by CBA and C3H mice. Thus, at least two allelic forms of the T15V_H gene occur in laboratory mice. The polymorphism of the V_k21D-E gene segments is more complex, since restriction endonuclease,[26] as well as IEF analyses (see below), has clearly demonstrated the existence of at least three allotypic forms of these genes.

Initially, therefore, our main concern was that the two anti-V_HT15 and anti-V_k21D-E reagents would not recognize all the "allotypic" forms of the relevant V gene segment. This is apparently not the case as, firstly, all sera studied contained molecules capable of inhibiting both the V_HT15-TC54 and the 14.4.4-H106-131 interactions, and, secondly, all sera inhibited these interactions with similar slopes (Figure 1).[27]

All the sera studied contained higher levels of V_k21D-E molecules than V_HT15-positive immunoglobulins, but the ratio of V_k21D-E/V_HT15 varied widely in the different strains (Table 1). These variations are mainly due to the content of V_HT15-positive molecules which can fluctuate over a 300-fold range from one strain to another, i.e., BAB.14 and NZB. Although, as a general rule, we could not detect any clear linkage between the serum level of V_HT15 and V_k21D-E$^+$ molecules to loci linked either to H-2 or to Igh, we further investigated the abnormally low level of V_HT15 molecules observed in the sera of NZB mice by analyzing the quantity of these molecules in the normal sera of seven NX8 recombinant strains.[28] This analysis, which is shown in Table 2, demonstrates that the abnormally low level of the V_HT15 gene segment in the serum of NZB animals cannot be traced to the allelic form of the coding gene.

Taken together, these data show that the levels of V_HT15 fluctuate considerably in thc sera of the different strains tested and there is apparently not direct correlation between the level of V_HT15$^+$ molecules and the Igh or the H-2 loci. This particular point is documented by the observation that the level of V_HT15$^+$ molecules was more than 24 times higher in C.B20 than in C57BL/6. Since the amount of V_HT15$^+$ Igs was remarkably constant among individuals of a given strain, these data strongly suggest that genes other than H-2 and Igh play an important role in the selection of the available repertoire. The validity of this conclusion is further supported by experiments in which we analyzed the IEF spectrotypes

Table 1
THE LEVELS OF V_HT15 AND V_k21 D-E GENE PRODUCTS IN THE NORMAL SERA OF INBRED MOUSE STRAINS

Strains	H-2	Igh-V[a]	Igh-C	V_HT15 Ig (μg/mℓ)	V_k21 D-E Ig (μg/mℓ)
BALB/c	a	a	a	51	202
BALB.B	b	a	a	36	383
BALB.K	k	a	a	29	360
C.B20	d	b	b	17	312
BAB.14	d	a	b	112	1200
RIII	r	a	j	10	500
C58	k	a	a	28	100
C57BL/6	b	b	b	0.7	312
C57BL/6 H-2^k	k	b	b	28	350
C57BL/6 Igh^a	b	a	a	82	315
SJA	s	a	a	28	314
SJL	s	b	b	8.4	500
PL	u	j	j	28	400
LP	b	b	b	28	900
NZB	d	j/d	n	0.3	900
C3H	k	j	j	13	450
AKR	k	j/d	d	0.9	350

Note: The values are expressed as 14.4.4. (V_k21E) and MOPC T15 (V_HT15) equivalent and determined by the ability of pooled sera from each strain to inhibit the H106-131 (anti-V_k21D-E)-14.4.4. and MOPC511-TC54 (anti-V_HT15) interactions.

[a] According to Brodeur and Riblet.[5]

Table 2
THE LEVEL OF V_HT15 Ig IN THE NORMAL SERA OF N × 8 RECOMBINANT INBRED STRAINS

Strain	H-2	Igh-1	Igh-Dex	V_HT15 Ig (μg/mℓ)[a]
C58	k	a	a	26
NZB	d	n	j	0.4
NX8 4	8	8	8	21
NX8 9	N	8	8	19
NX8 13	8	8	8	26
NX8 15	N	N	N	24
NX8 16	8	8	8	16
NX8 18	N	8	8	15
NX8 20	N	8	8	19

Note: The table entries have the following meanings: 8 indicates that the particular strain has inherited the C58 allele at the designed locus; N indicates inheritance of the NZB allele.

[a] The level of V_HT15 was determined in pooled sera of the different strains.

of the heavy chains of V_k21D-E-positive immunoglobulins isolated from normal sera.[29] Figure 2 shows the result of this analysis obtained with V_k21 Igs obtained from several inbred strains. All samples showed considerable heterogeneity, suggesting, therefore, that V_k21(D-E) can associate with multiple V_H segments. As expected, Igh polymorphism strongly influenced heavy chain IEF-banding pattern, however, considerable differences were also found between allotype-matched strains, i.e., between C.B20 and BAB.14 and between B6, LP, and SM, as well as between the H-2 congenic strains BALB/c and BALB.B. These differences could not be traced to differences in isotypic determinants, since radioimmunoassay analysis revealed that 90% of the isolated V_k21D-E-positive Igs belongs to the IgG1 subclass. It should also be stressed that the differences in the cathodic band observed in the IEF spectra between BALB/c and BALB.B animals have been repeatedly detected in several independent experiments and with sera obtained from different animals. Molecules isolated from F_1 between B6 and BALB/c sera showed an IEF-banding pattern which was the sum of those observed with the two parental strains, and this strongly suggests that the images obtained with the different samples reflect conserved repertoires rather than individual differences. The possibility that the B-cell repertoire is also controlled by genes other than those linked to the H-2 and Igh-loci was further verified by analyzing recombinant inbred strains. Figure 3 shows the IEF pattern of V_k21(D-E)-associated heavy chains isolated from the normal sera of nine RI strains. The BXH series of recombinant inbred strains consists of several strains derived from crossing C3H with C57BL/6 mice. Several loci have now been typed and among them H-2 and Igh, respectively, on chromosome 17 and 12. If control of heavy chain expression should be due to H-2 and Igh-linked loci only, it should then be expected that progenitor phenotypes should be recovered in those strains in which both loci segregated from the same parent. This is clearly not the case, as the IEF mobility of heavy chain of C57BL/6, (BXH)8, and (BXH)10 strains, all with identical H-2 and Igh haplotype, varied considerably. The peculiar phenotypes of the recombinant strains were further analyzed in the sera of C57BL/6 and BXH8 individual animals. Figure 4 shows the IEF patterns of V_k21-associated heavy chains isolated from individual mice of a given strain are highly conserved and reproducible. This redundancy is quite surprising and may imply that the expression of the preimmune repertoire is strictly controlled by internal pressures which reflect genetic polymorphism. The results obtained with the analysis of the level of expression of the V_HT15 product, together with the IEF analysis of V_H genes associated with the V_k21 segment, synergize, therefore, in suggesting that the repertoires observed in normal sera are highly conserved among individuals of the same strains and that these repertoires are also controlled by genes other than those linked to the Igh and H-2 loci. The nature and the numbers of these regulatory loci, however, have still to be determined.

B. Antigen-Independent Selection of V Genes Expression in the Preimmune Repertoire

The analysis presented above addressed a repertoire of immunoglobulins selected by internal and environmental antigens. Although these studies have provided us with direct evidences for the existence of multigenic control of this selection, this analysis did not provide direct information concerning mechanistic perspective relevant to the influence of genetic polymorphism of V_H and V_k expression. To begin to understand these processes, it is mandatory to have an understanding of the probability of expression of individual V_H and V_k gene product in the preimmune B-cell population. The usual characterization of preimmune B-cell repertoires involves the analysis of antibodies secreted by polyclonally activated B cells. Although the complete representation of the pool of antibody specificities among mitogen reactive B-cell subsets has been questioned,[30-32] this methodology remains, at the present time, the best available one for the analysis of the unselected B-cell repertoire. With this reservation in mind we determined, by limiting dilutions analysis, the frequency of B cells from several mice strains, competent to produce V_k21D-E or V_HT15-positive immu-

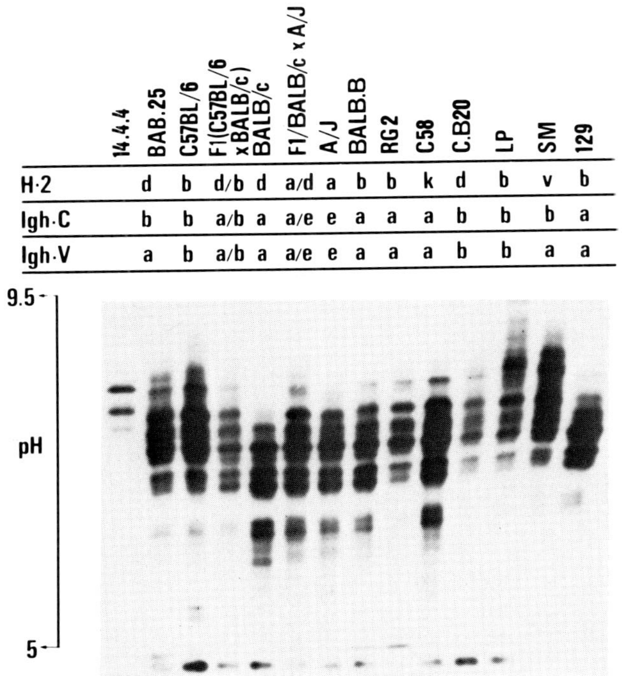

FIGURE 2

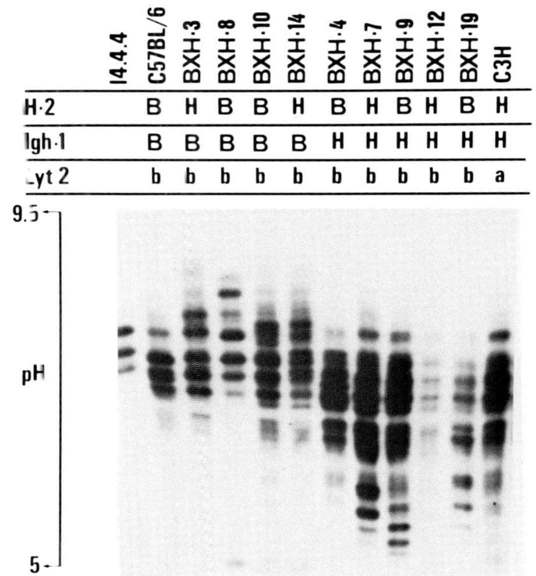

FIGURE 3

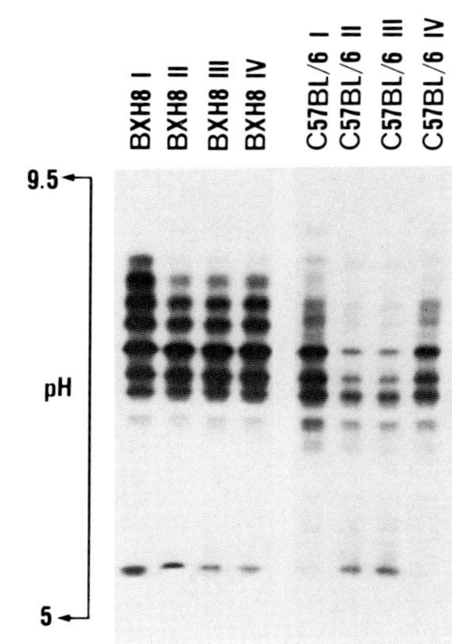

FIGURE 4

FIGURE 2. IEF analysis of H chains of V_k21^+ immunoglobulins isolated from the sera of the indicated mice. (From Primi, D., Devaux, C., Pierres, M., Barbier, E., and Cazenave, P.-A., *Eur. J. Immunol.*, 16, 518, 1986. With permission.)

FIGURE 3. IEF analysis of H chains of V_k21^+ immunoglobulins isolated from the sera of the indicated recombinant mouse strains. (From Primi, D., Devaux, C., Pierres, M., Barbier, E., and Cazenave, P.-A., *Eur. J. Immunol.*, 16, 518, 1986. With permission.)

FIGURE 4. IEF analysis of H chains of V_k21^+ immunoglobulins isolated from the sera of the indicated individual recombinant mice. (From Primi, D., Devaux, C., Pierres, M., Barbier, E., and Cazenave, P.-A., *Eur. J. Immunol.*, 16, 518, 1986. With permission.)

Table 3
FREQUENCIES OF V_HT15 and V_k21 D-E SEGMENTS UTILIZED IN PREIMMUNE B-CELL CLONES

Strain	Frequency of LPS-sensitive cells	Absolute frequencies of V_HT15 clones	Absolute frequencies of V_k21 clones	Absolute frequencies of anti-PC clones
BALB/c	1/20	1/160	1/22	1/50
BALB.B	1/22	1/283	1/30	1/60
BALB.K	1/19	1/253	1/26	1/69
C.B20	1/26	1/1600	1/20	1/60
C3H	1/6	1/1100	1/25	1/55
C57BL/6	1/6	1/1300	1/28	1/80
C57BL/6 H-2^k	1/8	1/800	1/30	1/50
C57BL/6.Igh^a	1/5	1/100	1/22	1/60
SJL	1/30	1/1600	1/31	1/90
C58	1/4	1/380	1/29	1/100
A/J	1/15	1/600	1/22	1/70

Note: Frequencies were determined as described in Reference 27. Absolute frequencies were determined by dividing the observed frequencies by the frequencies of LPS-sensitive cells.

noglobulins in response to LPS. As V_HT15 has been found to be associated with the immune response to phosphorylcholine (PC),[33-35] we also correlated the number of V_HT15 precursors to one of the B-cell clones with anti-PC activity. All values were corrected for the frequency of LPS-reactive cells in the spleen of the various strains tested. As shown in Table 3, the frequency of B cells utilizing V_HT15 varies from 1/110 in C57BL/6 Igh^a to 1/1300 in C.B20 mice. It is also evident, from the results obtained with BALB/c and C.B20 as well as with C57BL/6 and C57BL/6 Igh^a, that the polymorphism of the V_HT15 gene strongly influences its frequency of expression. It is also noteworthy that the ratio of V_HT15 anti-PC-specific B-cell precursors varies from a minimum of 1:26 in C.B20 mice to a maximum of 1:3.8 in the C58 strain. First this observation demonstrates that even in BALB/c mice, a considerable proportion of clones utilizing the V_HT15 segment is devoid of anti-PC activity, and, secondly, they suggest that a large proportion of anti-PC clones in C.B20 mice do not utilize V_HT15. The frequency analysis of B cells expressing the V_k21D-E gene products, on the other hand, gave a completely different picture than the one obtained with V_HT15. The number of V_k21D-E-positive precursors was, in fact, found to be remarkably similar, if not identical, in the splenocytes of all the strains tested. This highly conserved number of precursors, together with the findings that the level of V_k21D-E-positive immunoglobulins is also dominant over those molecules encoded by V_HT15 even in the selected repertoire, suggests either a nonrandom utilization of V_H genes or, alternatively, that the number of V_H genes is by far superior to the one of their V_k counterpart. The V_k gene pool is currently estimated to consist of about 100 genes.[6] If one assumes that all V_k genes have an equal probability of expression, one should expect, in the nonselected repertoire, a frequency of 0.1% for any given V_k gene. Considering that the H106-131 monoclonal antibody recognizes both V_k21D and V_k21E, the observed frequency of V_k21(D-E) precursors (0.3%) is highly compatible with this expected value. The possibility that all V_k genes have the same probability of expression is further supported first by the remarkably conserved frequency of expression observed in the splenocytes of all the strains tested and, secondly, by the fact that our estimates of the numbers of V_k21D-E-positive precursors is very similar to the one observed for B cells expressing the V_k6 gene segment.[36]

The strict correlation observed between the probability of expression of the V_HT15 and the allotypic form of the structural gene observed in the nonselected repertoire defines a selection mechanism which asymmetrically controls the expression of alleles of the same gene. A possible explanation for this antigen-independent selection can be traced at the level of H-L chain pairing during B-cell development. It is now well established that the intracellular immunoglobulin assembly follows an ordered sequence of events in which functional heavy chains are expressed before light chains.[37-40] As the degree of H-L chain interactions must primarily depend on the nucleotide sequence of the respective V_H and V_L genes, it follows that L chains must interact with different strengths with the various polymorphic forms of the same V_H gene product. In our particular case, V_HT15^a could, for instance, interact with a larger number of V_k gene products than V_HT15^b. Since apparently V_k gene segments are expressed at the same frequency and since accumulation of intracellular H chain appears to be toxic, the end result would necessarily be different frequencies of expression of the various allelic forms of the same gene.

Since we had specific probes for both the V_HT15 and V_k21D-E gene segments, we could directly test this hypothesis by analyzing whether V gene polymorphism could affect the expression of immunoglobulins utilizing the V_HT15-V_k21D-E pairs.

C. Structural Polymorphism of V_k21D and V_k21E Gene Products

Since we wanted to compare the probability of the two allelic forms of V_HT15 to be coexpressed with the V_k21D-E gene segments, it was essential to determine whether these V_k genes are also allelic. To this end we isolated V_k21D-E positive immunoglobulins on H106-131 immunoabsorbant from the normal sera of several inbred strains of mice and analyzed their IEF-light chain spectra. Figure 5 shows the results of this analysis. Two phenotypes were clearly distinguishible: the first one is shared by most laboratory mouse strains and the second one, which is characterized by two major bands that migrate more cathodal than those of the first phenotype, identifies V_k21D-E light chains of C58, AKR, and PL mice. A survey of V_k21D-E light chains of a larger number of laboratory mouse strains revealed, in addition, the existence of a third phenotype shared by SJA and SJL mice[41] (Figure 6). This third phenotype is characterized by a larger number of cathodic bands than the other two phenotypes. In order to establish whether the polymorphism observed was, indeed, solely due to loci mapping on chromosome 6, we analyzed the IEF pattern of light chains isolated from several congenic and double congeneic strains (Figure 7). The BALB/c phenotype was replaced by the C58 and AKR phenotype in the Ly.2-3-Igk-V congeneic strains C.C58, C.AKR, C.C58.AL20, C.AKR.AL20, and C.AKR. The IEF-banding pattern of V_k21D-E high chains from the Ly.2-3 congeneic strain C58.CE, on the other hand, was similar to the BALB/c one. The phenotype of V_k21D-E light chains of (C58 × BALB/c)F_1 was similar to the sum of the two parental phenotypes suggesting, therefore, codominance of the two traits. Taken together, the data reported above establish that the IEF pattern observed, indeed, reflects polymorphism at the k locus and that this polymorphism is not affected by genes mapping at other chromosomes than those on chromosome 6. Thus, three allelic forms of the V_k21D-E genes appear to exist. The first one is expressed by most strains of mice, the second one is shared by C58, PL/J, and AKR, and the third one defines SJL and SJA V_k21D-E chains. We have respectively assigned to these haplotypes the following nomenclature:[41] V_k21^b, V_k21^a, and V_k21^c.

D. Antigen-Independent Selection Is Caused by V Gene Polymorphism

The existence of two V_HT15 allotypes (V_hT15^a and V_HT15^b) and of three allelic forms of the V_k21D-E gene products (V_k21D-E^a, V_k21D-E^b, and V_k21D-E^c) and the availability of the probes which identify them provided us with an excellent opportunity to test the hypothesis postulated above according to which the antigen-independent V gene selection observed would result from posttranscriptional and/or posttranslational incompatibility between certain V_H and V_k genes. More precisely, we could directly analyze whether the three allelic forms of the V_k21D-E gene products could equally be coexpressed with the two alleles of the

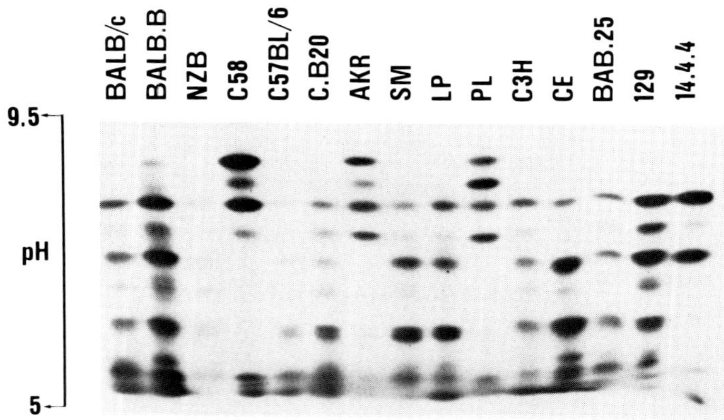

FIGURE 5

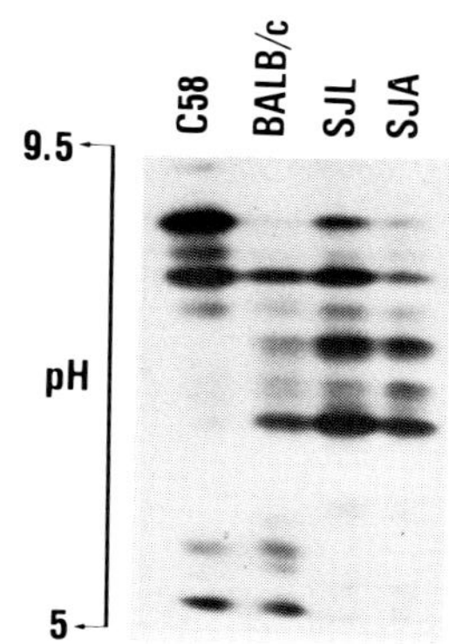

FIGURE 6

STRAIN	*Igh*	*Igk*
BALB/c	BALB/c	BALB/c
F1(BALB/c xC58)	BALB/c C58	BALB/c C58
C58	C58	C58
BALB/c-C58-C.AL20	AL/N	C58
BALB/c-C58	BALB/c	C58
BALB/c-AKR-C.AL20	AL/N	AKR
C.AL20	AL/N	BALB/c
BALB/c-AKR	BALB/c	AKR
AKR	AKR	AKR
C58-CE	C58	CE
CE	CE	CE
PL	PL	PL
NZB	NZB	NZB
14.4.4		

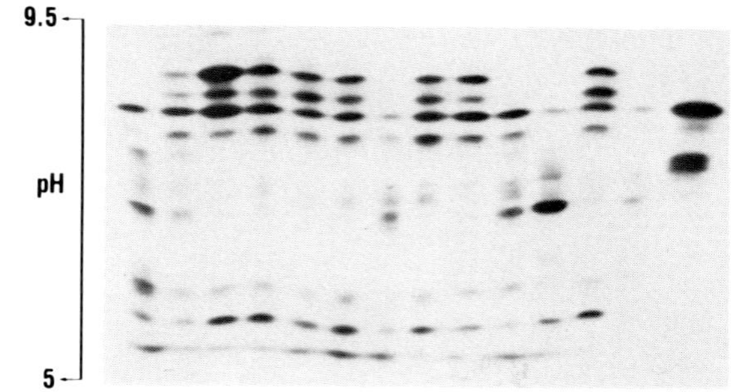

FIGURE 7

FIGURE 5. IEF analysis of $V_{\kappa}21E^{+}$ and $V_{\kappa}21D^{+}$ light chains isolated from the sera of the indicated strains of mice. (From Primi, D., Barbier, E., and Cazenave, P.-A., *Eur. J. Immunol.*, in press. With permission.)

FIGURE 6. IEF analysis of $V_{\kappa}21E^{+}$ and $V_{\kappa}21D^{+}$ light chains isolated from the sera of BALB/c, C58, SJL, and SJA mice. (From Primi, D., Barbier, E., and Cazenave, P.-A., *Eur. J. Immunol.*, in press. With permission.)

FIGURE 7. IEF analysis of $V_{\kappa}21E^{+}$ and $V_{\kappa}21D^{+}$ light chains isolated from the sera of the indicated congenic and double congenic mouse strains. (From Primi, D., Barbier, E., and Cazenave, P.-A., *Eur. J. Immunol.*, in press. With permission.)

V_HT15 gene segment. If V_H-V_L interactions in normal lymphocytes are independent of the subgroup of variability, then it should be expected that the various allelic forms of the V_HT15 segment should combine with equal probabilities to the $V_\kappa 21D$-E gene products. Thus, the level of V_HT15-$V_\kappa 21D$-E combined expression in normal sera should solely depend on the absolute amounts of the two gene products. The results in Figure 8 clearly show that this is not the case, since normal sera of SJL mice, which have low amounts of V_HT15^+ Igs, contained the highest amount of V_HT15-$V_\kappa 21D$-E^+ molecules.[42] Although these data do not elucidate the factors that determine the basis of the preferential V_L-V_H combinations, they strongly suggest that the immunoglobulin repertoire in normal serum is composed of molecules which utilize a highly biased combination of V_H-V_L gene products. In order to study this phenomenon with a more defined analysis, we isolated $V_\kappa 21D$-E-positive immunoglobulins on Sepharose^R H106-131 and determined the amount of the isolated molecules by their property to inhibit the 14.4.4.-H106-131 interaction. This procedure enabled us to analyze the levels of V_HT15 segments among defined amounts of 14.4.4 equivalent molecules isolated from several sources. The results obtained (Figure 9) are compatible with those observed with normal sera and they further suggest that V_H-V_L combinations are highly selective and depend primarily on V_H polymorphism. Our results establish that the $V_\kappa 21D$-E^b segments are found more preferentially associated with the V_HT15^a than with the V_HT15^b gene product. In clear contrast, $V_\kappa 21D$-E^c is expressed in association with the V_HT15^b, but not with the V_HT15^a segment. In order to gain information concerning the combinatorial property of $V_\kappa 21^a$, we studied the level of V_HT15-$V_\kappa 21D$-E molecules in congenic and double congeneic mice.[42] The data shown in Figure 10 strongly suggest that, contrary to $V_\kappa 21D$-E^c, $V_\kappa 21D$-E^a can perfectly reassociate with V_HT15^a, but not with V_HT15^b. In these experiments, in fact, the only limiting factor determining V_H-V_L association was the haplotype of the V_HT15 segment. Thus, although $V_\kappa 21^a$ and $V_\kappa 21^b$ are clearly different in their structure, they behave similarly with respect to their capacity to reassociate with the various allelic forms of the V_HT15 segment.

It can still be possible that our results simply reflect selected specificities which, in turn, can be influenced by V gene polymorphism. To distinguish whether truly mechanistic or selective processes account for our data, we analyzed the frequency of clones which can produce the various allelic combinations of V_HT15-$V_\kappa 21$ pairs. Our previous analysis reported above revealed that the frequency of LPS-sensitive clones expressing the V_HT15 segment varied from 1/160 to 1/600 depending on the strains studied. The frequency of $V_\kappa 21D$-E^+ clones, on the other hand, varied much less among the various strains and was approximately of one cell every 30 LPS-responsive lymphocytes. Assuming that V_H-V_L combinations are random, it should then be expected that the frequency of V_HT15-$V_\kappa 21D$-E-positive clones should be, in the best of cases, $1/100 \times 1/30 \times$ the fraction of LPS-sensitive cells. These considerations do not allow a direct estimation, by limiting dilution analysis, of the frequency of V_HT15-$V_\kappa 21D$-E clones, because the necessary number of input cells would be too large to allow clonal expansion. To avoid this problem, we set up large numbers of cultures containing a number of cells so that no more than 25% of the cultures would contain a precursor giving rise to a V_HT15 clone. The optimal cell input number for these conditions was calculated from our previously estimated frequencies. At the time of testing, each culture supernatant was split in two and added to TC54-precoated plastic microwells. Total V_HT15 molecules and V_HT15 molecules associated with $V_\kappa 21D$-E segments were then revealed either with ^{125}I-labeled TC54 or with ^{125}I-labeled H106-131 antibodies. Figure 11 shows that 10% of polyclonally activated BALB/c-V_HT15^+ clones coexpresses the $V_\kappa 21D$-E segments, while the V_HT15-$V_\kappa 21$ pair was never detected among 106 V_HT15-positive clones of the congeneic strain C.B20. Similar results were also obtained with clones from RIII and C57BL/6 strain (Figure 12). Thus, C57BL/6 and C.B20 mice contain the $V_\kappa 21$ homolog, but this product is never or very rarely coexpressed with the V_HT15^b segment. Eleven percent of

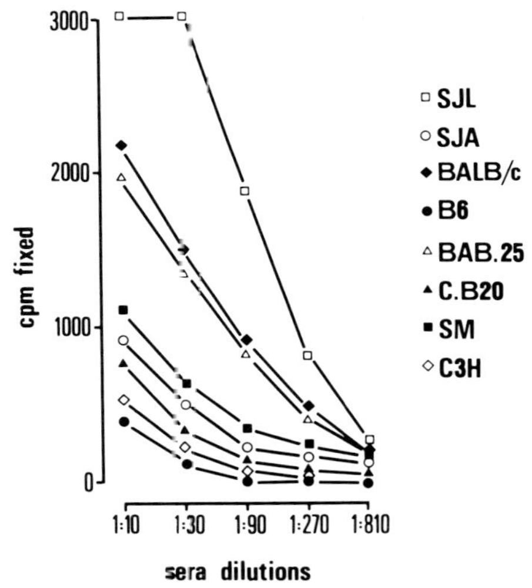

FIGURE 8

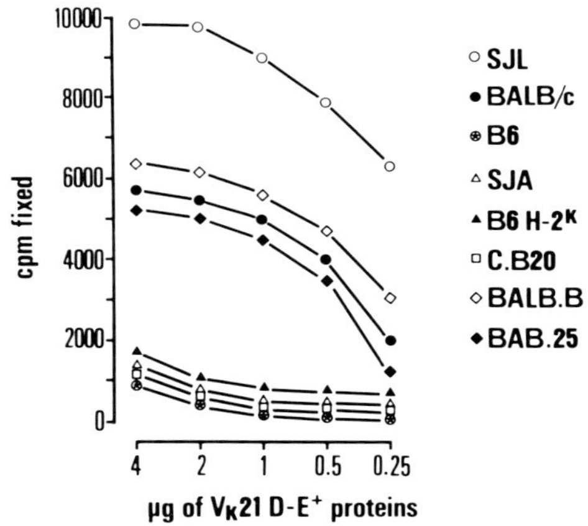

FIGURE 9

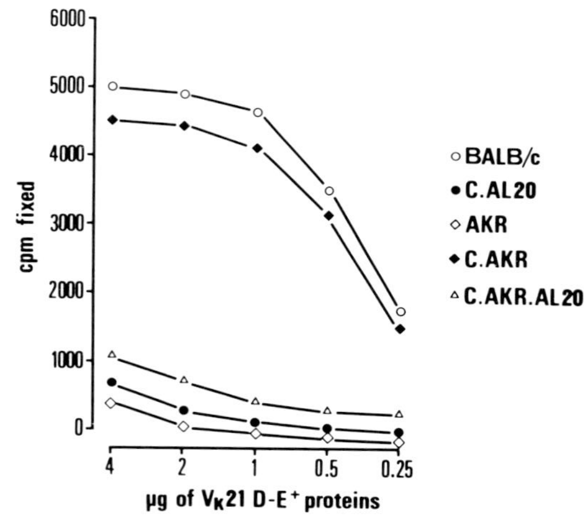

FIGURE 10

FIGURE 8. Analysis of the level of immunoglobulins simultaneously expressing the V_κ21D-E and the V_HT15 segments. Different dilutions of pooled normal sera of the indicated strains were added to TC54 (anti-V_HT15) precoated plastic wells. After washing, the V_HT15-V_κ21 molecules were revealed by incubating the plates with the ^{125}I-labeled H106-131 (anti-V_κ21 D-E) monoclonal antibody.

FIGURE 9. Analysis of V_HT15$^+$ immunoglobulins among V_κ21D-E$^+$ immunoglobulins isolated on H106-131 from the normal sera of the indicated mouse strains.

FIGURE 10. Analysis of V_HT15$^+$ immunoglobulins among V_κ21D-E immunoglobulins isolated from the normal sera of the k congenic (C.AKR) and k,Igh double congenic (C.AKR.AL20) mouse.

SJL V_HT15-positive clones, on the other hand, could coexpress the V_k21D-E segment, but this V_H-V_k pair was never detected among the 106 V_HT15-positive clones of SJA mice (Figure 13). These results, which fully confirm the data obtained with serum immunoglobulins, demonstrate that V_H-V_k combinations can be controlled both by the Igh and the Igk loci. In addition, since these data have been obtained in the absence of antigen, they also establish that this control is not the result of selection, but rather reflects mechanistic constraints consequent to the high degree of structural polymorphism of the interacting gene segments.

III. CONCLUSIONS

The experiments summarized in this chapter were carried out in order to better understand the laws that govern repertoire selection. In particular, we wanted to gain information on one apparently paradoxical aspect of the immune system which, on the one hand, tends to maintain an extremely diversified potential repertoire and, on the other hand, utilizes only a small proportion of its possibilities. Our studies revealed that during the time from which a pre-B cell becomes committed to Ig V gene rearrangement to the phase in which it matures to full immunocompetence, B lymphocytes undergo two severe cycles of selection. The first one is posttranscriptional and antigen independent and is due to V_H and V_k polymorphism that strongly affects the property of the various V_H gene products to recombine with a given V_k subgroup. The second step of B-lymphocyte selection probably works at the periphery of the immune system through the control of as yet not identified genes which map at loci other than H-2 and Igh.

Preferential and specific reassociation of homologous H and L chains isolated from myelomas proteins is well documented.[40-54] Particularly interesting is the case of the myeloma cell line S107 which expresses two rearranged k genes, but can secrete only one of these products.[46,47] In addition, studies of noncovalent association of H and L chains derived from human myeloma proteins have suggested that recombination involves specific interactions between C_k and C_H domains as well as V_H and V_L domains.[44] The novelty with the results reported here is that they have been obtained at the clonal level with normal nontransformed cells and, therefore, establish that this phenomenon is, indeed, of physiological relevance and that it can affect both V_H and V_L expression.

It is now well established that the intracellular immunoglobulin assembly follows an ordered sequence of events in which heavy chains are expressed before light chains. Further, acquisition of a productive rearrangement at both H and L chain loci has been postulated to be a signal for the cessation of all further rearrangements.[48] Since H and L chains are not genetically linked, it is reasonable to assume that V_H and V_L genes rearrange independently from each other. The antigen-independent step of selection for H-L chain pairing, consequently, must be a posttranscriptional event which occurs at the protein level and depends primarily on the sequences of the V_H and V_L genes that are productively rearranged and translated in a given clone. One prediction of our results is that a considerable number of newly arising bone marrow cells would never express functional immunoglobulins and would die as a consequence of lack of clonal expansion. It is difficult to estimate, at the present time, the level of reduction in the number of potential clones imposed by the selection of V_H and V_L pairs, but our quantitative determinations of the independent and combined expression of V_HT15 and V_k21D-E segments in various mouse strains indicate that such an antigen-independent selection may, indeed, affect a large proportion of newly arising B cells.

Our data, therefore, demand serious reconsiderations of the currently accepted estimates of the antibody repertoire size, which assume that V_H and V_L segments recombine randomly. These calculations must now take into account the probability of expression of each V gene as well as the probability of each V_H gene to recombine with each V_k segment. We believe

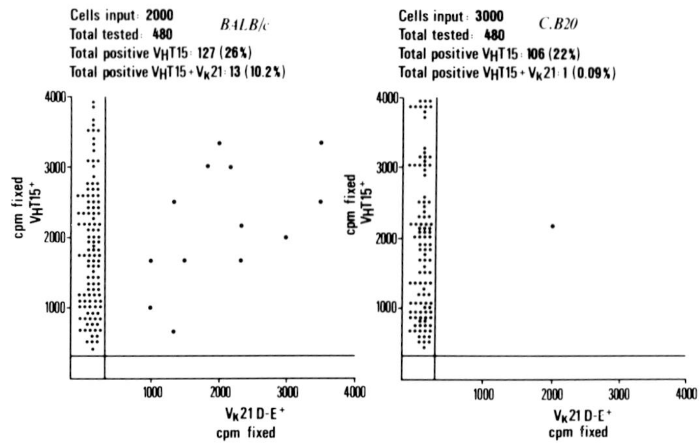

FIGURE 11. Clonal analysis of B cells simultaneously expressing the $V_{\kappa}21D$-E and the V_HT15 segments. For these experiments 480 cultures were set up, in the presence of LPS, containing a given number of B cells so that no more than 26% of cultures would contain a precursor, giving rise to a clone of V_HT15^+ immunoglobulin-producing cells. After 8 days of culturing each supernatant was split in two and added to TC54-precoated plastic wells. After an onvernight incubation the plates were washed, and bound immunoglobulin revealed either with ^{125}I-labeled TC54 monoclonal antibodies or with ^{125}I-labeled H106-131 proteins. Those supernatants that were negative in both tests are not shown.

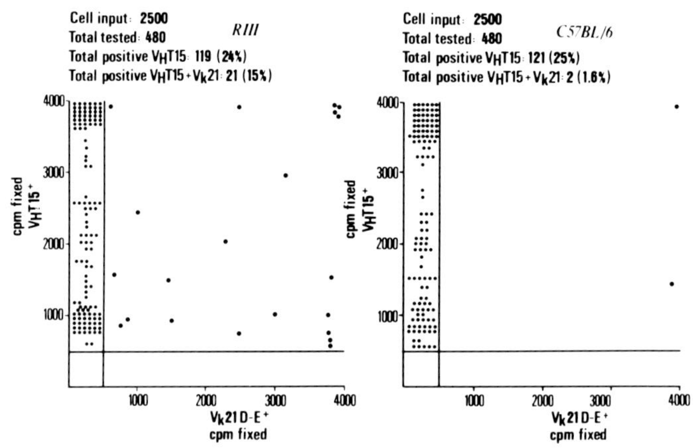

FIGURE 12. Same as Figure 11, but the clonotypes tested were from RIII and C57BL/6.

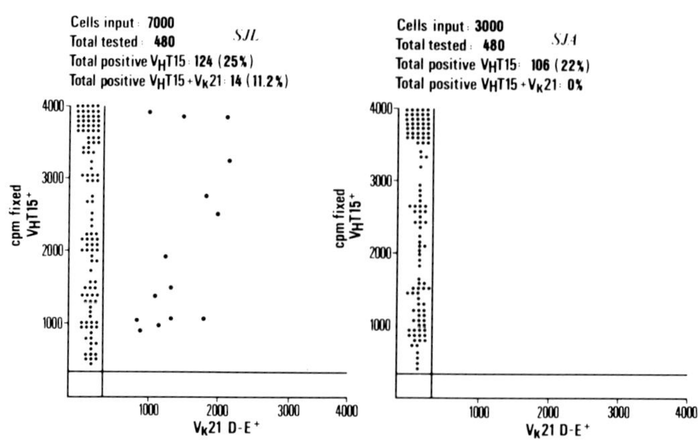

FIGURE 13. Same as Figure 11, but the clonotypes tested were from SJL and SJA animals.

that the considerations of these variables will strongly limit our repertoire estimates and will provide new and more realistic insight for the evolutionary necessity of somatic mutations in the generation of diversity.

We started this assay by asking why the immune system tends to maintain such a diversified potential repertoire when, in effect, it only utilizes a fraction of it. The results presented here synergize in suggesting that the answer for this uneconomical phenomenon can be traced to V gene polymorphism. Polymorphism of V genes is probably a necessity for mammalian life, but, in the case of immunoglobulins, this allelism can also be dangerous inasmuch as it may influence the number of productive V_H-V_L pairs. Thus, the necessity to maintain V gene polymorphism must have provided the evolutionary pressure for the maintenance of a large number of V genes, so that whatever alleles are inherited at a given V_H or V_L locus, there will always be a V_H or V_L gene counterpart to match it and to make a functional immunoglobulin.

Finally, the data summarized in this chapter have strong implications for our understanding of clonal dominance and for the repeated findings demonstrating that certain clonotypes are unusually highly represented in newly generated B-cell populations even before surface immunoglobulin expression.[49-53] These preferential clonal expressions may, in fact, be a direct consequence of the antigen-independent selection described here, which favors the asymmetric expansion of certain clones selected for their property to provide productive V_H-V_L combinations.

ACKNOWLEDGMENTS

We thank Drs. M. Pierres and M. Scharff for the gift of the H106-131 and TC54 antibodies.

REFERENCES

1. **Adams, J. M., Kemp, D. J., Bernard, O., Gough, N., Webb, E., Tyler, B., Gerondakis, S., and Cory, S.,** Organization and expression of murine immunoglobulin genes, *Immunol. Rev.*, 59, 5, 1981.
2. **Honjo, T., Nakai, S., Nishida, Y., Tatoaka, T., Yamawaki-Katoaka, Y., Takahashi, N., Obata, M., Shimizu, A., Yaoita, Y., Nikaido, T., and Ishida, N.,** Rearrangements of immunoglobulin genes during differentiation and evolution, *Immunol. Rev.*, 59, 33, 1981.
3. **Wood, C. and Tonegawa, S.,** Diversity and joining segments of mouse immunoglobulin heavy chain genes are closely linked and in the same orientation: implications for the joining mechanism, *Proc. Natl. Acad. Sci. U.S.A.*, 80, 3030, 1983.
4. **Kemp, D. J., Tyler, B., Bernard, O., Gough, N., Gerondakis, S., Adams, J. M., and Cory, S.,** Organization of genes and spacers within the mouse immunoglobulin V_H locus, *J. Mol. Appl. Genet.*, 1, 245, 1981.
5. **Brodeur, P. H. and Riblet, R.,** The immunoglobulin heavy chain variable region (Igh-V) locus in the mouse. I. One hundred Igh-V genes comprise seven families of homologous genes, *Eur. J. Immunol.*, 14, 922, 1984.
6. **Cory, S., Tyler, B. M., and Adams, J. M.,** Sets of immunoglobulin V_k genes homologous to ten cloned V_k genes, *J. Mol. Appl. Genet.*, 1, 103, 1981.
7. **Gearhart, P. J.,** Effect of somatic mutations on antibody affinity, *Ann. N.Y. Acad. Sci.*, 418, 171, 1983.
8. **Tonegawa, S.,** Somatic generation of antibody diversity, *Nature*, 280, 370, 1983.
9. **Sickevitz, M., Huang, S. Y., and Gefter, M. L.,** The genetic basis of antibody production: a single heavy chain variable region gene encodes all molecules bearing the dominant anti-arsonate idiotype in the strain A mouse, *Eur. J. Immunol.*, 13, 123, 1983.
10. **Reth, M., Bothwell, A. L. M., and Rajewsky, K.,** Structural properties of the hapten binding site and of idiotypes in the NP^b antibody family, in *Immunoglobulin Idiotypes and Their Expression*, Janeway, C., Wigzell, H., and Fox, C. F., Eds., Academic Press, New York, 1981, 169.

11. **Crews, S., Griffin, J., Huang, H., Calame, K., and Hood, L.,** A single V_H gene segment encodes the immune response to phosphorylcholine: somatic mutation is correlated with the class of the antibody, *Cell,* 25, 59, 1981.
12. **Schiff, C., Milili, M., and Fougereau, M.,** Immunoglobulin diversity: analysis of the germ-line V_H gene repertoire of the murine anti-GAT response, *Nucl. Acids Res.,* 11, 4007, 1983.
13. **Cosenza, H. and Kohler, H.,** Specific inhibition of plaque formation to phosphorylcholine by antibody against antibody, *Science,* 176, 1027, 1972.
14. **Sher, A. and Cohn, M.,** Inheritance of an idiotype associated with the immune response of inbred mice to phosphorylcholine, *Eur. J. Immunol.,* 2, 319, 1972.
15. **Claflin, J. L., Wolfe, J., Maddalena, A., and Hodak, S.,** The murine antibody response to phosphorylcholine. I. Idiotypes, structures and binding sites, in *The Biology of Idiotypes,* Green, M. I. and Nisonoff, A., Eds., Plenum Press, New York, 1984, 171.
16. **Augustin, A. and Cosenza, H.,** Expression of new idiotypes following neonatal suppression of a dominant clone, *Eur. J. Immunol.,* 6, 497, 1976.
17. **Elīnger, H. M. and Heusser, C. H.,** Expression of a distinct clonotype profile after recovery from antigen-induced unresponsiveness, *Eur. J. Immunol.,* 12, 530, 1982.
18. **Du Pasquier, L. and Wabl, M. R.,** Antibody diversity in amphibians: inheritance of isoelectric focusing patterns in isogenic frogs, *Eur. J. Immunol.,* 8, 433, 1978.
19. **Weiss, S., Lehmann, K., Raschke, W. C., and Cohn, M.,** Mice completely suppressed for the expression of immunoglobulin k light chain, *Proc. Natl. Acad. Sci. U.S.A.,* 81, 211, 1984.
20. **Meek, K., Jeske, D., Slaoui, M., Leo, O., Urbain, J., and Capra, J. D.,** Complete aminoacid sequence of heavy chain variable regions derived from two monoclonal anti-p-arophenylarsonate antibodies of BALB/c mice expressing the major cross-reactive idiotype of the A/J strain, *J. Exp. Med.,* 160, 1070, 1984.
21. **Devaux, C. A., Cabit, C., Marchetto, S., and Pierres, M.,** Shared idiotope on monoclonal anti-Ia7 antibodies reactive with determinants in a structural domain of the I-E molecule, *J. Immunol.,* 132, 1353, 1984.
22. **Devaux, C., Moinier, D., Mazza, G., Guo, X., Marchetto, S., Fougereau, M., and Pierres, M.,** Preferential expression of V_k21E light chains on Idx Ia7 positive monoclonal anti-I-E antibodies, *J. Immunol.,* 134, 4024, 1985.
23. **Devaux, C., Pierres, M., Epstein, S., and Sachs, D. H.,** Xenogeneic antibodies with apparent idiotypic specificities for anti-Ia7 antibodies are directed in part against V_k21E and D subgroup markers, *J. Immunol.,* in press.
24. **Desaymard, C., Giusti, A. M., and Scharff, M. D.,** Rat anti-T15 monoclonal antibodies with specificity for V_H and V_H-V_L epitopes, *Mol. Immunol.,* 21, 961, 1984.
25. **Rudikoff, S. and Potter, M.,** Allelic forms of the immunoglobulin heavy chain variable region, *J. Immunol.,* 124, 2089, 1980.
26. **Huppi, K., Marche, E. J., Scott, C., Potter, M., and Weigert, M.,** Genetic polymorphism at the k chain locus in mice: comparison of restriction enzyme hybridization fragments of variable and constant region genes, *Immunogenetics,* 21, 445, 1985.
27. **Primi, D., Drapier, A. M., and Cazenave, P.-A.,** Differential expression of sets of highly homologous V gene products in the selected and preimmune repertoire of inbred mouse strains, *J. Exp. Med.,* 163, 1051, 1986.
28. **Riblet, R., Claflin, L., Gibson, D. M., Mathieson, B. J., and Weighert, M.,** Antibody gene linkage studies in (NZBxC58) recombinant inbred lines, *J. Immunol.,* 124, 787, 1980.
29. **Primi, D., Devaux, C., Pierres, M., Barbier, E., and Cazenave, P.-A.,** Analysis of immunoglobulins expressing the V_k21E and V_k21D gene products. Evidence for multigenic control of the expression of V_H-V_L combinations, *Eur. J. Immunol.,* 16, 518, 1986.
30. **Mosier, D. E., Mond, J. J., and Goldings, E. A.,** The ontogeny of thymic independent antibody response in vitro in normal mice and mice with an X-linked B cell defect, *J. Immunol.,* 119, 18784, 1977.
31. **Press, J. L.,** The CBA/N defect defines two classes of T cell-dependent antigens, *J. Immunol.,* 126, 1234, 1981.
32. **Primi, D., Mami, F., Le Guern, C., and Cazenave, P.-A.,** Mitogen reactive B cell subpopulations selectively express different sets of V regions, *J. Exp. Med.,* 156, 181, 1982.
33. **Köhler, H.,** The response to phosphorylcholine, dissecting an immune response, *Transplant. Rev.,* 27, 24, 1975.
34. **Gearhart, P., Johnson, N. D., Douglas, R., and Hood, L.,** IgG antibodies to phosphocholine exhibit more diversity than their IgM counterparts, *Nature (London),* 291, 29, 1981.
35. **Gearhart, P. J., Sigal, N. H., and Klinman, N. R.,** Heterogeneity of the BALB/c anti-phosphorylcholine antibody response at the precursor cell level, *Proc. Natl. Acad. Sci. U.S.A.,* 72, 1707, 1975.
36. **Zhu, D., Lefkovits, I., and Köhler, G.,** Frequencies of expressed immunoglobulin light chain in lipopolysaccharide stimulated BALB/c spleen cells, *J. Exp. Med.,* 160, 971, 1984.

37. **Levitt, D. and Copper, M. D.,** Mouse pre-B cells synthesize and secrete μ heavy chains but not light chains, *Cell,* 19, 617, 1980.
38. **Burrow, P., LeJune, M., and Kearney, T. F.,** Evidence that murine pre-B cells synthesize μ heavy chain but no light chains, *Nature (London),* 280, 838, 1979.
39. **Raff, M. C., Megson, M., Owen, J. J. T., and Cooper, M. D.,** Early production of intracellular IgM in B lymphocyte precursors in the mouse, *Nature (London),* 259, 224, 1976.
40. **Baltimore, D.,** Synthesis of immunoglobulin μ chain gene products precedes synthesis of light chains during B lymphocyte development, *Proc. Natl. Acad. Sci. U.S.A.,* 78, 1823, 1981.
41. **Primi, D., Barbier, E., and Cazenave, P.-A.,** Structural polymorphism of V_k21E and V_k21D gene products in laboratory mice, *Eur. J. Immunol.,* 16, 292, 1986.
42. **Primi, D., Drapier, A. M., and Cazenave, P.-A.,** Highly preferential V_H-V_L pairing in normal B cells results in antigen independent selection of the available repertoire, *J. Immunol.,* 138, 1607, 1987.
43. **De Praval, C. and Fougereau, M.,** Specific interaction between V_H and V_L regions of human monoclonal immunoglobulin, *J. Mol. Biol.,* 102, 657, 1976.
44. **Watt, R. M. and Voss, E. W., Jr.,** Recombination of heavy and light chains immunoglobulins. Use of specific variable and constant region probes to monitor reassociation reactions, *J. Biol. Chem.,* 254, 7105, 1979.
45. **Kranz, D. M. and Voss, E. W., Jr.,** Restricted reassociation of heavy and light chains from hapten-specific monoclonal antibodies, *Proc. Natl. Acad. Sci. U.S.A.,* 78, 5807, 1981.,
46. **Bernard, O., Gough, N., Mond, J., and Adams, M.,** Plasmocytomas with more than one immunoglobulin RNA: implications for allelic exclusion, *Proc. Natl. Acad. Sci. U.S.A.,* 78-9, 5812, 1981.
47. **Kwuan, S. P., Max, E. E., Seidman, J. G., Leder, P., and Scharff, M. D.,** Two kappa immunoglobulin genes are expressed in the myeloma S107, *Cell,* 26, 57, 1981.
48. **Coleclough, C., Perry, R. P., Karjalainen, K., and Weigert, M.,** Aberrant rearrangements contribute significantly to the allelic exclusion of immunoglobulin gene expression, *Nature,* 290, 372, 1981.
49. **Klinman, N. R., Wylie, D. W., and Cancro, M. P.,** Mechanisms that govern repertoire expression, *Proc. Int. Congr. Immunol.,* 4, 123, 1980.
50. **Zharhary, D., Riley, R. L., Froscher, B. G., and Klinman, N. R.,** Genetic and environmental control of B cell idiotype expression, in *The Biology of Idiotypes,* Greene, M. I. and Nisonoff, A., Eds., Plenum Press, New York, 1983, 249.
51. **Zharhary, D. and Klinman, N.,** Antigen responsiveness of the mature and generative B cell populations of aged mice, *J. Exp. Med.,* 157, 1300, 1983.
52. **Riley, R. L., Wylle, D. E., and Klinman, N. R.,** B cell repertoire diversification precedes immunoglobulin receptor expression, *J. Exp. Med.,* 158, 1733, 1983.
53. **Klinman, N. R., Riley, R. L., Stone, M. R., Wylie, D. E., and Zharhary, D.,** The specificity repertoire of pre-receptor and mature B cells, *Ann. N.Y. Acad. Sci.,* 418, 130, 1983.
54. **Klinman, N. R. and Stone, M. R.,** The role of variable region gene expression and environmental selection in determining the antiphosphorylcholine B cell repertoire, *J. Exp. Med.,* 158, 1948, 1984.
55. **Nishikawa, S., Toshidata, T., and Rajewsky, K.,** The expression of a set of antibody variable regions in lipopolysaccharide-reactive B cells at various stages of ontogeny and its control by anti-idiotypic antibody, *Eur. J. Immunol.,* 13, 318, 1983.
56. **Juy, D., Primi, D., Sanchez, P., and Cazenave, P.-A.,** The selection and maintenance of the V region determinant repertoire is germ-line encoded and T cell independent, *Eur. J. Immunol.,* 13, 326, 1983.

Chapter 6

EXPRESSION OF IDIOTYPES AND ANTI-IDIOTYPES DURING DEVELOPMENT: FREQUENCIES AND FUNCTIONAL SIGNIFICANCE IN THE ACQUISITION OF THE ADULT B-CELL REPERTOIRE

M. Vakil and J. F. Kearney

TABLE OF CONTENTS

I. INTRODUCTION

The variable regions of immunoglobulin genes have the potential to generate a large number of antibody specificities by a variety of recombinatorial, combinatorial, and somatic processes occurring during B-cell development.[1,2] These variable regions must also encode for the idiotypic (Id) determinants of immunoglobulins that are proposed to be involved in the regulation of the immune system.[3] There has been an accumulation of indirect supportive evidence for this theory in the past.[4-7] However, the immunoregulatory mechanisms responsible for the uniform development of T- and B-cell repertoires during ontogeny, as well as the processes that result in the expression of dominant clonotypes in immune responses to certain antigens, are not well understood. Most of the in vivo studies addressing these issues have involved antigen or Id priming of T or B cells, or the use of monoclonal antibodies that were derived from rigorously immunized adult mice,[6,7] in a variety of ways and as such represent rather artificial and nonphysiological situations. Nevertheless, the effects of these agents in adult or neonatal recipients have been interpreted as representative of these mechanisms occurring during normal immunoregulation. These deliberate distortions of the normal immune system by extrinsic agents while providing a wealth of insight into the cellular mechanisms of immunomodulatory processes offer few conclusions as to the physiological parameters of regulatory processes. These shortcomings which of necessity accompany such experimental approaches have emphasized the need for reexamination of the immune system from a different perspective.

There has been increasing evidence in recent years that the fetal immune system consists of a limited number of B-cell clonotypes and shows extensive auto-anti-idiotypic (auto-anti-Id) activity,[8,9] which, however, appears to diversify during development to give rise to a more heterogeneous adult B-cell repertoire with an apparent accompanying disappearance of self-reactivity.[9] As a further approach to facilitate the analysis of the ontogeny of the B-cell repertoire, we have generated hybridomas from normal B cells in the livers and spleens of perinatal BALB/c mice. The stable hybridomas obtained should, thus, result from the "rescue" of B cells that exist at the time of fusion in a naturally activated state. We have also generated hybridomas from mitogen-stimulated fetal liver-derived cells. These hybridomas represent a pool of B lymphocytes that were artificially activated and should, presumably, include the naturally activated B cells as well as others which might not normally be fused in the absence of mitogenic stimulation. Hybridomas were also constructed from splenic B cells of normal unmanipulated adult mice. Specificity analysis of monoclonal antibodies derived from these panels of hybridomas showed that a high proportion of the neonatal B cell-derived antibodies was reactive towards a wide range of self and nonself molecules.[10] In contrast, the monoclonal antibodies derived from adult mice displayed more restricted binding characteristics.

These perinatally derived hybridomas, thus, provided us with a collection of antibodies from B-cell clonotypes representative of a very early stage of development. In vitro analyses of the monoclonal antibodies secreted by these hybridomas facilitated the characterization of their distinct binding properties. Functional analyses of some of these antibodies with respect to the modulation of certain antibody responses in syngeneic mice suggest that these early-appearing B cells exert a maximal influence on precursor B cells during the postnatal stages and also appear to play a significant role in the establishment of the adult B-cell repertoire, by the Id selection of appropriate B-cell clones.

II. IN VITRO ACTIVITIES OF PERINATAL ANTIBODIES

A. Reactivity with Conventional Antigens and Id

It has been shown by the use of splenic focus assays that in mice the functional maturation

Table 1
OCCURRENCE OF CONVENTIONAL SPECIFICITIES IN THE PERINATAL B-CELL REPERTOIRE

Antigen	Source[a] and number[b] of clones			
	FL	2DL	3DL	3DS
NP-BSA	2(0.05)	0	0	0
NIP-MSA	0	0	0	0
DNP-OVA	6(0.14)	3(0.07)	0	1(0.02)
TNP-BSA	8(0.21)	2(0.04)	0	1(0.02)
OX-BSA	7(0.18)	6(0.14)	1(0.02)	1(0.02)
PC-BSA	0	0	0	0
DEX-BSA ($\alpha 1 \rightarrow 3$)	0	0	0	0
DEX-BSA ($\alpha 1 \rightarrow 6$)	0	0	0	0
NAG-BSA	0	0	0	0
IN-BSA	0	0	0	0
Levan	0	0	0	0

[a] FL, fetal liver: 2DL, 2-day liver; 3DL, 3-day liver; 3DS, 3-day spleen.

[b] Numbers represent total antigen-reactive clones in each fusion; figures in parentheses represent frequencies of such clones.

of the specificity repertoire proceeds in a programed fashion. While B cells specific for DNP and other haptens can be detected in the fetal liver,[11] cells responding to PC are not found before 4 to 5 days after birth,[12] and B cells that specifically react with $\alpha 1 \rightarrow 6$ dextran appear even later.[13] Although precursor B cells reactive with $\alpha 1 \rightarrow 3$ dextran and expressing the M104E Id can be detected during the first week of life, these do not seem to expand to significant numbers in adult mice. Instead, the J558 Id bearing precursors which appear around days 12 to 15 rapidly develop to become the most dominant clonotype within the adult precursor B-cell population specific for this antigen.[14] Monoclonal antibodies from our panel of perinatal hybridomas were screened for binding to the conjugates of bovine serum albumin (BSA) or other protein with haptens such as 4-hydroxy-nitrophenyl-acetyl (NP); iodonitrophenyl (NIP); 2,4 dinitrophenyl (DNP); 2,4,6 trinitrophenyl (TNP); oxazalone (OX); phosphorylcholine (PC); $\alpha 1 \rightarrow 3$ dextran (DEX,B1355); $\alpha 1 \rightarrow 6$ dextran (DEX,B512); *N*-acetyl glucosamine (NAG), and inulin (IN), as well as to bacterial levan. As predicted from the studies mentioned above, a significant number of hybridomas with specificity for DNP and TNP were derived from the fetal liver (Table 1). Some of these were also found to cross react with OX. Hybridomas with specificity for DNP, TNP, or OX were also found in the 2-day liver and, less frequently, in the 3-day spleen. However, until 3 days after birth, no reactivities with any of the other antigens could be detected, suggesting that the appropriate precursor B cells specific for these antigens had either not been generated by immunoglobulin gene rearrangements or were not activated and could not be rescued by cell fusion. We and others have previously reported that during ontogeny, there appears to be a preponderance of the expression of V_H genes from the M21 and Q52 families in the early B lineage lymphocytes.[15] Apart from this striking bias towards usage of M21 and Q52 V_H genes which happen to be located most proximal to the D-J_H locus early in development, there does not appear to be a temporal order for the frequency of V_H rearrangement with respect to age that progresses from the genes that are most proximal to this locus towards those that map distal to this locus.[16] Nevertheless, the V_H genes that are required for the expression of specificities like PC, DEX, and IN are found to be infrequent in perinatal pre-B- and B-cell hybridomas.[16,17] Furthermore, preliminary evidence based on the IEF patterns

Table 2
OCCURRENCE OF ANTI-ID (Ab_2 AND Ab_3) ACTIVITY IN THE PERINATAL B-CELL REPERTOIRE

Conventional antigens	No. of total ligand reactive clones[a]				
	DNP/TNP	OX	PC	DEX	BL
Ab_1 used as ligand	M460	NQ12	T15 M167 M603[b]	J558 M104E[b]	J606 UPC10
Ab_2 clones detected	0	0	2	1	8
Ab_2 used as ligand	FD5-1	—	GB4-10	EB3-7 SJL-18[b]	—
Ab_3 clones detected	14	ND	2	8	ND

[a] Ligands consisting of either hapten-protein conjugates or purified Ab_1 or Ab_2 antibodies were immobilized on polyvinyl at 1—2 μg/mℓ.
[b] No reactivity towards these Id was detectable.

of light chains expressed by perinatal hybridomas suggests that the light chain repertoire in newborn mice may also be restricted.[18] The absence of reactivity towards PC, DEX, and IN in the panel of perinatal hybridomas may, therefore, result from the absence of rearrangement of appropriate V_H and/or V_L genes and/or a lack of appropriate combinatorial associations of heavy and light chain pairs required to generate the appropriate specificities and Id.

The perinatal hybridomas were also screened for reactivity towards a large number of mouse monoclonal antibodies. Some of these, e.g., T15, J558, J606, and M460, represent major Id found in the sera of BALB/c mice undergoing primary responses to the antigens mentioned above.[19-22] Others were anti-Id antibodies directed against such dominant Id and were constructed by using conventional immunization protocols.[23] The design of this specificity screening procedure facilitated the detection of Ab_2- and Ab_3-like activities in the neonatal hybridoma collection, and these findings are summarized in Table 2. None of the hybridomas tested were found to react with the anti-DNP antibodies MOPC315 and MOPC460. In contrast, we were able to detect anti-T15, anti-J558, anti-J606, and anti-UPC10 antibodies. Screening for binding to previously defined monoclonal anti-Id antibodies revealed the presence of Ab_3 activity in the panel of perinatal B-cell hybridomas. Several hybridomas tested positive for binding to FD5-1 (anti-MOPC460). These were all placed in one group, since FD5-1 has been found to define an idiotope expressed by antibodies to DNP, TNP, and OX.[24] Two hybridomas were found to react with GB4-10 (anti-T15Id) and nine with EB3-7 (anti-J558Id). The high incidence of Ab_2 and Ab_3 antibodies suggested that as far as polysaccharide antigens such as PC, DEX, and IN are concerned, the expansion of auto-anti-Id B cells precedes that of corresponding Id during ontogeny. These results are supported by our previous observations[25] and those of others[26,27] that the ontogenic appearance of anti-T15 B cells parallels or precedes slightly that of T15 Id-bearing precursors.

B. Multiple Reactivity: A Characteristic of Perinatal B Cells

The specificity analysis of hybridoma antibodies also led to another interesting finding. Sixty percent of the antibodies placed in the Ab_2 and Ab_3 categories were found to be multispecific. As shown in Figure 1, anti-T15 BD2 reacted with J558, while two of the anti-J606 reacted with UPC10 and three with EB3-7. Of the 14 FD5-1 reactive antibodies, MD6 reacted with DNP alone and KA5 with OX, while PB2 was found to react with the

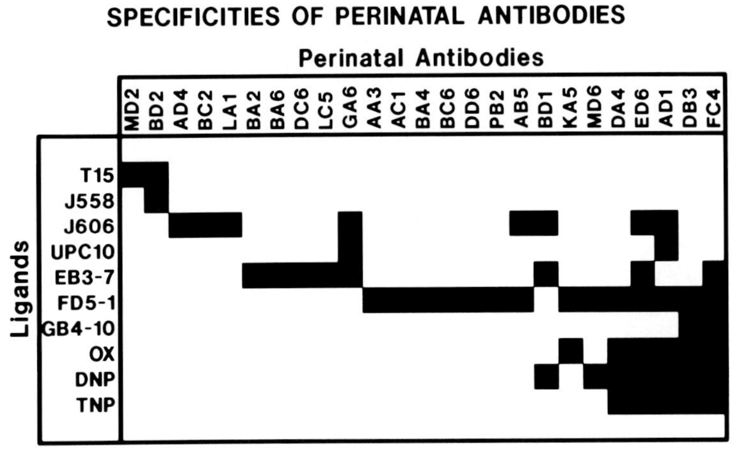

FIGURE 1. The binding of each purified monoclonal antibody to 50 different polyvinyl immobilized antigens was tested in a direct binding ELISA. The reactivities of the most interesting clones are shown. T15, J558, J606, and UPC10 represent dominant Id in responses to PC, $\alpha 1 \rightarrow 3$ DEX, and levan respectively. EB3-7 is an anti-J558, FD5-1 and anti-MOPC-460, and GB4-10 an anti-T15. The antigens DNP, TNP, and OX are included to illustrate the multispecific reactivity of certain anti-Id antibodies.

pathogen *Pasteurella pneumotropica* and DA4 with DNP, TNP, and OX. Seven of the remaining 12 bound Id determinants on one or more immunoglobulin molecules and most of these also reacted with DNP, TNP, and OX. These results indicated that reactivity with more than one antigen as well as with self-idiotopes was characteristic of perinatal antibodies.

Results of direct binding ELISA assays and their interpretations have frequently been regarded with skepticism in the past, particularly with respect to antibodies that are found to bind to several apparently structurally unrelated molecules in a "nonspecific" manner. Because such antibodies offer little solace to believers of the "one antibody one specificity" hypothesis and because their multispecific nature complicates biochemical and functional analyses, the relevance of these antibodies to our ideas on antibody production and/or immune regulation has been neglected in the past. Recently, a high proportion of monoclonal antibodies isolated from neonatal B-cell hybridomas was shown by Holmberg and co-workers to bind a number of immunoglobulin molecules, cytoskeletal proteins, and haptens in similar assays,[9,28] confirming that multispecific reactivity is, indeed, a characteristic of early appearing B-cell clones. The set of Ig and non-Ig target molecules selected for analysis of binding specificities and the results obtained allowed us to go one step further in the characterization of these V region epitopes involved in the apparent Id-specific interactions. Anti-Id antibodies have been classified into various categories with respect to the association of idiotopes on the variable regions of the respective Ab_1 antibodies and these have been described in detail in Chapters 1 to 4. We, therefore, investigated the idiotope-directed binding properties of some of these multispecific antibodies in competitive inhibition ELISA. These have been reported previously, and based on these results, a summary description of some of the striking features of perinatal antibodies follows.

As shown in Figure 2, the binding of each anti-Id (Ab_2) antibody to the respective Id antibody (Ab_1) was inhibited in the presence of appropriate antigen, viz. PC, DEX, or IN/levan. The binding of anti-anti-Id (Ab_3) antibodies such as DB3 and FC4 to the respective Ab_2 antibodies such as GB4-10 or EB3-7 was also inhibited in the presence of the appropriate Ab_1, i.e., T15 or J558. Since the Ab_2 or Ab_3 activity was shown to be displaced by the appropriate antigen or Ab_1, the Ab_2 antibodies resembled the internal images of conventional

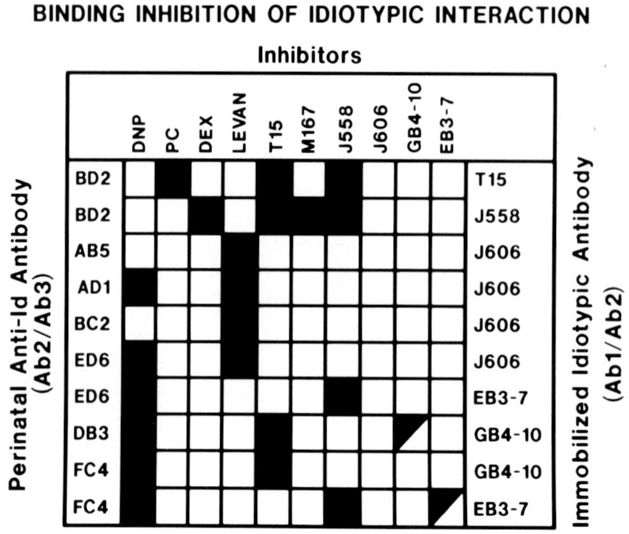

FIGURE 2. The binding of Ab_2 and Ab_3 antibodies to polyvinyl immobilized Ab_1 or Ab_2 antibodies was determined in the presence of inhibitors. Filled squares represent 50% inhibition at equimolar concentrations of test antibody and inhibitor, except for DNP-ϵ-aminocaproate, in which case a concentration of 10^{-5} *M* was used for inhibitory index. Half-filled squares indicate 50% inhibition under these conditions.

antigens, and Ab_3 antibodies, those of the dominant Id elicited in response to these antigens. Furthermore, BD2 binding to T15 or J558 was inhibited by both T15 as well as J558, whereas the binding of anti-J606 antibodies to J606 was inhibited only in the presence of antigens such as free inulin, IN-BSA, and levan, and additionally by DNP in the case of ED6 and AD1, but not by J606. These results suggest that the epitopes on the J606 molecule recognized by these antibodies are binding site related, but are recognized only if the latter is immobilized on polyvinyl. The binding of the Ab_3 antibodies DB3, FC4, and ED6 to their respective Ab_2 antibodies was also only partially inhibited by homologous Ab_2, suggesting that these Id determinants were also sensitive to changes in conformation and were exposed following adsorption on a solid support.

The binding of antibody BD2 to T15 was inhibited in the presence of J558 and enhanced in the presence of MOPC167,[18] whereas the binding of the same antibody to J558 was inhibited by both T15 and MOPC167 (Figure 2). This complex phenomenon will be discussed later with reference to clonal selection through Id. This observation, however, demonstrates that BD2 recognizes T15 and J558 through distinct, but closely related, binding sites.

Antibodies DB3 and FC4 were found to react with GB4-10 (anti-T15). In addition, FC4 was found to react with EB3-7 (anti-J558) and DB3 reacted with BD2. Both DB3 and FC4 are, therefore, Ab_3 with respect to T15 and J558. Both DB3 and FC4 also react with DNP, TNP, OX, and FD5-1 (anti-M460). Such antibodies can, therefore, be characterized as examples of antihapten antibodies (Ab_1) with T15 and J558 acting as their Ab_3 antibodies as shown in Figure 3. The terminology Ab_1, Ab_2, Ab_3, ...etc. is merely operational, used by investigators that biased their experiments by characterizing antibodies which were raised by immunization against, and selected for reactivity with, a given antigen or Id. However, as will become clearer from in vivo expriments described later, the role of the early appearing B cells in the functional development and/or maturation of the later-appearing idiotope-positive B cells is suggestive of a directionality in the progression of idiotope-directed signals during neonatal development. We, therefore, chose to designate the antihapten antibodies such as DB3 and FC4 as Ab_3 rather than Ab_1.

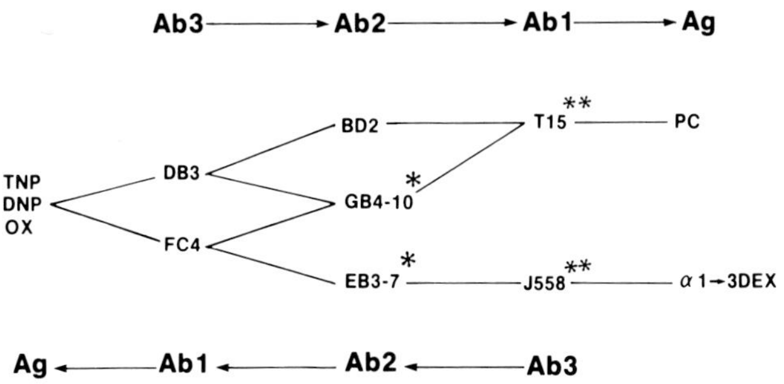

FIGURE 3. Examples of Ab_1, Ab_2, and Ab_3 activity: GB4-10 and EB3-7 (*) are monoclonal A/J antibodies raised against the myeloma proteins T15 and J558 (**), respectively.

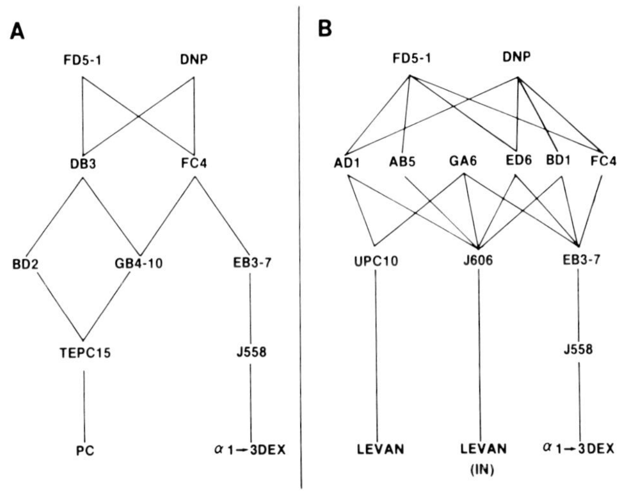

FIGURE 4. Schematic of Id connections among distinct Id. The antibodies shown in this figure are of myeloma or hybridoma origin. The connections were made on the basis of reactivities shown in Figure 1.

C. Interconnections in the B-Cell Compartment

On the basis of in vitro binding characteristics of the perinatally derived antibodies outlined above, it was possible to connect disparate antigen-antibody systems via Id determinants. Hypothetical ''paper'' networks such as those shown in Figure 4 are based on the information obtained from hybridoma antibodies and are, therefore, limited and probably incomplete. Nevertheless, these limited interactions have proven to be useful in the design of in vivo experiments and in the interpretation of results obtained. It was shown that while FC4 reacts with both GB4-10 and EB3-7, and not with BD2, DB3 reacts with GB4-10 and BD2, but not with EB3-7 (Figure 4A). Since BD2 reacts with both T15 and J558, both antibodies DB3 and FC4 are anti-anti-Id to T15 as well as J558. All eight anti-J606 antibodies appeared to be distinct from each other with respect to their binding characteristics in ELISA. Only two of these cross react with UPC10, which does not bind inulin but is reactive towards the $\beta2 \rightarrow 6$ linked portion of levan.[21] Three of them also react with EB3-7 and are, thus, anti-anti-Id to J558. Only the anti-J606 antibodies that connect distinct Id are shown in Figure 4B. The bottom line to these observations is that the perinatal B-cell repertoire of BALB/c mice appears to be highly connected through Id determinants. Consequently, there is a high probability that the corresponding B cells interact in vivo in appropriate microenvironments,

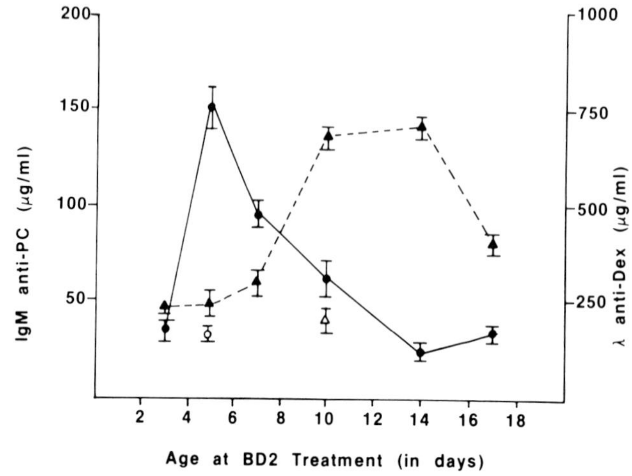

FIGURE 5. BD2-induced enhancement of anti-PC and anti-DEX responses: (—●—), anti-PC and (—▲—), anti-DEX antibodies in response to PC or DEX challenge, respectively, in mice treated with BD2. ⌀ and ▲ represent responses to PC and DEX in age-matched control mice.

and that these interactions may have significant influences on the developing B-cell repertoire. The rest of this chapter is devoted to a discussion of the experimental evidence favoring a functional role of perinatal multispecific B cells in the selective expansion of appropriate clones as they arise during development and their eventual constitution of the normal adult B-cell repertoire.

III. IN VIVO ACTIVITIES OF PERINATAL ANTIBODIES

A. T15 and J558 B Cells Share Regulatory Signals during Development

Anti-Id antibodies have been shown to modulate the expression of appropriate Id(s) in a positive or negative fashion.[29,30] These reports are discussed in Chapter 10. There have been frequent reports suggesting that enhancement or suppression of a target Id by a given anti-Id antibody may be largely a dose-dependent phenomenon.[31] Other reports imply that such modulatory effects, particularly those of the Id-specific suppression, are more pronounced if the anti-Id antibodies are introduced during neonatal stages, due to the high susceptibility of neonatal B cells, compared to that of adult B cells, to cross-linking of their immunoglobulin receptors resulting in their permanent inactivation.[32-34] Most of these experiments have used either monoclonal or heterologous IgG class antibodies. Since these antibodies are of the IgM class and were obtained from perinatal mice, we have argued that the effects of administration of these antibodies during the perinatal stages, while still nonphysiological, would more closely mimic the actual function of their in vivo B-cell counterparts.

1. Positive Regulation by Passively Transferred Antibody

Antibody BD2, as described above, is an anti-Id to both T15 and J558. This antibody was injected into neonatal mice at various ages between days 1 and 17, and the mice were tested for the production of anti-PC and anti-DEX antibodies in response to appropriate antigen challenges, following a rest of 6 to 8 weeks. As shown in Figure 5, treatment with BD2 on days 5 and 7 primed the response to the antigen PC, whereas treatment on days 10 and 14 caused a comparable increase in the anti-DEX titers. When the time of effective enhancement of both responses by this antibody was compared to the developmental appearance of specific precursors, it was clear that these narrow windows coincide with the time of first appearance of functional T15- and J558-like B cells, respectively.[10] These observations, therefore, not only ascribe a function to the antibody BD2, but strongly suggest that normal BD2-like B cells generate signals for Id-bearing precursors which the passively transferred antibody may serve to amplify or exaggerate. Such positive idiotope-directed signals had been previously proposed to play a role in the development of anti-PC responsiveness.[35] Here we have shown that such B cells exist during development for both PC and DEX systems and that signals generated by the interaction between complementary pairs of B cells and/or their products may result in an expansion and/or differentiation of the appropriate target B cells. Such a proposal is directly supported by our demonstration of negative regulation of these antigen systems and is presented in the next section.

The modulatory effects of the antibodies DB3 and FC4 were also investigated in similar experiments and have been described in detail elsewhere.[10] It was shown that if DB3 was introduced into newborn mice 36 hr after birth, that is at a time when the interaction between DB3- and BD2-like B cells is proposed to occur, it led to an enhancement of both anti-PC and anti-DEX responses. However, if FC4 was introduced at about the same time, it enhanced the anti-DEX response but failed to increase the anti-PC titers in the recipient mice. There are two major implications from these results. Firstly, Ab_3 is capable of effecting a positive regulation of Id, and for this to occur the involvement of an intermediate Ab_2 is necessary. With the observed expansion of anti-T15 B cells in adult mice in response to treatment with MM60 (an anti-anti-T15) sets a precedent for such a mechanism.[25] Secondly, FC4 appears to prime the J558-like B cells via anti-Id B cell(s) distinct from those represented by BD2, demonstrating the existence of anti-J558 activity so far not isolated in our panels by hybridoma formation. It is, therefore, reasonable to argue that passively transferred DB3 and FC4 may cause an expansion of anti-T15 and/or anti-J558 B cells. Such an expansion may then have an additive effect on the normal function of anti-Id B cells and results in the enhancement of responses to PC and DEX. In summary, the neonatally activated Ab_2- and Ab_3-like B cells in neonatal mice appear to function as the positive modulators of Ab_1-like B cells that appear several days later in development.

2. *Negative Regulation by Suppression of Auto-Anti-Id*

While the demonstration of *additive* positive modulation by auto-anti-Id implies a possible functional role for the perinatal B cells through interactions, it does not confirm whether such interactions are absolutely necessary for the development of the adult B-cell repertoire, and, in fact, so far our results may be interpreted as yet another set of aritificial situations produced by the introduction of extrinsic antibodies. To answer this question more directly, we chose to selectively *inactivate* certain early appearing B cells and then test if the development of appropriate connected Id(s) was affected. From in vitro binding assays, it was known that antibodies such as DB3 and FC4 shared an Id defined by the monoclonal antibody FD5-1. Although this antibody was not derived from perinatal mice, it is of the IgG1 subclass and it could, therefore, be used as a tool to inactivate B cells which express this idiotope. As shown in Table 3, introduction of FD5-1, indeed, caused a suppression of responses to PC and DEX. Earlier observations implied that DB3- and FC4-like antibodies expanded intermediate Ab_2 B cells in order to cause enhancement of responses to PC and DEX. We, therefore, propose that following FD5-1 treatment, the interaction between Ab_3 and Ab_2 B cells was abrogated at least temporarily, resulting in a reduction in the frequency of Ab_2 B cells and, subsequently, that of Ab_1. This is reflected in the mice receiving such a treatment, by a decrease in the frequency of FD5-1^+ as well as $T15^+$ precursors, and in a more functional sense by a drastic reduction of antibody titers, when such mice are challenged with the appropriate antigen.[24]

FD5-1 induces the suppression of both anti-PC and anti-DEX responses, however, the time of administration of FD5-1 is crucial to the demonstration of such an effect. Treatment

Table 3
INDIRECT SUPPRESSION OF UNRELATED RESPONSES BY FD5-1

Age at time of treatment	Dose of FD5-1	Percent control response[a]	
		Anti-PC	Anti-DEX
−21 (IU)[b]	200 μg	88.0	ND
−6 (IU)	200 μg	93.41	ND
−3 (IU)	200 μg	7.29	134.4
3 (IP)	50 μg	14.60	147.82
4 (IP)	50 μg	35.11	97.99
6 (IP)	50 μg	37.93	78.68
9 (IP)	50 μg	105.36	5.43
11 (IP)	50 μg	66.80	13.94
15 (IP)	50 μg	146.31	15.96
17 (IP)	50 μg	106.88	105.57
42 (IP)	50 μg	86.95	119.56

[a] Geometric means of antibody in μg/mℓ for each group were compared to those of a group of mice given saline at birth and challenged following 8 weeks.

[b] Route of introduction: IU, in utero; IP, intraperitoneal.

3 days before birth and up to 3 days of age causes a reduction of anti-PC response, while treatment on days 9 through 15 suppresses the anti-DEX response. These observations support our previous hypothesis that T15- and J558-like B cells are regulated through similar processes, but at distinct time points during development. Furthermore, these periods of effective treatment overlap with those when BD2 was shown to positively modulate responses to either PC or DEX. The interpretation of these results is that FD5-1-induced suppression is a result of interference with interactions between Ab_2- and Ab_1-like B cells at critical times during B-cell developmental stages rather than as a result of the establishment of suppressor circuits in the mice receiving the treatment.

B. Negative Regulation of Id during Neonatal Stages

1. Anti-J606 Delays the Appearance of J606 Id

In the preceding section we presented evidence for B-cell elements that are involved in the positive regulation of certain clonotypes which dominate the adult responses to PC and DEX. The web of interacting lymphocytes in perinatal mice also appears to contain a population of B cells that limits the development of other idiotypically linked B cells temporarily. It has been shown previously that the response to the polysaccharide antigen bacterial levan consists of two distinct sets of antibodies. One set, represented by the myeloma protein J606, is directed towards the β2 → 1-linked fructosan inulin (IN) portion of levan and is dominated by the J606Id, while the other, represented by the myeloma UPC10, binds levan but fails to react with IN.[21] UPC10-like B cells develop early during ontogeny,[37] however, J606-like B cells do not become functional until about 3 weeks after birth.[35] In our in vitro binding assays, we could identify a large number of perinatal hybridoma-derived antibodies with anti-J606 activity. Only two of these were found to cross react with UPC10. Two of these anti-J606 antibodies were tested for modulation of the antilevan response by administration to neonatal mice. BC2 or AD1 were introduced into BALB/c mice 19 or 21 days after birth with a bias that these may maximally influence the developing J606-like B cells at a time when the latter appeared to develop into functional antibody secreting cells. The mice were rested for 3 to 4 weeks and challenged with levan. In contrast to the BD2-

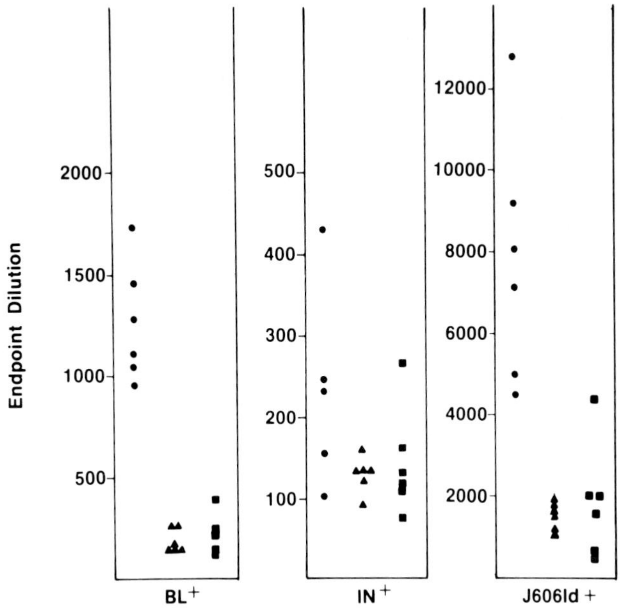

FIGURE 6. Mice were treated with either PBS on day 21 (●), 50 μg BC2 on day 19 (▲), or 50 μg AD1 on day 21 (■). They were rested for 3 weeks, challenged with 10 μg levan extracted from Aerobacter levanicum, and bled on day 10. The titers of serum antibody binding to levan (BL), inulin (IN), and goat anti-J606 were determined in an ELISA.

induced enhancement of T15 and J558, treatment with either BC2 or AD1 induced a marked reduction of the antilevan response as well as a suppression of the J606 Id (Figure 6), assuming that the passively transferred anti-Id antibodies supplemented the effects of endogenous anti-Id. The results of these experiments suggest that the function of naturally occurring anti-J606 is, perhaps, to suppress the expression of J606 early during ontogeny.

Since the frequency of hybridomas reactive towards J606 was found to be very high (shown in Table 2), it may reflect an expansion of anti-J606 B cells during neonatal stages. It is probable that such expanded B cells or the antibodies secreted by them block the levan binding sites on the receptors of J606-like B cells, resulting in a state of IN-specific unresponsiveness. The population of anti-J606 B cells may eventually diminish by internal selection against multispecific antibody products. As a result, the J606-like B cells are relieved of their suppression and can then respond to the antigen. Previous observations that B cells bearing J606 Id are present in neonatal mice but fail to participate in the response following challenge by bacterial levan,[36] support the idea that such B cells are rendered unresponsive by negative regulation. The need to maintain an overall balance in the developing repertoire may require that certain B cells be negatively regulated. This phenomenon may also ensure the generation of such specificities which may be required for protection against potential pathogens such as *Pasteurella pneumotropica* and *Streptococcus pneumoniae*. Since a part of the antilevan response develops early during ontogeny, newborn mice are protected against levan-containing bacteria. Furthermore, since our knowledge about the mechanisms that generate Id directed regulatory signals is limited, it is difficult to justify a bias for the programed development of the B-cell repertoire.

2. Passive T15 Induces a Suppression of the T15 Id

In the context of the observations in the IN-J606 system, another phenomenon deserves mention. We have consistently observed that the introduction of T15 by maternal routes or within the first week of life drastically reduces the ability of these mice, when adults, to mount an anti-PC response.[37] Two alternative mechanisms are proposed for such indirect suppression. The extrinsic T15 antibody may induce an expansion of BD2-like anti-T15 B cells. Such an expansion of anti-Id may cause a blockade of the PC binding sites of receptors on T15-like B cells, thereby abrogating their development. On the other hand, extrinsic T15 may itself bind to the receptors on anti-T15 B cells and block the interaction between the proposed stimulator anti-T15 B cells and intrinsic T15, consequently blocking the development of the latter. Which of these two mechanisms is responsible for the observed suppression of responsiveness to PC is unclear. Experiments designed to study the effects of varying doses and different isotype subclasses of antibodies bearing the T15 Id, as well as other relevant antibodies on the expression of both T15 and J558 Id, are currently in progress in our laboratory. These studies are expected to shed more light on the mechanisms by which positive or negative regulatory signals may be generated between sets of complementary B lymphocytes.

IV. THE DEVELOPMENT OF THE SPECIFICITY REPERTOIRE

A. The Id Cascade and the Progression of Signals

The studies described in this and other reports[10,24] on the functional characterization of early appearing anti-Id B cells provide strong evidence for a major contribution of these cells in the development of the normal B-cell repertoire in BALB/c mice with respect to the acquisition of responsiveness to various antigens. They also suggest that for antigens such as PC and DEX, the development of specific B cells appears to be under a positive regulatory control, while that of IN-specific B cells is under a negative control during neonatal stages. Such regulatory processes may be secondary and complementary to the genetic mechanisms that lead to a nonrandom pattern of expression of variable region genes in perinatal B cells. In previous studies, we and others have reported that the early-appearing autoreactive or anti-Id B cells utilize V_H genes from the MOPC21 and Q52 families which are located proximal to the D-J_H locus.[16,17,24] It appears, therefore, that genes in these families may have been retained in this chromosomal location to function in the regulation of B cells expressing V_H genes positioned more distal to the C_H locus and which are utilized more frequently in antibody responses in adult mice. Encoded in this latter group are the specificities for several polysaccharide antigens commonly found as major immunogenic determinants on pathogenic or opportunistic organisms,[38,39] whereas early-appearing B-cell receptors encode for haptens such as DNP, TNP, and OX for which no microorganism counterparts have yet been described.

In accord with these observations, we would propose that the development of the B-cell repertoire proceeds in a cascade-like fashion from the early appearing B cells to those that appear later and which are characterized by more restricted binding properties, by the progression of signals via appropriate intermediate B-cell connections. These signals may be produced by distinct populations of newly generated B cells and may be positive or negative. However, they occur through idiotope-directed interactions and control the development of distinct B-cell clonotypes in a programed fashion indicative of a very tight regulation.

B. Selection of Appropriate Clones and Clonal Dominance

In light of these observations, we further propose that the phenomenon of clonal dominance of certain Id, which has been shown to be linked to the *Igh*-C locus,[40] may also be programed early during development through idiotope-directed processes prior to antigenic exposure. We and others[37,41] have observed that the first PC-specific precursor that can be detected during ontogeny in functional assays does not express the normally dominant T15 Id. Our observation that antibody MOPC167 enhances the binding of anti-Id BD2 to T15 while inhibiting that between BD2 and J558 in a solid phase assay is intriguing. Moreover, there is no demonstrable reciprocal enhancement of binding of BD2 towards MOPC167 in the presence of either T15 or J558. Perhaps intrinsic MOPC167-like B cells or their antibody products serve to enhance the interaction between BD2-like and T15-like B cells, thereby skewing the stimulatory processes in a direction that favors the expansion of T15 Id-bearing B cell over their competitors, resulting in their eventual dominance.

We are currently in the process of testing this idea by asking whether introduction of MOPC167 at appropriate times during development would prime the recipient mice for enhanced responses to PC, DEX, or both. We would also ask whether treatment with J558 would abolish the dominant expression of T15 Id and vice versa, since each of these antibodies inhibits the binding of BD2 to the other, and, therefore, these Id may possibly compete for the intrinsic anti-Id in vivo. It is of note that the first few DEX-specific precursors detected in functional assays express M104E Id rather than J558.[14] However, once J558 Id is expressed, the transition to its dominant expression is rather quick, suggestive of strong Id directed selective forces that may participate in the development of J558 dominance.

V. CONCLUDING REMARKS

In summary, the processes leading to the uniform acquisition and establishment of the BALB/c adult B-cell repertoire involve complex idiotope-directed interactions that appear to proceed from the early-appearing B cells to the later-appearing ones in a cascade of Id-directed signals. Interference with any of these circuits at an early stage results in the occurrence of major deficiencies in the adult immune repertoire. The cellular mechanisms involved in these proposed B-cell-activated cascades are not clear, but one speculation is warranted and relates to the recent definition of a novel B-cell subset expressing the "Lyl" differentiation marker.[42-44] We would suggest that the B cells found in fetal and neonatal lymphoid organs belong to this subset and may have special properties such as secretion of autocrine-like factors, which may facilitate the apparent expansion of appropriate B cells as a result of the proposed interactions. Studies involving the biochemical dissection of these Id-directed interactions will be helpful in providing a better understanding of these complex mechanisms that bring about a uniform development of the immune system as well as in the elucidation of abnormalities that result in the manifestation of certain immune disorders.

ACKNOWLEDGMENTS

We would like to thank Ms. Ann Brookshire for her assistance in the preparation of this manuscript. This work was supported by NIH grants CA 16673, CA 13148, and AI 14782.

REFERENCES

1. **Hood, L., Campbell, J. Y., and Elgin, S. C. R.,** The organization, expression, and evolution of antibody genes and other multigene families, *Annu. Rev. Genet.*, 9, 305, 1975.
2. **Adams, J. M.,** The organization and expression of immunoglobulin genes, *Immunol. Today,* 1, 10, 1980.
3. **Jerne, N. K.,** Towards a network theory of the immune system, *Ann. Immunol. (Inst. Pasteur),* 125C, 373, 1974.
4. **Pawlak, L., Hart, D., and Nisonoff, A.,** Requirements for prolonged suppression of an idiotypic specificity in adult mice, *J. Exp. Med.*, 137, 1442, 1973.
5. **Weiler, I., Weiler, E., Sprenger, R., and Cosenza, H.,** Idiotype suppression by maternal influences, *Eur. J. Immunol.*, 7, 531, 1977.

6. **Rajewsky, K. and Takemori, T.,** Genetics, expression and function of idiotypes, *Annu. Rev. Immunol.*, 1, 569, 1983.
7. **Kearney, J. F., Barletta, R., Quan, Z., and Quintans, J.,** Monoclonal vs. heterogeneous anti-H8 antibodies in the analysis of the anti-phosphorylcholine response in BALB/c mice, *Eur. J. Immunol.*, 11, 877, 1981.
8. **Lymberi, P., Dighiero, G., Ternynck, T., and Avrameas, S.,** A high incidence of cross-reactive idiotypes among murine natural autoantibodies, *Eur. J. Immunol.*, 15, 702, 1985.
9. **Holmberg, D., Forsgren, S., Ivars, F., and Coutinho, A.,** Reactions among IgM antibodies derived from normal, neonatal mice, *Eur. J. Immunol.*, 14, 435, 1984.
10. **Vakil, M. and Kearney, J. F.,** Functional characterization of monoclonal auto-anti-idiotypic antibodies isolated from the early B cell repertoire of BALB/c mice, *Eur. J. Immunol.*, submitted.
11. **Press, J. L. and Klinman, N. R.,** Frequency of hapten-specific B cells in neonatal and adult murine spleens, *Eur. J. Immunol.*, 4, 155, 1974.
12. **Sigal, N. H., Pickard, A. R., Metcalf, E. S., Gearhart, P. J., and Klinman, N. R.,** Expression of phosphorylcholine-specific B cells during murine development, *J. Exp. Med.*, 146, 933, 1977.
13. **Fernandez, C. and Moller, G.,** Immunological unresponsiveness to native dextran B512 in young animals of dextran high responder strains is due to lack of Ig receptor expression. Evidence for a non-random expression of V-genes, *J. Exp. Med.*, 147, 645, 1978.
14. **Stohrer, R. S. and Kearney, J. F.,** Ontogeny of BALB/c precursors responding to alpha 1 → 3 dextran, *J. Immunol.*, 133, 2323, 1984.
15. **Yancopoulos, G. D., Desiderio, S. V., Paskind, M., Kearney, J. F., Baltimore, D., and Alt, F. W.,** Preferential utilization of the most J_H-proximal gene segments in pre-B cell lines, *Nature*, 311, 727, 1984.
16. **Perlmutter, R. M., Kearney, J. F., Chang, S. P., and Hood, L. E.,** Developmentally controlled expression of immunoglobulin V_H genes, *Science*, 227, 597, 1985.
17. **Holmberg, D.,** personal communication.
18. **Kearney, J. F., Vakil, M., and Nicholson, N.,** Non-random V_H gene expression and idiotype anti-idiotype expression in early B cells, in *Evolution and Vertebrate Immunity: The Antigen Receptor and MHC Gene Families*, Kelsoe, G. and Schulze, D., Eds., Texas University Press, Austin, 1987, 175.
19. **Claflin, L. and Davie, J. M.,** Clonal nature of the immune response to phosphorylcholine. IV. Idiotypic uniformity of binding site-associated antigenic determinants among mouse anti-phosphorylcholine antibodies, *J. Exp. Med.*, 140, 673, 1974.
20. **Hansberg, O., Perlmutter, R. M., Briles, D. E., and Davie, J. M.,** Analysis of the diversity of murine antibodies to dextran B1355. III. Idiotypic and spectrotypic correlations, *Eur. J. Immunol.*, 8, 352, 1978.
21. **Lieberman, R., Potter, M., Humphrey, W., Jr., Mushinsky, E. B., and Vrana, M.,** Multiple individual and cross-specific idiotypes on 13 levan-binding myeloma proteins of BALB/c mice, *J. Exp. Med.*, 142, 106, 1975.
22. **Dzierzak, E. A., Rosenstein, R. W., and Janeway, C. A., Jr.,** Expression of an idiotype (Id-460) during in vivo anti-DNP responses. II. Transient idiotypic dominance, *J. Exp. Med.*, 154, 1432, 1981.
23. **Kearney, J. F.,** Isolation of hybridomas secreting monoclonal anti-idiotypic antibodies, *Fed. Proc. Fed. Am. Soc. Exp. Biol.*, 38, 1421, 1979.
24. **Vakil, M., Sauter, H., Paige, C., and Kearney, J. F.,** In vivo suppression of perinatal multispecific B cells results in a distortion of the adult B cell repertoire, *Eur. J. Immunol.*, 16, 1159, 1986.
25. **Pollok, B. A. and Kearney, J. F.,** Identification and characterization of an apparent germline set of anti-idiotypic regulatory lymphocytes, *J. Immunol.*, 133, 114, 1984.
26. **Augustin, A. and Cosenza, H.,** Expression of new idiotypes following neonatal suppression of a dominant clone, *Eur. J. Immunol.*, 6, 497, 1976.
27. **Strayer, D. S. and Kohler, H.,** Immune response to phosphorylcholine. II. Natural "auto"-anti-receptor antibody in neonatal BALB/c mice, *Cell. Immunol.*, 25, 294, 1976.
28. **Holmberg, D., Wennerström, G., Andrade, L., and Coutinho, A.,** The high idiotypic connectivity of "natural" newborn antibodies is not found in adult mitogen-reactive B cell repertoires, *Eur. J. Immunol.*, 16, 82, 1986.
29. **Bona, C.,** Regulatory idiotypes, in *Idiotypy in Biology and Medicine*, Kohler, H., Urbain, J., and Cazenave, P.-A., Eds., Academic Press, New York, 1984, 29.
30. **Trenkner, E. and Riblet, R.,** Induction of anti-phosphorylcholine antibody formation by anti-idiotypic antibodies, *J. Exp. Med.*, 142, 1121, 1975.
31. **Takemori, T. and Rajewsky, K.,** The immune response against anti-idiotype antibodies. I. Induction of idiotope bearing antibodies and analysis of the idiotope repertoire, *Eur. J. Immunol.*, 12, 1040, 1982.
32. **Metcalf, E. S. and Klinman, N. R.,** In vitro tolerance induction of neonatal and adult bone marrow cells: a functional marker for B cell maturation, *J. Immunol.*, 118, 2111, 1977.

33. **Kearney, J. F., Pollok, B. A., and Stohrer, R. S.,** Selective alteration of the humoral response to alpha 1 → 3 dextran and phosphorylcholine by early administration of monoclonal anti-idiotype, in *Idiotypy in Biology and Medicine,* Kohler, H., Urbain, J., and Cazenave, P.-A., Eds., Academic Press, New York, 1984, 187.
34. **Kohler, H.,** Clonal dominance — a product of idiotype-specific interaction, in *Strategies of Immune Relation,* Sercarz, E. and Cunningham, A. J., Eds., Academic Press, Orlando, 493, 1980.
35. **Bona, C., Mond, J. J., Stein, K. E., House, S., Lieberman, R., and Paul, W. E.,** Immune response to levan. III. The capacity to produce anti-inulin antibodies appears late in ontogeny, *J. Immunol.,* 123, 1484, 1984.
36. **Bona, C. and Victor, C.,** Ontogeny of anti-levan and inulin antibody responses, in *Idiotypy in Biology and Medicine,* Kohler, H., Urbain, J., and Cazenave, P.-A., Eds., Academic Press, New York, 1984, 173.
37. **Vakil, M. and Kearney, J. F.,** unpublished observations.
38. **Briles, D. E., Forman, C., Hudak, S., and Claflin, L.,** Anti-phosphorylcholine antibodies of the T15 idiotype are optimally protective against Streptococcus pneumoniae, *J. Exp. Med.,* 156, 1177, 1982.
39. **Kearney, J. F., McCarthy, M. M., Stohrer, R. S., Benjamin, W., and Briles, D. E.,** Induction of germ-line anti-α1 → 3 dextran antibody response in mice by members of the Enterobacteriaceae family, *J. Immunol.,* 135, 3468, 1985.
40. **Stall, A. M., Quintans, J., and Loken, M. R.,** T15 idiotype expression in murine response to phosphorylcholine is actively regulated by genes linked to the Igh-C locus, *J. Immunol.,* 136, 2689, 1986.
41. **Fung, J. and Kohler, H.,** Analysis of the early non-regulated germline precursor repertoire for PC, in *B Lymphocytes in the Immune Response: Functional, Developmental and Interactive Properties,* Klinman, N. R., Mosier, D. E., Scher, I., and Vitetta, E. S., Eds., Elsevier/North-Holland, Amsterdam, 1981, 69.
42. **Hayakawa, K., Hardy, R. R., Parks, D. R., and Herzenberg, L. A.,** The "Ly-1" B subpopulation in normal, immunodefective and autoimmune mice, *J. Exp. Med.,* 157, 202, 1983.
43. **Dorf, M. and Sherr, D. H.,** An idiotype-specific helper population that bears immunoglobulin, Ia and Lyt-1 determinants, *J. Exp. Med.,* 159, 1189, 1984.
44. **Okumura, K., Hayakawa, K., and Tada, T.,** Cell-to-cell interaction controlled by immunoglobulin genes: role of Thy-1$^-$, Lyt-1$^+$, Ig$^+$ (B) cell in allotype-restricted antibody production, *J. Exp. Med.,* 156, 443, 1982.

Chapter 7

AUTO-ANTI-IDIOTYPE ANTIBODIES*

K. A. Knisley and L. S. Rodkey

TABLE OF CONTENTS

* Supported, in part, by National Institutes of Health grant AI 20590.

I. INTRODUCTION

This paper will review data accumulated in this laboratory over the last 10 years which give some insight into the behavior and interrelationship between antibodies and the anti-idiotypic (anti-Id) antibodies which appear in this experimental system, and in systems studied by others, to regulate the appearance of B-cell clonal products in the serum. It seems nearly dogmatic by now that the immune system has the ability to recognize and respond to both foreign and self-epitopes. Numerous mechanisms seem to be triggered as a result of these recognition events when the idiotope is the element of recognition. Early in these studies the outbred rabbit was selected deliberately as the animal of choice for these studies, as it may be a model system more nearly similar to humans, in many respects, than the available inbred strains of mice and because of the well-defined allotypic markers available on rabbit Ig molecules which allow the idiotype (Id)/anti-Id assays to be controlled in quite sensitive ways. In particular, the *a* locus allotypic markers a1, a2, and a3 are particularly useful because they are known to be V-region markers and are heterogeneous, with each set apparently possessing several discrete subsets of molecules that may share some allotype epitopes within the subset but possessing unique markers in each subset.

II. ARTIFICIAL INDUCTION OF AUTO-ANTI-IDIOTYPIC ANTIBODIES

Studies were begun in an effort to determine if normal outbred animals were capable of mounting antibody responses specific for their own previously synthesized antibody Id.[1] Rabbits were immunized over a long period with the hapten trimethylammonium coupled to keyhole limpet hemocyanin. Antihapten antibodies were specifically purified and the pepsin fragments of these antibodies were prepared. These rabbits were reinjected later with pepsin fragments of their own previously synthesized antibodies after polymerizing the fragments with glutaraldehyde and emulsifying the polymer in complete Freund's adjuvant. The general protocol for artificial induction of auto-anti-idiotypic (auto-anti-Id) antibodies is shown diagrammatically in Figure 1. A quantitative radioimmunoassay was used to measure the reactivity of auto-anti-Id antibodies in sera collected after reinjection of these rabbits with their own previously synthesized antibody pepsin fragments. The data, shown in Table 1, show that each rabbit made antibodies specific for its own antibody Id, but these sera were completely unreactive with antibodies of the same specificity collected from other rabbits. Closer examination of the data shows that only a subset of the total antibody population-born idiotopes could be recognized by auto-anti-Id antibodies. In these results, only 17 to 40% of the molecules with antihapten specificity were recognized by auto-anti-Id sera from different individuals. These results were initially interpreted to mean that the heterogeneity of the antihapten response was so great that only 17 to 40% of the molecules were present in a concentration sufficient to elicit an auto-anti-Id response and that the other 83 to 60% of the molecules consisted of a large number of clonotypes that were not present in concentrations sufficient to elicit a response. This interpretation is now being questioned based on more recent data (see below) which suggest that certain crucial structures may be necessary for expression of some idiotopes. Other data from this initial study showed that the Id-auto-anti-Id reactions that were detected could be partially inhibited with hapten. The results showed, however, that only 60% of the reaction could be inhibited. Therefore, there was a subpopulation of approximately 40% of the Id-auto-anti-Id complexes that could not be inhibited with free hapten, even at very high hapten concentrations.

This study satisfactorily confirmed that normal outbred animals possessed the genetic and biosynthetic capacity to mount auto-anti-Id antibody responses specific for the individual's own, previously synthesized antibody Id when they are suitably stimulated. This study verified the crucial prerequisite for the network concept which requires that the network

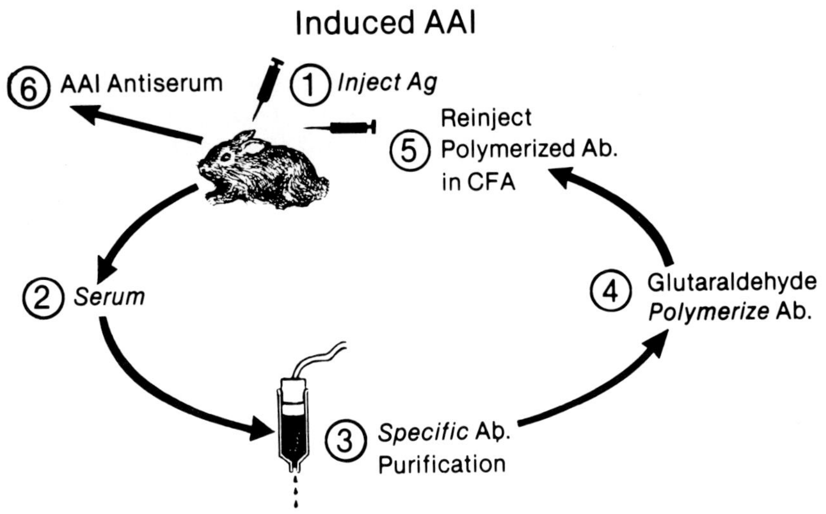

FIGURE 1. Artificial induction of auto-anti-Id antibodies. (1) Rabbits are injected with an antigen; (2) serum is collected; (3) specific antibodies are purified on an antigen-coupled Sepharose[R] column; (4) the antibodies are polymerized with glutaraldehyde; (5) these antibodies are reinjected into the original antibody-producing rabbit in complete Freund's adjuvant; (6) the rabbit is bled to collect auto-anti-Id antiserum.

Table 1
REACTIONS OF INDUCED AUTO-ANTI-ID ANTISERA

	Labeled $F(ab')_2$ source				
Antiserum source	**B-18**	**B-19**	**B-21**	**B-22**	**B-26**
B-18	17.0	2.3	0.6	2.3	2.7
B-19	0.9	39.3	1.6	2.0	2.4
B-21	0.6	3.4	40.7	1.3	2.3
B-22	0.1	0.7	0.3	23.3	0.7
B-26	0.2	1.6	0.1	0.3	23.3
Preinoc[a]	0.8	1.3	1.5	2.3	2.3

[a] Preinoculation serum from each individual.

Reproduced from *The Journal of Experimental Medicine*, 1974, 139, 715, by copyright permission of The Rockefeller University Press.

function within the individual in which the initial immune response is triggered. The network concept requires that the individual not be permanently tolerant of their own antibody idiotopes and this study supported that requirement.

Numerous studies have used anti-Id antisera elicited in other species, or in nonsyngeneic strains of the same species to measure different properties of idiotopes on Ig and on T-cell receptors. The demonstration of auto-anti-Id-synthesizing abilities by the same individual that synthesized the Id antibodies initially led us to question whether the idiotopes that were recognized within the individual were the same set as those that might be recognized by another individual. These studies[2] were done by immunizing rabbits with hapten and using the specifically purified antibodies to elicit auto-anti-Id antibodies in the same individual that synthesized the antibodies and eliciting isologous anti-Id antibodies in an allotype-matched recipient rabbit that had not been immunized with the hapten initially. The auto-

Table 2
SEQUENTIAL PRECIPITATION OF ID USING AUTO-ANTI-ID PRECIPITATION FOLLOWED BY ISOLOGOUS ANTI-ID PRECIPITATION OR USING ISOLOGOUS ANTI-ID PRECIPITATION FOLLOWED BY AUTO-ANTI-ID PRECIPITATION

^{125}I F(ab′)$_2$	First antiserum	Counts precipitated (%)	Second antiserum	Counts precipitated (%)
R5	R5 (auto-anti-Id)	12	R9 (isologous anti-Id)	9
R5	R9 (isologous anti-Id)	25	R5 (auto-anti-Id)	3
R10	R10 (auto-anti-Id)	18	R12 (isologous anti-Id)	45
R10	R12 (isologous anti-Id)	67	R10 (auto-anti-Id)	0
R11	R11 (auto-anti-Id)	28	R13 (isologous anti-Id)	35
R11	R13 (isologous anti-Id)	61	R11 (auto-anti-Id)	1

From L. S. Rodkey, Studies of idiotypic antibodies: reactions of isologous and autologous anti-idiotypic antibodies with the same antibody preparations, *J. Immunol.*, 117(3), 986-989. Copyright by Williams and Wilkins, 1976. With permission.

Table 3
FREE HAPTEN INHIBITION OF AUTO-ANTI-ID AND ISOLOGOUS ANTI-ID REACTIONS WITH THE SAME ID

^{125}I F(ab′)$_2$	Antiserum	5.8×10^{-3} M[a] (%)	6.4×10^{-2} M[a] (%)
R5	R5 (auto-anti-Id)	90	62
R5	R9 (isologous anti-Id)	78	55
R10	R10 (auto-anti-Id)	75	63
R10	R12 (isologous anti-Id)	92	85
R11	R11 (auto-anti-Id)	86	66
R11	R13 (isologous anti-Id)	87	66

[a] Hapten molarity at concentration of free hapten before adding the goat anti-Fc reagent to the tubes. Percentage results presented as percentage of an uninhibited control.

From L. S. Rodkey, Studies of idiotypic antibodies: reactions of isologous and autologous anti-idiotypic antibodies with the same antibody preparations, *J. Immunol.*, 117(3), 986-989. Copyright by Williams and Wilkins, 1976. With permission.

anti-Id and isologous anti-Id reagents were then used in radioimmunoassay inhibition experiments to determine if the idiotopes recognized by both were identical. The results of this study are shown in Table 2 and show that auto-anti-Id reagents consistently recognized smaller subsets of Id than did the isologous anti-Id reagents. Further, the smaller subset of Id recognized by auto-anti-Id reagents was always included within the set of Id recognized by the isologous auto-Id reagents. Experiments were set up in an attempt to determine if the observed differences in the sets of Id recognized by the isologous anti-Id and auto-anti-Id reagents were related to affinity of the different subsets of antibodies for the immunizing hapten. The rationale for these studies was the well-known affinity maturation of immune responses in which early antibodies of low affinity are replaced with antibodies of higher average affinity for hapten during the course of the response. For these studies,[2] the reactions of both auto-anti-Id and isologous anti-Id reagents with the same antibody F(ab′)$_2$ were inhibited with free hapten. The results of three of these reactions are shown in Table 3. The

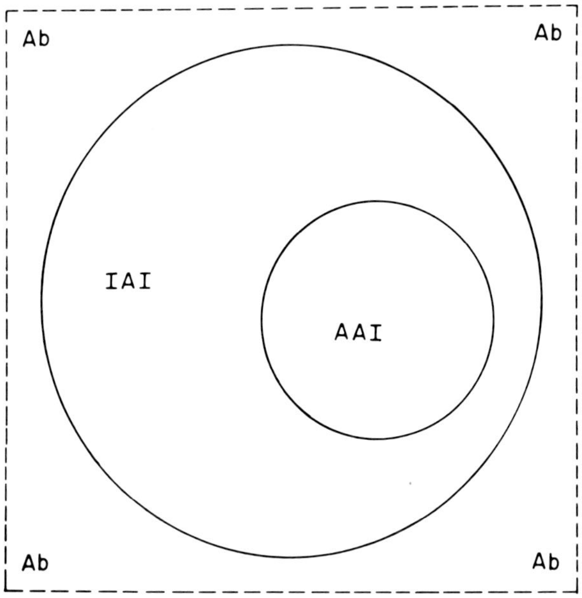

FIGURE 2. Relationship of Id recognized by isologous anti-Id antibodies and auto-anti-Id antibodies. Both are subsets of the total antibody population (the square) and all Id recognized by auto-anti-Id are contained within the population recognized by isologous anti-Id.

results showed that greater hapten inhibition was shown with auto-anti-Id in one case, greater hapten inhibition was shown with isologous anti-Id in a second case, and in the third case, auto-anti-Id and isologous anti-Id were similarly inhibited Thus, there is no consistent finding relating to the affinity of the antibodies subsets recognized by auto-anti-Id vs. isologous anti-Id reagents. Schematically, the subsets of antibodies in a given antiserum which are recognized isologous anti-Id and auto-anti-Id antibodies can be represented as in Figure 2. All molecules recognized by auto-anti-Id antisera were also recognized by isologous anti-Id antibodies. Thus, there is not any fundamental difference in the populations recognized by each different antiserum except that smaller subsets of molecules are recognized at each different level of recognition.

III. NATURAL OCCURRENCES OF AUTO-ANTI-ID ANTIBODIES

The Id network concept originally described by Jerne[3] requires that the network be Id-driven. The implicit assumption of the Id network concept is that this system functions naturally during the course of an immune response to limit the immune response in either a quantitative or qualitative way. Although the data described above clearly showed that normal outbred animals were competent to mount auto-anti-Id responses under the right circumstances, they did not suggest whether the system could function naturally. Further, if the system, indeed, functions naturally, is it effective in limiting the immune response quantitatively and/or qualitatively? These questions led us to design experiments which could detect the presence of natural auto-anti-Id responses and to measure the immunoregulatory effect of these responses. The general experimental approach used was to induce immune responses, purify the resulting antibodies by specific immunoadsorption and elution, rest the animals, and to then look for the presence of immunoregulatory auto-anti-Id antibodies during this rest period. For these experiments, we chose to work with a vaccine preparation of the Gram-positive bacterium *Micrococcus lysodeikticus*. Earlier work by Wikler, Urbain,

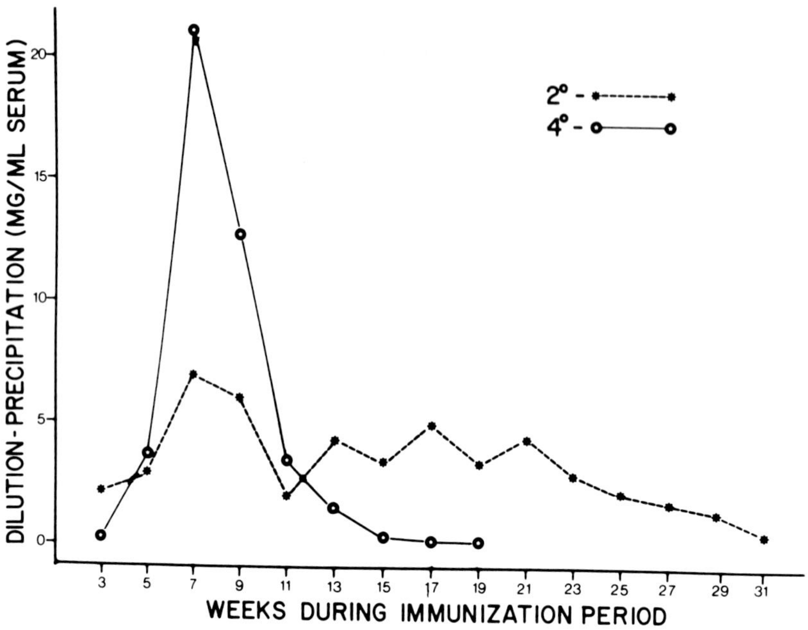

FIGURE 3. Dilution-induced precipitation results of sera from rabbit 102. Serum samples from indicated dates were diluted and the collected precipitate was measured for content of antibody. Samples from the second round (2°) and fourth round (4°) of injections were assayed.

and Strosberg had shown that the micrococcal carbohydrate antigen on these organisms is an extremely potent immunogen in rabbits. The working hypothesis was that the auto-anti-Id response might be very similar to other antibody responses in being dose dependent. Therefore, we expected that the micrococcal vaccine might elicit a strong immune response which, in turn, might elicit a detectable auto-anti-Id response without the necessity of artificial reinjection of the antibodies. Further, we felt that the previously noted limitation to the clonality of the antimicrococcus antibody responses might tend to elicit larger quantities of auto-anti-Id.

The first group of experimental animals was immunized with micrococcus vaccine three times weekly for a 3-week period followed by a rest period. A second round of injections was followed by a rest period. A total of four rounds of injections was administered to these rabbits. Studies of this group of rabbits identified one that mounted a strong auto-anti-Id response which was then shown to functionally modify the subsequent responses to the micrococcal vaccine.[4]

Studies of the response of this animal, rabbit 102,[4] were initiated because unusual behavior of the serum collected during the second round of immunization. Simple dilution of these sera at ratios between 1:10 to 1:30 in buffered saline consistently produced copius amounts of precipitate. Ultracentrifuge studies of the whole sera showed the presence of large amounts of circulating complexes in various size ranges in second-round sera. Numerous precipitation inhibition and coprecipitation experiments verified that the dilution-induced precipitation reaction observed in the second- and fourth-round sera from rabbit 102 was mediated by triplex reaction of Id/auto-anti-Id/reumatoid factor (IgG specific). The Id/auto-anti-Id part of this reaction was weakly hapten inhibitable. The amounts of precipitate detected appeared to cycle during the second round of immunization, suggesting that the concentrations of Id or auto-anti-Id were varying in a cyclic manner. Figure 3 shows the cycling of the quantities of precipitate found in the second-round antiserum. Cycling was not seen in fourth-round

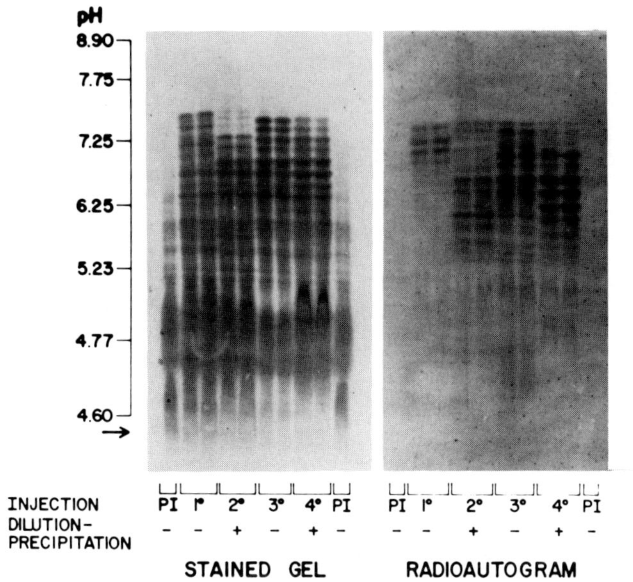

FIGURE 4. Isoelectric focusing analysis of sera from rabbit 102 thorugh 4 rounds of antigen injections. The stained gel (left) and the resulting radioautogram (right) show the differences in antibody clonotypes in the four rounds of responses to Micrococcus vaccine injections. Sera exhibiting dilution-induced precipitation are indicated. The pH gradient is shown on the left.

sera, although a dramatic increase in precipitate quantity was found as compared to second-round sera. This was highly suggestive of an anamnestic-like response.

An intriguing finding was made during the studies of 102 which has been exploited in more recent studies in our laboratory to identify sera which may have undergone auto-anti-Id down-regulation. When the sera from the four rounds of immunization were compared side-by-side on an isoelectric focusing plate and the electrophoretic separation of the sera was followed by exposure of the plate to radioactive micrococcal carbohydrate in order to localize antibody clonotypes that bind micrococcal carbohydrate antigen, the clonotype patterns of the antigen-binding clonotypes were strongly dependent on the presence or absence of auto-anti-Id antibodies. These data (Figure 4) show that first-round antimicrococcal antibodies are clustered at pIs between pH 7 and 8. Second-round antimicrococcal antibodies, in the presence of auto-anti-Id antibodies reactive with first-round antibodies, are located at pIs of 6.5 to 7.4. Following a 1-year rest, the third-round immunization was given and the resulting clonotypes included all representatives of first- and second-round sera. Later, a fourth immunization with micrococcal vaccine elicited antibodies once again lacking the clonotypes representative of the first-round pattern, and the fourth-round sera contained substantial amounts of auto-anti-Id antibodies. Thus, the appearance of auto-anti-Id antibodies comes at a time when a dramatic shift of clonotypes synthesized in response to micrococcal carbohydrate is occurring. Further, this apparent suppressive function of auto-anti-Id antibodies is reversible. First-round clonotypes that are suppressed in the second round reappear in the third round. This reversibility has clear implications for any proposed therapeutic use of Id suppression protocols. A further point is that, for example, in the second round of immunizations, although the first-round clonotypes have been successfully suppressed, new sets of clonotypes with specificity for the vaccine antigens have been mobilized to synthesis so that there is a strong antimicrococcal antibody response even in the absence of the first-round antibody clones.

Table 4
EFFECT OF DIFFERENT IODINATION METHODS ON ANTIMICROCOCCAL ID

	^{125}I F(ab')$_2$ labeling method	
Antiserum	**IC1**	**Chloramine-T**
89-7	11.8[a]	4.9
91-7	20.7	9.1
95.7	23.5	8.5

[a] Numbers are percentage of molecules bound.

Reprinted with permission from *Mol. Immunol.*, 20, Binion, S. B. and Rodkey, L. S., Destruction of antibody idiotopes with ultra-low concentrations of reducing agents, Copyright 1983, Pergamon Press, Ltd.

Several other groups of rabbits were immunized in an attempt to verify the results we found with 102 and to attempt to study several other aspects of naturally induced auto-anti-Id immunoregulation. The general approach was to immunize the rabbits with micrococcal vaccines, rest the rabbits, and to collect sera during the rest period to attempt to detect auto-anti-Id antibodies reactive with antibodies collected during the peak of the antibody response. Consistent failure to detect auto-anti-Id antibodies over a long period of time led us to alter the method of labeling the pepsin fragments of the antibodies from the Chloramine-T method[5] to the Macfarland ICI method.[6] In these studies[7] aliquots of the purified antimicrococcal antibody pepsin fragments were iodinated using either the Chloramine-T method or the IC1 method. Late sera from several animals were assayed for the presence of auto-anti-Id antibodies using both labeled preparations. These results showed (Table 4) that auto-anti-Id antibodies were, indeed, present in these late sera, but that the idiotopes that are recognized by the auto-anti-Id antibodies were being destroyed by the Chloramine-T iodination method. We showed[7] that the destruction was not due to the oxidation potential of Chloramine-T, but due to the reduction step of metabisulfite addition which is used to stop the oxidizing action of Chloramine-T. This was confirmed when experiments were done showing the destructive capacity of mercaptoethanol on these idiotopes. The effective range of reducing agent action on these idiotopes was found to be 1 to 5 $\times$ 10^{-5} *M*. It is interesting to note that this concentration is the one originally described by Click[89] and by Chen and Hirsh[10,11] which enhanced the production of antibodies in vitro. Since this concentration of reducing agent enhances secondary responses in vitro, but not primary responses,[2,13] it is highly likely that the reductive destruction of idiotopes that are recognized by immunoregulatory auto-anti-Id antibodies would prevent the in vitro recognition of these idiotopes by either Id-specific T suppressor cells or by auto-anti-Id antibodies. Either scenario would show enhanced in vitro immune response to the antigen.

In further studies using the IC1 protocol for iodination of pepsin fragments from specifically purified antibodies, we surveyed a group of 19 rabbits that had been immunized for several rounds with micrococcal vaccine[14] for the production of natural auto-anti-Id antibodies. Forty-two percent of the rabbits studied showed the presence of auto-anti-Id antibodies following an initial antibody response to micrococcus. Assays for individual specificity of the auto-anti-Id antibodies gave unexpected results. As shown in Table 5, cross reactions

Table 5
CROSS REACTIONS OF NATURALLY INDUCED AUTO-ANTI-ID ANTISERA

Auto-anti-Id	Radiolabeled $F(ab')_2$ source 89-7	91-7	93-7	95-7	80-8	80-4	102
89-7	16.1[a]	15.4	4.1	16.4	9.6	15.1	24.2
91-7	12.2	31.6	9.5	16.4	13.7	19.2	29.0
93.7	17.5	33.3	17.4	30.8	23.3	24.4	38.4
95.7	9.8	15.3	3.6	25.7	6.3	13.3	35.1
80-8	7.7	11.9	0.7	11.2	11.2	15.7	19.2
80-4	4.9	8.9	1.0	10.0	15.4	28.9	33.1
102	4.5	6.7	0.5	11.4	5.2	15.6	41.6

[a] Numbers indicate percentage of each labeled antimicrococcal $F(ab')_2$ that was bound by each natural auto-anti-Id antiserum.

Reproduced from *The Journal of Experimental Medicine*, 1982, 156, 863, by copyright permission of The Rockefeller University Press.

in this group of animals were extremely strong between antimicrococcal antibodies from each rabbit and the late auto-anti-Id-containing sera from other rabbits. Numerous quantitative inhibition studies were carried out in this group of rabbits in an attempt to determine if the cross reactions were due to identical idiotopes carried on the antibodies or if the cross reactions were mediated by structurally similar, yet nonidentical, idiotopes. The results of these studies[14] showed that the cross reactions noted were due to structurally identical idiotopes synthesized in different outbred rabbits. These data were in direct contrast to the data usually obtained in studies of outbred animals, because such sera normally are found to have only individually specific Id. Our data are supportive of the concept of regulatory idiotopes being the mediators of natural auto-anti-Id immunoregulation.[15]

The data collected to this point generally convinced us that naturally occurring auto-anti-Id responses were a normal aspect of many, if not most, immune responses as defined by our experimental protocol. The practical significance of these data for attempting to understand the role of auto-anti-Id-mediated immunoregulation was questioned by us because of the hyperimmunization protocols used to elicit the initial immune responses in these animals and because the antibody levels were substantially above those normally encountered in most artificially induced immune responses. Therefore, we searched for an experimental model system for inducing immune responses which did not involve hyperimmunization and that involved the minimal amount of experimental intervention.

Steinberg and Wilson[16] first described the immune response occurring in humans in which offspring of a mother who is heterozygous for two Ig allotypes and of a father who is homozygous for a different allotype coded at the same locus can usually be shown to eventually develop a natural immune response to the uninherited maternal allotype. They showed that such offspring make immune responses to these allotype markers that could be detected as early as 7 months and for as long as 35 years. This work defined an immunological system in which the antigenic exposure was a normal consequence of development and required no external manipulation and, thus, seemed useful for studies of natural auto-anti-Id antibody responses.

Several subsequent studies showed that a similar response can be expected in rabbits in which heterozygous females are mated with homozygous males. Adler and Noelle,[17] Hagen et al.,[18] and Adler and Adler[19] have shown that this experimental design frequently induced natural production of antiallotype antibodies in the offspring to the maternal allotype that was not inherited by the offspring.

For these studies,[20] a heterozygous rabbit of allotype a1a2b4b5 was mated with a homozygous male of allotype a3a3b4b4. The resulting offspring were first test bled on day 78 after birth, with small serum samples being taken approximately every 14 days thereafter for more than a year. These sera were all tested in a sensitive radioimmunoassay in an attempt to detect antibodies specific for the allotype which was missing from each individual. The a2a3b4b4 offspring were assayed for anti-a1 antibodies and also for anti-b5 antibodies. The a2a3b4b5 offspring were tested for anti-a1 and the a1a3b4b4 were tested for anti-a2 and anti-b5. All offspring were found to make antibodies to one or both of the noninherited allotype markers at some time after birth, with the time of onset of the natural antiallotype response varying from as early as day 78 to as late as day 176. This property was, thus, found to be highly variable even among littermates of the same mating. These responses were studied in a variety of ways in order to determine the specificity characteristics of this response. Radioimmunoassay titration experiments showed that all anti-b5 responses detected were similar in that each anti-b5 serum contained at least one antibody specificity for the b5 epitopes as expected. They varied in antibody concentration with time, but no variations in specificity could be related to the concentration variations. This was not unexpected, since the available data suggest that each *b* locus allotype bears a set of characteristic epitopes that are the same as the epitopes on all other molecules coded by that particular allele. A very different picture emerged when the sera were tested by radioimmunoassay to determine the properties of the anti-a1 responses. The initial experiments to study anti-a1 responses showed that the anti-a1 response seemed to vary quantitatively even when the experiment was set up using a binding assay which usually resulted in the ratio of reagents being in the zone of gross antibody excess. Since the results of the assays persisted in showing what appeared to be quantitative variation, a second set of experiments was done which was designed to titrate the natural anti-a1 to assure that antibody excess over the included iodinated a1 target molecules was achieved. The titration experiments showed that the first experiment had given accurate results in which only subsets of a1 molecules were recognized by the anti-a1 antisera taken at different times after birth and that the later sera recognized a smaller subset of a1 molecules than did the sera collected earlier in the natural anti-a1 responses. Additionally, this variation occurred in cycles whereby the peak number of a1 molecules recognized in a later cycle always consisted of a smaller subset of a1 molecules than did the antibodies in an earlier cycle. These results showed that the anti-a1 antibody responses were varying with time in their specificities for different subpopulations of a1 molecules, suggesting that populations of anti-a1 molecules specific for distinct subpopulations of a1 molecules were being systematically deleted. This type of specificity deletion is what is predicted by the Id network concept. In order to determine if auto-anti-Id antibodies might be present during the times in the responses in which the specificities of the anti-a1 responses were changing, anti-a1 antibodies from the first cycle of anti-a1 response were purified by affinity chromatography, digested with pepsin, and labeled with ^{125}I. These molecules were used in quantitative radioimmunoassays and mixed with aliquots of each bleeding which was taken after the time when the antibodies used for digestion were synthesized. These assays showed unequivocally that at a period in which the anti-a1 specificity dropped, the animal made a natural anti-I antibody specific for anti-a1 molecules made earlier. This response was confirmed for total of five cycles of anti-a1 production from two rabbits. The naturally induced auto-anti-Id antibodies peaked during valleys of anti-a1 production and the auto-anti-Id antibodies dropped to low levels during peaks of anti-a1 production. These data are remarkably similar in all characteristics, except the time frame of the responses to the data reported by Kelsoe and Cerny for in vitro studies of T15 antibodies and auto-anti-Id responses to T15.[21] It is of great interest to determine what effect such auto-anti-Id responses have on subsequent responses to the same antigen. For this reason these rabbits were deliberately reinjected with a1 molecules to determine if the earlier auto-anti-Id production would have any effects on later anti-a1 production. These rabbits were injected with a1 molecules and the responses were monitored for specificities of antibodies synthesized for a1 subpopulations. The data showed that the earlier auto-anti-Id responses had no observable effect on the overall anti-a1 response, because anti-a1 antibodies of all specificities were detected after deliberate injection. Thus we conclude that natural auto-anti-Id regulation may be reversible in its function. This cannot be concluded in an unequivocal manner, however, since it was not determined if the clonotypes of the anti-a1 antibodies made after deliberate injection were identical to the clonotypes which were deleted during the naturally occurring auto-anti-Id modulation of the response. In agreement with earlier data collected studying the response to micrococcus vaccines (above), the idiotypes that elicited the regulatory auto-anti-Id response were cross reactive and the idiotopes involved were highly reduction sensitive.

In an effort to further characterize auto-anti-Id antibodies, studies have been initiated in our laboratory to investigate some of the physicochemical properties and reaction characteristics of natural auto-anti-Id antibodies. We have taken advantage of the development of a nitrocellulose blotting technique developed in the lab in which antibodies are separated by isoelectric focusing and then immobilized on nitrocellulose paper. Following this binding to nitrocellulose, biotinylated antigen can be added followed by peroxidase-labeled avidin to locate antibody clonotypes. Some recent work has shown this to be a powerful method for studying the make-up of precipitates or of sera containing aggregates of antibody with antigen or antibody with auto-anti-Id by separating the components of the precipitate or serum in an isoelectric focusing gel made up in 8 *M* urea. Following blotting of the separated components onto nitrocellulose, the urea can be easily washed away and the separated components can be probed. This technique has been used to study the natural auto-anti-Id-containing second-round serum from rabbit 102.[4] These results, shown in Figure 5, have given some further insight into natural auto-anti-Id regulation. Figure 5 shows the comparison of antimicrococcal antibodies in first- and second-round serum from rabbit 102 with natural auto-anti-Id antibodies by isoelectric focusing analysis. The figure shows that the auto-anti-Id antibodies bind antimicrococcal antibodies from 102 and, also, from 92-6, an unrelated rabbit. Further, some of the auto-anti-Id antibody binding the antimicrococcal antibodies is inhibited using micrococcal CHO and other auto-anti-Id clonotypes are not inhibited. The clonotype distribution patterns show that the antigen-inhibitable auto-anti-Id clonotypes are rather diffuse and markedly polyclonal in nature. The noninhibitable auto-anti-Id clonotypes which are found in second round, in marked contrast, are extremely restricted in their clonotype distribution patterns, which suggests the participation of a very small number of V-region genes contributing to synthesis of these molecules. These appear to be the clonotype representatives of the natural auto-anti-Id antibodies detected in earlier studies[14] which detect the same Id on antimicrococcal antibodies from many outbred rabbits. Thus, the high degree of restriction in the heterogeneity of auto-anti-Id clonotypes which recognize antimicrococcal Id from numerous outbred animals suggests that little somatic variation can be tolerated when these molecules are synthesized.

IV. CONCLUSIONS

Evidence has been accumulated in this, as well as several other experimental systems, which shows that the capacity to mount immunoregulatory auto-anti-Id responses is present in normal outbred animals and that this capacity seems to be mobilized regularly, even during natural immune responses. Such naturally induced auto-anti-Id antibodies can exert strong influences on subsequent responses to antigens, with substantial clonotype shifts

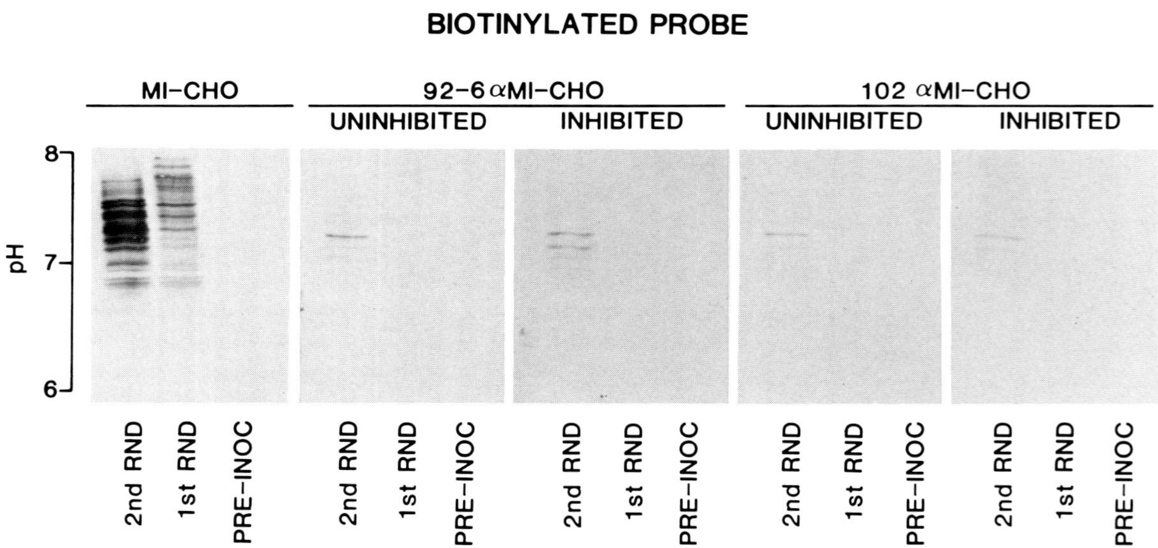

FIGURE 5. Isoelectric focusing analysis of preinoculation (pre-inoc), first round (1st rnd), and second round (2nd rnd) sera from rabbit 102. Antisera were electrofocused and blotted onto nitrocellulose paper. These antibodies were probed with biotinylated *Micrococcus lysodeikticus* carbohydrate (M1-CHO), anti-Micrococcus antibodies from rabbit 92-6 (92-6 αM1-CHO), and 102 anti-Micrococcus antibodies isolated from first-round sera (102 αM1-CHO). The reactions of 92-6 and 102 anti-micrococcal antibodies were done in the presence (inhibited) or absence (uninhibited) of free Micrococcus CHO.

occurring in some cases and demonstrable shifts in specificity occurring in other cases. It is still a debatable point whether the observed effects are due to the direct action of auto-anti-Id antibodies, to mechanisms that involve T suppressor cells, or to the action of auto-anti-Id antibodies on accessory cells such as T helper cells. Further studies will undoubtedly clarify the specific mechanisms involved.

One point that is potentially critical in trying to understand the basis of mechanisms of network-mediated immunoregulation has to do with the nature of idiotopes that can trigger these events. The basic question is whether all idiotopes are equal in their abilities to induce regulatory auto-anti-Id responses. Our earlier studies[1] suggested that even when antibodies were purified, pepsin digested, and glutaraldehyde polymerized and reinjected emulsified in complete Freund's adjuvant, only 40% or less of the antibodies bore idiotopes that could be recognized by the animal. The problems with interpretation of these data due to possible heterogeneity were mentioned earlier. The more recent data[14,20] lead us to suggest that the concept of unique idiotopes that elicit auto-anti-Id responses should be strongly considered. The extreme reduction sensitivity of the identical idiotopes made in 8 of 19 rabbits studied suggests that a specific disulfide bond may position certain idiotopes in such a way that they are unusually immunogenic. O'Donnell et al. have shown[22] that numerous Ig subpopulations exist in rabbits with variations in the number and location of cysteine residues in the N-terminal portion of the molecules. These sequence variants were present in low concentrations in normal IgG pools isolated from normal rabbits and could clearly be increased dramatically in concentration with immunization up to autoimmunogenic levels.

There is now ample evidence to be able to draw some preliminary conclusions about the possible biological implications of auto-anti-Id immunoregulatory events in the adult. In two studies presented here we have shown the reversible nature of these responses. Isoelectric focusing studies showed that the clonotypes characteristic of a first-round antibody response, deleted by some auto-anti-Id mechanism from a second-round response, reappeared in a third-round response. In a different system, deliberate injection of antigen elicited antibody specificities that had earlier been deleted by natural auto-anti-Id responses. These two lines of evidence are in complete agreement with studies done by Strayer et al.[23,24] in which anti-Id suppression of T15 responses in adults was shown to be a transient type of suppression. Thus the accumulated evidence strongly suggests that auto-anti-Id-mediated suppression in the adult outbred animal appears to be a transient rather than permanent type of suppression.

Further insight into this regulatory system has been provided by our recent studies of the extremely restricted heterogeneity of the nonantigen inhibitable auto-anti-Id antibodies which occur naturally during immune responses in outbred animals. The restriction of these antibodies to very few clonotypes suggests strong genetic or developmental restrictions on the expression of natural auto-anti-Id antibodies. Earlier studies[14] established strong cross reactivity between antibodies specific for micrococcal carbohydrate when assayed using natural auto-anti-Id antibodies, which was in contrast to other studies using induced auto-anti-Id antibodies[1] in which no Id-auto-anti-Id cross reactions were detected. This appears due in large part to reaction of a restricted set of natural auto-anti-Id antibodies with idiotypes shared on antimicrococcal antibodies from many outbred rabbits. The restricted auto-anti-Id antibodies are not internal image reactions because of the noninhibitability of the reactions with antigen. Further work should clarify the role of these molecules in natural autoregulation.

REFERENCES

1. **Rodkey, L. S.,** Studies of idiotypic antibodies. Production and characterization of autoantiidiotypic antisera, *J. Exp. Med.,* 139, 712, 1974.
2. **Rodkey, L. S.,** Studies of the idiotypic antibodies: reactions of isologous and autologous anti-idiotypic antibodies with the same antibody preparations, *J. Immunol.,* 117, 986, 1976.
3. **Jerne, N. K.,** Towards a network theory of the immune system, *Ann. Immunol. Inst. Pasteur (Paris),* 125C, 373, 1974.
4. **Brown, J. C. and Rodkey, L. S.,** Autoregulation of an antibody response via network-induced auto-anti-idiotype, *J. Exp. Med.,* 150, 67, 1979.
5. **Hunter, W. M. and Greenwood, F. C.,** Preparation of iodine-131 labeled human growth hormone of high specific activity, *Nature (London),* 194, 495, 1962.
6. **McFarlane, A. S.,** Efficient trace labelling of proteins with iodine, *Nature (London),* 182, 53, 1958.
7. **Binion, S. B. and Rodkey, L. S.,** Destruction of antibody idiotopes with ultra-low concentrations of reducing agents, *Mol. Immunol.,* 20, 475, 1983.
8. **Click, R. E., Benck, E. L., and Alter, B. J.,** Enhancement of antibody synthesis in vitro by mercaptoethanol, *Cell. Immunol.,* 3, 156, 1972.
9. **Click, R. E., Benck, L., and Alter, B. J.,** Immune responses in vitro. I. Culture conditions for antibody synthesis, *Cell. Immunol.,* 3, 264, 1972.
10. **Chen, C. and Hirsch, J. G.,** Restoration of antibody forming capacity in cultures of nonadherent spleen cells by meracaptoethanol, *Science,* 176, 60, 1972.
11. **Chen, C. and Hirsch, J. G.,** The effects of mercaptoethanol and of peritoneal macrophages on the antibody forming capacity of nonadherent mouse spleen cells in vitro, *J. Exp. Med.,* 136, 604, 1972.
12. **Luzzati, A. L. and Ramoni, C.,** Primary antibody response of rabbit blood lymphocytes in vitro, *J. Immunol. Methods,* 47, 210, 1981.
13. **Read, S. E. and Braun, D. G.,** In vitro antibody response of primed rabbit peripheral blood lymphocytes to group A variant streptococcal polysaccharide, *Eur. J. Immunol.,* 4, 422, 1974.
14. **Binion, S. B. and Rodkey, L. S.,** Naturally induced auto-anti-idiotypic antibodies. Induction by identical idiotopes in some members of an outbred rabbit family, *J. Exp. Med.,* 156, 860, 1982.
15. **Paul, W. E. and Bona, C. A.,** Regulatory idiotopes and immune networks: a hypothesis, *Immunol. Today,* 3, 230, 1982.
16. **Steinberg, A. G. and Wilson, J. A.,** Hereditary globulin factors and immune tolerance in man, *Science,* 140, 303, 1963.
17. **Adler, F. L. and Noelle, R. J.,** Enduring antibody responses in ''normal'' rabbits to maternal immunoglobulin allotypes, *J. Immunol.,* 115, 620, 1975.
18. **Hagen, K. L., Young, L. E., Tissot, R. G., and Cohen, C.,** Factors affecting natural antiallotype antibody production in rabbits, *Immunogenetics,* 6, 355, 1978.
19. **Adler, F. L. and Adier, L. T.,** Consequences of prenatal exposure to maternal alloantigens, *Ann. N.Y. Acad. Sci.,* 392, 266, 1982.
20. **Rodkey, L. S. and Adler, F. L.,** Regulation of natural anti-allotype antibody responses by idiotype network-induced auto-anti-idiotypic antibodies, *J. Exp. Med.,* 157, 1920, 1983.
21. **Kelsoe, G. and Cerny, J.,** Reciprocal expansions of idiotypic and anti-idiotypic clones following antigen stimulation, *Nature (London),* 279, 333, 1979.
22. **O'Donnell, I. J., Frangione, B., and Porter, R. R.,** The disulphide bonds of the heavy chain of rabbit immunoglobulin G, *Biochem. J.,* 116, 261, 1970.
23. **Strayer, D. S., Cosenza, H., Lee, W. M. F., Rowley, D. A., and Kohler, H.,** Neonatal tolerance induced by antibody against antigen-specific receptor, *Science,* 186, 640, 1974.
24. **Strayer, D. S., Lee, W. M. F., Rowley, D. A., and Kohler, H.,** Anti-receptor antibody. II. Induction of long-term unresponsiveness in neonatal mice, *J. Immunol.,* 114, 728, 1975.

Chapter 8

REGULATORY FUNCTIONS OF ANTI-IDIOTYPE ANTIBODIES: SUPPRESSIVE AND ENHANCING EFFECTS

C. B. Victor-Kobrin

TABLE OF CONTENTS

I. INTRODUCTION

The ability of the immune system to manifest as large an immune repertoire as it does is directly attributable to the enormous diversity of its resident lymphocyte population. The fact that all these lymphocytic clones are capable of achieving a harmonious coexistence in the same immune system is testimony for the operation of a very efficient means of autonomously regulating clonal expression. Jerne[1] was the first individual who possessed the insight to see that, in spite of their tremendous diversity, the immune system's clones could establish a network of constant communication between themselves which was based on idiotypic (Id) interactions. He further postulated that as a consequence of these interclonal Id interactions, immunoregulatory signals were relayed back to the clones, directing them to modulate their prevailing levels of expression accordingly. Subsequent experimentation has not only validated the basic tenets of Jerne's Network Theory,[1] but has also demonstrated the pivotal role which anti-idiotypic (anti-Id) antibodies play in modulating the expression of Id-bearing B- and T-cell clones in the immune system.

It is the goal of this chapter to report on the various experimental systems employed to study the immunoregulatory role of anti-Id antibodies. As this topic encompasses a vast body of literature which has been extensively reviewed by several authors,[2-4] the emphasis will lie on recent work in well-characterized murine systems which have contributed significantly toward furthering our understanding of this field, with earlier work cited as necessary to introduce this material.

II. THE EFFECTS OF THE AUTO-ANTI-IDIOTYPIC IMMUNE RESPONSE

The immunoregulatory role of the anti-Id antibody was first suggested by several investigators working in independent Id systems who observed that an auto-anti-idiotypic (auto-anti-Id) response coincided with a decrease in the Id-positive component of a humoral immune response. This was first demonstrated by Cosenza[5] who was studying the kinetics of the T15 Id-positive component of the antiphosphorylcholine (PC) immune response following a single immunization with a pneumococcal vaccine containing the haptenic determinant PC as a cell wall component. Coincidental with the peaking of the T15 Id^+ anti-PC plaque-forming cell (PFC) response at day 5 after immunization was a detectable rise in the auto-anti-T15-Id PFC response. While the T15 Id^+ anti-PC response steadily decreased 6 to 10 days after immunization, the auto-anti-T15 Id response continued its ascent toward its peak PFC response.

Bona et al.[6] showed that following immunization with the polyfructosan bacterial levan (BL), the number of levan-specific PFCs expressing the E109 cross-reactive Id (IdX) decreased between 15 and 30 days post immunization, while the number of auto-anti-E109 IdX PFCs simultaneously climbed.

In a similar fashion, Schrater et al.[7] demonstrated that the PFC response to the haptenic determinant trinitrophenyl (TNP) peaked at day 4, but declined quite rapidly already at day 7 following immunization with TNP-Ficoll in AKR mice. This decline in the anti-TNP titer was attributed to the appearance of auto-anti-Id antibodies which could be isolated by elution with TNP from the spleen cells of these day 7 immune mice.

The elicitation of auto-anti-T15 Id,[5] E109 IdX,[6] and TNP Id[7] antibodies as well as the corresponding decrease in the Id-bearing specific PFC responses were not observed in nude mice.

Two main points emerge from these observations. First is the fact that self-Id are immunogenic to the immune system. The ensuing auto-anti-Id response proceeds not only without the normally harmful side effects we've come to associate with anti-"self" responses, but, in fact, is quite beneficial if not necessary in carrying out immune system regulation.

Not surprisingly, the auto-anti-Id response is a T-dependent response which is consistent with the globular protein nature of the Id determinant. Second, the data from these three independent experimental systems collectively support the idea that anti-Id antibodies do operate under physiological conditions to down-regulate the expression of B cells producing antibody bearing the complementary Id. In these three systems which all utilize T-independent antigens to elicit expression of the Id-bearing antibody molecules, it has been shown that the anti-Id is interacting directly with the B cell through the Id-bearing membrane immunoglobulin.

III. THE EFFECTS OF EXOGENOUSLY ADMINISTERED ANTI-ID ANTIBODIES

Only after studying Id expression in the immune system which has been experimentally manipulated by exogenous administration of anti-Id antibody can one fully appreciate the entire spectrum of effects which anti-Id antibodies can elicit. It is worthwhile mentioning at this point that the source of the anti-Id reagent is an important parameter to consider in evaluating these experiments. All anti-Id antibodies can be classified according to the genetic relatedness of the animal in whom the anti-Id was raised, to the animal who produced the Id-bearing antibody. There are three such classifications which are defined as follows: (1) xenogeneic or heterologous-anti-Id is produced in an animal of a different species, (2) allogeneic or homologous-anti-Id is produced in a genetically different member of the same species (e.g., another inbred strain of mouse not expressing the Id); (3) syngeneic anti-Id is produced in a genetically identical member of the same species (e.g., another member of the same inbred strain of mouse expressing the Id).

While they are the most difficult to raise, the syngeneic or autologous anti-Id is the preferred reagent to use in these experiments for two main reasons. First, the primary goal behind all of these experiments is to administer the anti-Id antibody in the least obtrusive way as possible such that the only perturbation which should be introduced into the immune system should be solely due to the interaction of the anti-Id antibody with its target Id. However, if the anti-Id is particularly of xenogeneic or even of allogeneic origin, it will be unavoidable for the anti-Id antibody to draw attention to itself as an immunogenic foreign entity. The second more compelling reason lies in the specificity of the syngeneic reagent. Several investigators have shown that Id are most immunogenic in a xenogeneic immunization protocol, less so in an allogeneic one, and least immunogenic in a syngeneic situation. While it is clear that the xenogeneic anti-Id contains antibodies to more individual Id than either the allogeneic or syngeneic reagent, one can't be sure how many of those idiotopes actually participate in immune regulation under physiological conditions. This point is particularly relevant in light of Bona's recent observations that in a syngeneic situation, the immune system does not recognize all idiotopes as regulatory idiotopes.[8] Among the various properties which an idiotope must possess to be a bona fide regulatory idiotope is that it obviously must be immunogenic in a syngeneic situation. Hence, administering anti-Id antibodies other than syngeneic ones introduces into the immune system antibodies to nonregulatory idiotopes which may elicit effects which do not normally occur under physiological conditions.

A. Suppressive Effects of Anti-Id Antibodies

1. Adult Id Suppression

The parenteral administration of monoclonal or polyclonal anti-Id antibodies to adult animals can transiently suppress B-cell synthesis of Id-bearing antibody during the course of an immune response. The effects elicited by these antibodies are similar to those observed during an immune response when an Id-bearing antibody evokes an auto-anti-Id immune response.

Cosenza and Kohler[9] were two of the earliest investigators to induce Id suppression in the adult animal by administering allogeneic A/HE anti-T15 Id antibodies to BALB/c mice. The T15 Id is borne by over 90% of the antibodies induced during the immune response to the haptenic determinant PC.[10] Upon immunization with PC-containing pneumococcal vaccine, the treated animals showed a >90% suppression of the plaque-forming cells (i.e., B cells) synthesizing anti-PC antibodies bearing the T15 Id. The suppression was of a relatively short duration (6 weeks), but, nevertheless, was 100% Id specific, since the synthesis of anti-PC antibodies bearing non-T15 Id was totally unaffected throughout this period. The mechanism of this suppression was shown to be the anti-Id antibodies directly interacting with the B cells through their Id-bearing membrane immunoglobulin (mIg). Two observations support this mechanism:

1. A fluoresceinated rabbit anti-T15 Id antibody stained 25 to $35/10^4$ splenocytes from a normal adult BALB/c, but only $<1/10^4$ in the suppressed BALB/c. However, if the splenocytes from the suppressed animal were incubated in vitro under conditions which allowed them to shed and regenerate their mIg, then the number of cells stained by the anti-T15 Id reagent was comparable to the normal animal.[11] Furthermore, regeneration in vitro of the mIg appeared to relieve this population of splenocytes of its Id suppression, since it could now mount a PC-specific immune response which was quantitatively and qualitatively similar to that of the normal mouse.[12-13]
2. The splenocytes of the suppressed mouse could not transfer the Id suppression to normal recipients who were immunized with a pneumococcal vaccine.[12]

Suppression of a population of PC-specific antibodies in adult BALB/c mice bearing a single idiotope of the T15 Id was achieved using monoclonal anti-Id antibodies.[14] Animals were treated with GB4-10, an allogeneic monoclonal anti-T15 idiotope, immunized 7 days later with pneumococcal vaccine, and bled 7 days after the antigenic challenge. This cycle of antigen immunization and bleeding was repeated for a total of 77 days. The titer of anti-PC-specific antibodies remained at levels comparable to those observed in the preimmune bleeds of the animals (which were collected before the experiment was initiated) until 49 days after administration of the anti-Id. At that point, the levels of anti-PC antibodies rose until they were quantitatively indistinguishable from untreated pneumococcal vaccine-immunized animals. However, in sharp contrast to this latter group, none of those antibodies bore the GB4-10 idiotope. The levels of GB4-10 bearing anti-PC antibodies in the suppressed animal remained at preimmune levels for the duration of the experiment (70 days). Furthermore, not only were the levels of another family of anti-PC antibodies bearing the unrelated $Ab_{1\text{-}2}$ idiotope unaffected by this suppression, their levels showed a compensatory increase such that they accounted for all the anti-PC antibodies in the animals. Normally, it is the GB4-10 Id^+, $Ab_{1\text{-}2+}$ subset which is expressed by the vast majority of the anti-PC antibodies in the untreated animal and the GB4-10^-, $Ab_{1\text{-}2+}$ subset is a very minor component.

Kelsoe et al.[15] demonstrated that the dosage of the anti-Id antibody is an important factor in establishing Id suppression in adult C57BL/6 mice which were treated with a monoclonal anti-idiotope in amounts ranging from the nanogram to microgram quantities. The allogeneic anti-idiotope, AC146, was generated in CBA/n mice and recognizes a hapten-inhibitable idiotope on B1-8, a C57BL/6 monoclonal specific for the haptenic determinant nitrophenylacetyl (NP). The AC146 idiotope is consistently expressed in the humoral anti-NP response of mice bearing the $IgCh^b$ allotype. Mice treated with 10 ng, 100 ng, or 1 μg of AC146 actually showed enhanced levels of AC146 Id^+ anti-NP antibodies following antigenic challenge with NP-chicken gammaglobulin (CGG). Suppression of 50 to 70% of the AC146 Id^+ component of this immune response was achieved only in animals treated with 10 μg of the anti-idiotope. Upon immunization with NP-CGG, AC146 idiotope-suppressed mice mounted an anti-NP response which quantitatively was indistinguishable from that of untreated mice. This suppression lasted only for 4 weeks, and by 8 weeks these animals fully regained the ability to mount an AC146$^+$ anti-NP response.

Bona et al.[16] succeeded in inducing a very short suppression of the E109 Id$^+$ component of the anti-inulin (100% β2,1 fructosan linkages) immune response in BALB/c mice. Adult mice were treated with an allogeneic A/J anti-E109 Id antibody and then challenged with bacterial levan, a branched polyfructosan containing a backbone of β2,6 linked fructosans with the same β2,1 fructosan linkage which inulin has, at its branch points. For a period of 20 days after treatment with the anti-Id, the E109 Id$^+$ anti-inulin response was completely inhibited as assayed by a PFC assay, by isoelectric focusing assays, and hemagglutination titers on the sera of these animals. Recovery from this suppression was achieved between 50 and 120 days when these animals regained the ability to mount an E109 Id$^+$ anti-inulin response. The suppression appears to result from the direct interaction of the anti-Id antibodies with the E109 Id-bearing mIg of the B cell, since this suppression could be induced in nude mice.

Parenterally administered anti-Id antibodies can also induce Id suppression by activating a population of Id-specific suppressor T cells. By administering xenogeneic rabbit anti-ars Id antibodies, Hart et al.[17] succeeded in inducing an Id-specific suppression in adult A/J mice of the IdX-positive component of the antibody response to the hapten azophenylarsonate (ars CRI). The suppression was long lasting; only half of the mice recovered from the suppression 12 to 22 weeks after treatment. In this system the suppression could be transferred to ars-KLH immunized recipients by the splenocytes or peritoneal cells of suppressed mice.[18] The cellular population responsible for effecting the suppression was a Lyt2,3$^+$ T cell[19] which comprised a substantial 8 to 14% of the T-cell population in the suppressed animal, and was specific for and bound to the CRI of anti-ars antibodies. These Id-specific suppressor T cells were thought to induce the Id suppression by interacting with CRI-bearing helper T cells, although these investigators never rigorously excluded the possibility that they are interacting with the ars-specific B cells through CR1$^+$ mIg.

The subsequent demonstration by Hirai et al.[20] of T cells with receptors bearing the ars CRI, as well as those exhibiting the anti-ars CRI configuration in in vitro spleen cell cultures derived from these ars CRI-suppressed mice, allowed these investigators to speculate that the anti-Id induced its suppressive effects by first activating a population of Id-bearing T cells. These T cells, in turn, would activate the anti-Id effector suppressor T cell. This scheme is consistent with and could explain earlier puzzling observations that suppression could also be transferred with Lyt1$^+$2$^-$ T cells.[19] If the Id-bearing T cell has the Lyt1$^+$2$^-$ phenotype, it would be an inducer cell, thus, seemingly tranferring suppression by inducing the final anti-Id suppressor Ly2$^+$3$^+$ T cell.

Interestingly enough, experiments using a monoclonal anti-idiotope showed that T cells are not always necessary to induce suppression of the Id borne by ars-binding antibodies. Rothstein et al.[21] induced suppression to the MB idiotope in T cell-depleted A/J mice using an allogeneic (derived from BALB/c mice) anti-idiotope. The MB idiotope is borne by a family of ars-binding antibodies and is prototypically expressed by the heavy chain of HP36-65, a monoclonal anti-ars antibody whose V_H is encoded by an A/J germline V_H gene. Following administration of the anti-MB idiotope, the animals were challenged with ars-KLH in complete Freund's adjuvant (CFA) on day 14, in incomplete Freund's adjuvant (ICFA) on days 28 and 45, and after a 24-week rest, in CFA on day 216. In bleeds taken on day 215 and day 228, the levels of anti-ars antibodies were comparable to those elicited from untreated mice comparably immunized with ars-KLH. In sharp contrast to the untreated animal, however, antibodies bearing the MB idiotope were simply not detectable.

Hornbeck[22] showed an interesting difference between the responses of B-cell clones which share Id, but not antigenic specificities to a parenterally administered monoclonal anti-idiotope in adult strain A mice. In these mice, Id sharing exists between antibodies specific for the hapten ars and a population of non-ars-specific antibodies which are part of a naturally occurring ongoing immune response to environmental antigens. The stimulus for this endogenous response is not known. AD8, a rat monoclonal anti-idiotope, recognizes one of these shared idiotopes between these two types of antibodies. AD8 administered to adult mice according to the same protocol used by Hart et al.[17] to induce ars CRI suppression in A/J mice did, indeed, suppress the AD8 Id^+ component of the ars immune response in these mice. However, animals treated according to the same protocol with AD8, but who were never immunized with ars-containing antigens, contained enhanced levels of AD8-bearing molecules in their sera which did not bind ars. The mechanisms by which the endogenous immune response escapes the suppression of the hapten-specific portion of the repertoire, and even benefits from it, are presently under investigation by these investigators.

The other instance where anti-Id antibodies induced Id suppression in the adult by activating suppressor T cells was in the A5A Id system as described by Eichmann et al.[23] The A5A Id is borne by 30 to 35% of the antibodies specific for Group A streptococcal carbohydrate (A-CHO) following immunization with the bacterium in A/J mice. Administration of xenogeneic guinea pig anti-A5A Id to adult mice did not affect the animal's ability to mount an A-CHO response. However, in contrast to untreated animals, none of these antibodies bore the A5A Id. Depending on the dose of anti-Id used to treat the mice, the kinetics and mode of suppression differed quite dramatically. Mice treated with 10 ng to 3 μg (low zone suppression) of anti-A5A Id showed partial suppression at day 25, with complete suppression at day 85, the duration of the experiment. In animals treated with 10 μg (high zone suppression) of anti-Id, the converse was true. Furthermore, only in the former group of animals could the suppression be shown to be mediated by suppressor T cells. The target of this suppressor T cell was shown to be an A5A Id^+ helper T cell, which is consistent with the observation that in in vitro culture systems derived from the lymphocytes of low zone-suppressed animals under the appropriate conditions, the A5A Id^+ B cells will mount an A-CHO response, but the T cells will not participate in this response under any circumstance. In the high zone-suppressed animal both the B- and T-cell compartments are affected.[24]

Another interesting point to be raised by this experimental system was the role which the isotype of the anti-Id plays in inducing suppression. Eichmann[23] and colleagues showed that while both low and high zone A5A Id suppression could be induced with the whole IgG fraction of the guinea pig anti-Id reagent, only those antibodies belonging to the IgG_2 subclass were the actual effectors of suppression. In fact, the IgG_1 component of the same IgG fraction from which the suppressive IgG_2 portion was derived could enhance the expression of the A5A Id. Unfortunately, the correlation of isotype with function has not held up in other experimental systems. Using an allogeneic A/J anti-T15 Id antibody, Kohler et al.[25] showed that while the Fc portion of the antibody was necessary to induce suppression of the T15 Id^+ anti-PC response in an in vitro culture system, anti-Id antibodies belonging to the IgG_1, IgG_{2a}, IgG_{2b}, and IgG_3 subclasses could all induce a suppression which was identical to that of the unfractionated antibody. Using several spontaneous isotype switch variants of the monoclonal anti-idiotope AC146, Müller et al.[26] confirmed the demonstration of Kelsoe et al.,[15] that in this Id system, the dosage of the monoclonal anti-idiotope and not its isotype determines whether it will effect an idiotope-specific enhancement or suppression. Variants of the anti-AC146-Id hybridoma belonging to the IgG_1, IgG_{2a}, IgG_{2b}, or IgE isotypes all mediated AC146 idiotope enhancement when a 10-ng dose was administered to adult animals and suppression when a 10-μg dose was used.

The data presented in this section from the various experimental systems all solidly support the ability of anti-Id antibodies to exert a profound influence on Id expression in the adult immune system. While differences in the results obtained between the various systems do not permit us to describe the "typical" state of adult Id suppression, a general profile of the phenomena can be established. The suppression is induced by the parenteral administration of monoclonal or polyclonal, allogeneic or xenogeneic anti-Id antibody. While it is necessary for the anti-Id antibody to retain its Fc portion, the precise isotype of the anti-Id is not nearly as important as its dosage in establishing the suppression. While this mode of suppression is strictly Id specific, the degree to which the antigenic response will be affected will be determined by the proportion of that response bearing that Id. In the T15 and E109 Id systems, the vast majority of the anti-PC and inulin-specific antibodies, respectively, bears that Id. Hence, in the early phases of the suppression, the antigenic response will be temporarily depressed until other B-cell clones bearing different Id are allowed to emerge and expand. In some instances,[14,27] such clones have been shown to already exist in the repertoire, but are simply not expressed in the presence of those bearing a dominantly expressed Id. In other systems such as the ars CRI, A5A Id, and AC146 Id of anti-ars, A-CHO, and NP antibodies, respectively, virtually no effect will be observed on the immune response, since the suppressed Id accounts for only a minor proportion of those antibodies. The duration of suppression varied greatly between the systems. A very short suppression was induced for the E109 Id lasting only 20 days, while a temporary suppression of 4, 6, and 22 weeks was achieved in the AC146, T15 (induced by allogeneic polyclonal serum), and ars CRI (induced by xenogeneic anti-Id, respectively). Using allogeneic monoclonals, a more chronic suppression was achieved in the T15 Id (>70 days) and ars CRI (228 days). Interestingly, low zone Id suppression of the A5A Id which was to be mediated by suppressor T cells was of a more chronic nature (>7 weeks), while high zone suppression only lasted 3 to 4 days. What is consistently observed, however, regardless of the actual duration of the Id suppression, is that the animal fully regains the ability to synthesize Id-bearing antibody molecules once the suppression is relieved. The suppression does not effect a permanent change in the immune repertoire. Also, it is not clear when anti-Id antibodies will activate suppressor T cells to mediate Id suppression. It should be noted, however, that in the two systems where it was demonstrated (e.g., ars CRI and A5A Id systems), xenogeneic or heterologous rabbit and guinea pig anti-Id antibodies were, respectively, used to induce suppression. However, when no T-cell participation in the suppression was apparent (e.g., T15 Id, ars CRI, and E109 Id systems), allogeneic polyclonal on monoclonal anti-Id antibodies were used to induce suppression. This point is particularly evident in the ars CRI system where the difference between T-cell participation in the suppression was the usage of a xenogeneic vs. an allogeneic reagent. While it is possible that the allogeneic reagent, being a monoclonal antibody, did not possess the appropriate specificity to activate suppressor T cells, one can only speculate that with the xenogeneic nature of the anti-Id antibody in the ars CRI and A5A Id systems, perhaps an abnormally high content of nonantiregulatory Id antibodies might play an important role in this apparent paradox.

2. Neonatal and Maternally Induced Id Suppression

The effects of anti-Id antibodies on the development of the immune repertoire can be examined by exposing the developing immune systems of neonatal or even fetal animals to exogenously administered anti-Id. During fetal and neonatal development, an animal is naturally exposed to maternal antibody. Maternal IgG freely and continuously crosses the placenta.[28] Furthermore, milk is a rich source of maternal IgG for the suckling neonate which is rapidly absorbed into its circulation without denaturation.[29-31] Therefore, having already demonstrated the immunoregulatory capabilities by auto-anti-Id synthesized during the course of an immune response, it was conceivable that such maternal anti-Id antibodies could help shape the offspring's immune repertoire.

One of the earliest and most extensively studied experimental systems for neonatal Id suppression has been the T15 Id system of anti-PC antibodies. Augustin and Cosenza[32] chronically suppressed the expression of T15 Id^+ anti-PC antibodies in BALB/c mice treated within 24 hr of birth with allogeneic A/J anti-T15 Id serum. These mice were rendered completely unresponsive to any antigenic challenge with PC for the first 15 weeks of life, at which point some mice slowly regained this ability. What was striking, however, was that these animals who supposedly recovered from the Id suppression produced a predominantly T15 Id^- anti-PC response. The Id of this T15 Id^- anti-PC response was more closely examined by Berek et al.[33] who immortalized some of these B cells as hybridomas. Of the six IgM hybridomas analyzed, none fully displayed the T15 Id as defined by an allogeneic A/J anti-T15Id reagent; however, four did give an indication that they do display some of the idiotopes associated with the T15 Id. A/J anti-T15 Id antibodies could fully inhibit the plaque-forming abilities of these four hybridomas. However, not all the T15 idiotopes were being expressed by these hybridomas, since an eight-fold higher concentration of anti-Id serum was needed to inhibit these hybridomas than the concentration needed to inhibit other $T15Id^+$ PC binding hybridomas derived from untreated mice. The observation that these hybridomas express some T15 idiotopes was supported by the fact that A/J anti-15Id antibodies could inhibit 80% of the PC PFC response of neonatally T15-Id-suppressed mice, at a five-fold higher concentration than was needed to inhibit the PC PFC response of untreated mice. Finally, an IEF analysis of these four hybridomas showed they possessed a common heavy chain spectrotype with other heavy chains derived from T15 Id^+ hybridomas from untreated mice. Therefore, these data would indicate that only 20 to 40% of the anti-PC antibodies in neonatally suppressed mice are completely T15 Id^-. Furthermore, suppression of the dominant T15 Id does not result in the emergence in the response of another Id, since anti-Id sera generated to each of the six hybridomas derived from these mice showed that no major Id cross reactivity could be detected among them.

Induction of neonatal T15 Id suppression has been achieved both with and without the participation of suppressor T cells. Augustin and Cosenza[32] not only failed to transfer the suppression to 2-week-old syngeneic recipients by injection of purified T or B cells from the suppressed mice, but they also induced a chronic T15 Id suppression in thymectomized mice.[34] Du Clos,[35] Kim,[36] and Fung,[37] on the other hand, also used allogeneic A/J anti-T15-Id antibodies to induce a chronic neonatally induced suppression of the T15-Id, which appeared to be mediated by suppressor T cells. Du Clos[35] showed that the T cells derived from 8-week-old neonatally suppressed animals could drastically reduce the in vitro anti-PC response elicited from the spleen cells of untreated age-matched mice when they were cocultured together. Kim[36] confirmed these results and further characterized this population of T cells from the suppressed mice which could transfer the Id suppression in vitro as exhibiting the Lyt2 alloantigen and specifically binding to T15 Id-coated petri dishes. Fung[37] demonstrated in his system that the suppressor T cells deriving from 15-week-old neonatally Id-suppressed mice could, indeed, transfer suppression by severely depressing the T15 Id^+ anti-PC response in in vitro coculturing experiments as well as in in vivo adoptive transfer experiments. However, the suppression could be transferred only to immature neonatal and not adult spleen cells or animals. Furthermore, by adoptively transferring the T cells from untreated adult mice into adult neonatally suppressed mice, the suppression could be abrogated. Not only did these mice mount a quantitatively normal PC response relative to their untreated suppressed counterparts, but this response predominantly bore T15 Id determinants. Hence, it appears that the target of the T15 Id-specific suppressor T cell in neonatally suppressed animals is a helper T cell necessary for the expression and possibly the maturation of the T15 Id^+ B cells.

This scheme is supported by Fung's et al.[38] studies on the state of the T15 Id^+ B cell in neonatally suppressed mice. Using the splenic fragment culture technique, these investigators showed that the precursor frequency of B cells secreting T15 Id^+ anti-PC antibody was greatly reduced in 8-week-old suppressed mice. These data were consistent with their inability to mount a PC-specific immune response at this age. However, in 32-week-old suppressed mice, the frequency of these T15 Id^+ PC-specific B cells returns to normal values observed in unsuppressed controls. In spite of this, these animals can only mount a T15 Id^- anti-PC response at this age. Subsequent experiments showed that these B cells possessed characteristics which indicated that they were in a relatively immature state. First, the PC-specific precursors from 8-month-old suppressed mice showed an exquisite sensitivity to tolerance indirection to PC on a heterologous carrier which was comparable to what was observed with untreated neonatal cells. Secondly, the T15 Id^+ PC-specific B cells observed in 32-week-old suppressed mice could be stimulated to synthesize antibody if these mice were administered a PC-LPS conjugate, a TI-1 antigen which can stimulate immature B cells. Therefore, it appears that the T15 Id^+ anti-PC B cells exist in a state of arrested maturation, rendering them unable to participate in the PC immune response once the ability to respond to this antigen is regained in the neonatally suppressed animal.

Berek[39] and Kearney[14] used several different syngeneic and allogeneic monoclonal anti-T15 idiotopes to induce neonatal Id suppression in BALB/c mice. Similar to the suppression induced by allogeneic polyclonal anti-T15 Id antibodies, Kearney showed that neonatal exposure to the $Ab_{1\text{-}2}$ and GB4-10 anti-T15 idiotopes rendered the mice temporarily (2 months) unable to mount an immune response to PC and chronically suppressed (>5 months) for the expression of T15 Id^+ anti-PC antibodies. Berek observed that mice which were neonatally administered the 10/13 (a syngeneic anti-Id recognizing a binding site-associated idiotope), 16/16 (an allogeneic A/J anti-Id also recognizing a binding site-associated idiotope), or 32-65 (an allogeneic anti-Id recognizing a framework-associated idiotope) anti-idiotopes not only manifested their Id suppression after intentional immunization with PC, but they also showed greatly depressed levels of the endogenously occurring T15-Id^+ anti-PC antibodies which arise from environmental stimulation. More significant was the observation that mice suppressed by any one of the three anti-idiotopes were not necessarily idiotope suppressed. As a representative example, an animal who was suppressed with the 10/13 antibody actually had serum titers of 10/13 Id-bearing antibody which far exceeded those of the 32/65 or 16/16 Id-bearing population both prior to and after immunization with PC. Clones simultaneously bearing the 10/13, 32-65, and 16/16 idiotopes were preferentially suppressed over those bearing only the 10/13 idiotope. While the segregation of these three idiotopes is generally not detected among the T15-Id^+ anti-PC antibodies of untreated mice, hybridomas generated from the suppressed mice confirmed that clones arose in these suppressed animals which bear only the 10/13 Id.

This phenomenon of a monoclonal anti-idiotope preferentially suppressing antibodies bearing certain idiotopes which are associated with the complementary idiotope rather than suppressing all those antibodies which bear the complementary idiotope was again observed by Takemori[40] in the NP Id system. Two major Id subsets of anti-NP antibodies appear regularly and with equal frequency in C57BL/6 mice. They are the AC38 Id^+/AC146 Id^+ and AC38 Id^+/AC146 Id^- subsets. When mice are neonatally administered the AC38 monoclonal anti-idiotope, the anti-NP response is not affected; however, for a period of 14 weeks, the levels of both AC38 Id^+/AC146 Id^- and AC38 Id^+/AC146 Id^+ subsets are severely depressed. While the animals regain the ability to synthesize AC38 Id^+/AC146 Id^- antibodies at 14 to 16 weeks, synthesis of the other family is not observed. It should be noted that recovery of the IgM fraction of AC38 Id^+/146 Id^- antibodies preceded that of the IgG fraction until 9 weeks later. Adoptive transfer experiments indicate that the suppression in this system is on both the B- and T-cell compartments. When the B cells of 13-week-old treated mice were adoptively transferred with T cells from untreated animals into irradiated hosts which were subsequently immunized with NP-CCG, no difference is seen in the magnitude of the anti-NP response relative to the control which received untreated B and T cells. However, neither the AC38 Id^+/AC146 Id^+ or AC38 Id^+/AC146 Id^- antibodies were detectable. Interestingly, one does not observe the synthesis of any AC38

Id^+/AC146 Id^- antibodies which may have been anticipated, since the mice regain this ability at 13 weeks. Indeed, when the T cells from the 13-week-old manipulated animals are transferred with the B cells from untreated mice, it is only the AC38 Id^+/AC146 Id^+ subset of anti-NP antibodies which is severely depressed. As was previously noted when the mice recovered their expression of the AC38 Id^+/AC146 Id^- subset, in all the adoptive transfer experiments, the effects were more pronounced in the IgG fraction of Id-bearing anti-NP antibodies than in the IgM fraction. From these data, these investigators have constructed a generalized scheme to explain the paradoxical lack of idiotope suppression in animals treated with monoclonal anti-idiotopes. Initially, the anti-idiotope will interact with the Id-bearing mIg of B cells and render them unresponsive to antigenic stimulation. In addition, this Id-anti-Id interaction would also serve as a signal to activate a T-cell-mediated suppressive mechanism which would be specific for that V_H region, but depending on the specificity of the T-cell repertoire, not necessarily for the same idiotope which the monoclonal antibody sees. Hence, if the T-cell mediated suppression is more stable and long lived than the direct inactivation by the anti-idiotope of the Id-bearing B cells, it is reasonable to anticipate the earlier recovery from suppression of those B-cell clones which exclusively bear the complementary idiotope of the anti-idiotope used to treat the neonate. It follows that those B-cell clones which bear the idiotope recognized by the suppressor T cell, regardless now of whether or not they coexpress the idiotope seen by the monoclonal antibody, will be rendered nonresponsive for the duration of the suppression.

Rothstein et al.[41] used three different protocols to demonstrate that monoclonal anti-idiotopes can induce chronic idiotope-specific suppression. Two homologous anti-idiotopes were used in this study, MB and AI. They identify individual V_H determinants on the heavy chains of A/J anti-ars antibodies. While the AI idiotope is always coexpressed with the MB idiotope, the MB idiotope is not always coexpressed with AI. The first suppression protocol called for administering AI to neonatal mice followed by immunization with ars-KLH. Such animals showed at 116 days of age a complete suppression of AI-bearing antibodies with a depressed, but measurable, level of MB Id^+ antibodies and no effect on the anti-ars response. In the second protocol, neonates which were born to mothers who themselves were treated with MB or AI also were treated with the same anti-idiotope within 2 to 5 days after birth, immunized with ars-KLH, and analyzed at 116 days of age. While the anti-ars response was not affected in either case, mice treated with AI *in utero* and neonatally were suppressed completely for the AI idiotope and marginally for the MB idiotope. Mice treated with MB *in utero* and neonatally, on the other hand, were suppressed for both idiotopes, since AI is always coexpressed with MB. Finally, mice were studied whose only exposure to MB or AI was *in utero*. Again, these mice exhibited the same type of idiotope-specific suppression which was seen in the animals treated according to the first two protocols.

Bona et al.[16] observed several interesting phenomena in BALB/c mice neonatally suppressed for the E109 Id borne by anti-inulin antibodies. BALB/c mice treated with allogeneic A/HE anti-E109 Id antibodies show an 84-day-long suppression of not only antibodies bearing the E109 Id, but the entire anti-inulin response as well. This suppression was independent of T-cell influence. The fact that neonatally induced Id suppression can be obtained in this system is interesting, since Bona et al.[42] have previously shown that there is a substantial ontogenic delay (4 to 6 weeks of age) in the appearance of functional anti-inulin precursor cells. Therefore, the mechanism of this suppression must affect either immature members of this lineage which must already be present at birth or the administered anti-Id must persist until these precursors emerge and then suppress them.

This suppression of the inulin response is also curious, since normally no more than 50% of the response bears this Id. Furthermore, anti-E109 Id antibodies could selectively inhibit the in vitro polyclonal PFC response to BL and not to NWSM or TNP-BA, and the in vitro TNP response to TNP-BL and TNP-inulin, but not TNP LPS. Collectively, these results

Table 1
EFFECT OF NEONATAL ADMINISTRATION OF ANTIREGULATORY IDIOTOPE ANTIBODIES

Mouse strain	Anti-idiotope injected at birth	Description of anti-idiotope	Antibody response (μg/mℓ)		Id response (μg/mℓ)	
			α1-3 dextran	Levan β2-6, β2-1 fructosan	J558-IdX	J606-IdX
BALB/c	Nil		94.5 ± 39.4	118.6 ± 34.0	47.3 ± 5.1	20.7 ± 14.5
	AC146	Syngeneic MAb specific for B1-8 Id of anti-NP antibodies	34.0 ± 13.7	89.3 ± 20.7	7.3 ± 3.8	16.3 ± 8.9
	AIDA 23.2	Syngeneic anti(anti-A48 Id)antibody specific for IDA 23, an anti-A48 Id antibody	100.5 ± 18.3	40 ± 12.5	47.5 ± 11.8	18.0 ± 5.3
	SN3-9A	Syngeneic MAb specific for the PY206 Id of antiinfluenza strain X31 hemagglutinin-specific antibody PY206	1.0 ± (3)	126.0 ± 31.7	2.5(3)	43 ± 27
	CD3-2	Allogeneic MAb specific for the J558 IdX	<1	89.7 ± 37.6	<0.1	15.3 ± 6.8
	Anti-E109 IdX	Allogeneic polyclonal antibodies specific for the E109 Id	77 ± 2.6(4)	27.4 ± 44.4(4)	84.8 ± 35.6	3.0 ± 1.4(4)
			NP	Levan β2-6, β2-1 fructosan	B1-8-IdX	
C57BL/6	Saline		244 ± 48.3	93.4 ± 45.2	28.4 ± 6.2	
	AC146	See above	227.5 ± 67.5	83.2 ± 43.7	<0.3	
	AIDA23-2	See above	116.3 ± 17.1	89.0 ± 20.1	35.8 ± 5.3	
	SN3-9A	See above	192.0 ± 41.6	94 ± 33	13.9 ± 10.2	
	CD3-2	See above	177.3 ± 31.8	141.6 ± 20.1	10.6 ± 4.5	

Note: One-day-old BALB/c or C57BL/6 mice were injected on days 1, 3, and 5 with 100 μg of purified monoclonal anti-Id antibodies. After 6 weeks, the BALB/c mice were injected i.p. with 100 μg of dextran B1355S or with 20 μg of levan and the C57BL/6 mice were injected with 100 μg of NP-Ficoll and 20 μg of levan in saline. The mice were bled on day 7 after antigen challenge. The concentration of both antigen-specific antibodies as well as J558, B1.8, and J606 Id-bearing immunoglobulins was determined on the samples obtained from individual mice.

suggest that anti-E109 Id antibodies can suppress the response to several antigenic determinants borne on the same molecule, including those which are not determinants recognized by the Id-bearing antibody. Bona termed this phenomenon indirect suppression.

By inducing neonatal Id suppression with several monoclonal anti-idiotopes which recognized regulatory idiotopes encoded by the J558 germline V_H gene family, we could demonstrate suppression not only of the complementary Id and its corresponding antigens response, but also of other J558 V_H encoded Id and their immune responses (Table 1). BALB/c or C57BL/6 mice were treated with the AC146, AIDA23-2, SN3-9A, or CD3-2 monoclonals before immunization with dextran or NP-Ficoll, respectively. All four anti-idiotopes could recognize a cross-reactive idiotope, not only on NP or dextran binding antibodies, but also on monoclonal antibodies specific for the ars hapten, influenza virus hemagglutinin, the A48 Id, and several monoclonal antibodies with unknown antigen binding specificity. However, all derived their V_H gene from the J558 germline gene family. BALB/c mice immunized with either dextran or bacterial levan as a control (levan-binding antibodies derive their V_H genes from the V_H J606 or V_H X24 germline gene family and not J558) showed a specific inhibition of their expression of J558 IdX^+ antibodies and the corresponding dextran response when treated with the CD3-2 and SN3-9A anti-idiotopes, and a partial inhibition in animals treated with AC146 (Table 1).

The partial inhibition of the antibacterial levan response observed in BALB/c mice treated with AIDA23-3 can be attributed to the suppression of the A48-Id^+ component of this immune response by the activation of anti-A48-Id clones. AIDA23-3 antibodies have been previously shown to elicit the production of antibodies against A48 regulatory idiotopes.[8]

In C57BL/6 mice that were immunized with NP-Ficoll or bacterial levan, no significant differences were observed between the magnitudes of the anti-NP and antilevan responses among the various groups of animals. By contrast, a strong inhibition of the B1.8 Id was observed in animals treated at birth with AC146 and a weaker, but significant, inhibition with CD3-2 and SN3-9A monoclonal antibodies. No J606 IdX antibodies were detected in these mice, which is in agreement with a previous observation made by Lieberman et al.,[43] who demonstrated the linkage of IdX G, B, and A to the $IgC_H{}^a$ haplotype.

These findings demonstrate that parenteral administration of anti-idiotope antibodies against antibodies which derive their V_H genes from the V_H J558 germline gene family, but otherwise display different antigen specificities, can profoundly alter the antidextran response in BALB/c mice and the anti-NP response in C57BL/6 mice. This coregulation was specific for clones bearing a CRI encoded by V_H genes from the J558 V_H gene family, because the antifructosan antibody response was not affected. Id suppression obtained with some, but not all, anti-Id antibodies (i.e, SN3-9A for J558 IdX and CD3-2 for B1.8 IdX) could be related to the affinity of these anti-Id antibodies for this CRI or, alternatively, these antibodies recognize germline-encoded idiotopes. The observed neonatal Id suppression is probably related to a direct interaction of anti-Id antibodies with the immunoglobulin receptor of B-cell clones, as we demonstrated previously by an inability to transfer the suppression with T cells and by the fact that the suppression was also obtained by using nude mice.[16] Thus, these data demonstrate that Id-mediated cross-reactive regulation leads to cross-reactive inhibition of clones with different antigen specificities and that these CRI function as regulatory idiotopes.

Id suppression induced by maternal influence shares many characteristics with neonatally induced suppression, but also exhibits several unique properties. Cosenza[44] studied the expression of the T15 Id in BALB/c mice who were maternally suppressed for this Id. Because T15 Id-bearing antibodies constitute a naturally occurring immune response to environmental pathogens, high titers always exist in the sera of nonimmune mice, making any attempt to induce the production of syngeneic anti-T15 Id in adult mice practically impossible, unless a prevailing state of Id suppression inhibits this endogenous expression. Therefore, BALB/c females who were already neonatally suppressed for the expression of

T15 Id^+ antibodies were immunized with the PC binding myeloma protein T15 in order to generate syngeneic anti-T15-Id. When this activity was detected in their sera, they were mated to BALB/c males. As anticipated, the litters produced from this union were completely unresponsive to antigenic challenge by PC at 7 to 10 weeks of age and were chronically suppressed for T15 Id expression. What was surprising, however, was the exceedingly high serum anti-T15 titers which were observed in the 7-week-old suppressed animals. Given a measured half-life of 1 week for maternal immunoglobulin obtained from milk, these animals who were already weaned at 3 weeks of age should have less than 1/16 of the maternal anti-id titer in their sera which could be acquired from nursing, and certainly much less from placental transmission. Interestingly, at 10 weeks of age, though the mice are still suppressed, no anti-T15 titers are detected. It appears that some endogenous anti-T15-Id clones have been triggered in these animals, which reestablish their steady-state levels within the immune system once all maternal immunoglobulin disappears.

It should be mentioned that maternal anti-id is not the only entity which can induce maternal Id suppression.

T cells are involved in the suppression of anti-ars CRI_A^+ Id antibodies in adult A/J mice who are treated with xenogeneic anti-Id.[17] Kresina[45] showed that pregnant females receiving these T cells prior to mating or the sera from ars CRI_A suppressed mice 5 days prior to parturition, gave birth to litters which were also suppressed for this Id. The suppressive agent was shown not to be immunoglobulin and was transmitted only transplacentally and not through the milk. Therefore, since the issue of maternal transmission of cells transplacentally is still unresolved, the mechanism of this suppression would seem to involve the transplacental transmission of a T-cell factor. This explanation is strongly supported by the fact that not only the T cells, but a nonimmunoglobulin entity in a suppressed animal's serum, can also confer transplacental suppression in this system.

Bona et al.[16] also studied maternally induced suppression in the E109 Id system. CB20 females, a congenic strain of mouse which bears the C57BL/6 heavy chain immunoglobulin locus on a BALB/c background, were immunized with the BALB/c E109 myeloma protein to produce anti-Id antibodies, and then mated to BALB/c males. These F_1 progeny at 4 months of age exhibited complete unresponsiveness to inulin and, of course, a complete suppression of the E109 Id^+ anti-inulin antibody. It is important to emphasize here that despite the fact that the allotypic determinants were also immunogenic in this system (CB20 is $IgC_H{}^b$ and BALB/c is $IgC_H{}^a$), the suppression was Id specific. The F_1 progeny of CB20 females immunized with XRPC24, another BALB/c IgA (the heavy chain isotype of E109) which is, however, galactan specific, mounted normal E109 Id^+ anti-inulin responses. The interesting fact to emerge from these experiments is that titers of noninulin binding E109 Id^+ antibodies were detected in the sera of suppressed animals. While such clones are, in fact, detectable earlier in ontogeny than the inulin-specific ones, in this system again the suppression is established much earlier than the ontogenic emergence of these E109 Id^+ clones. The fact that the noninulin binding clones seem to overcome their suppression earlier than the inulin-specific ones can, perhaps, be explained by the anti-E109 Id-mediated diversion of a ''protoclone'' away from inulin specificity.

Weiler et al.[46] extensively studied the maternally induced Id suppression of J558 Id^+ antidextran antibodies in BALB/c mice. In order to produce an allogeneic anti-J558 Id, female SJL mice ($IgC_H{}^b$) were immunized with dextran-immune BALB/c ($IgC_H{}^a$) spleen cells. The membrane Ig of these cells served as a satisfactory immunogen in this system, since >95% of BALB/c antidextran antibodies bear the J558 Id. The F_1 progeny produced from the mating of these J558-immune SJL females and BALB/c males showed a transient unresponsiveness to dextran which is characteristic in all systems, such as the T15 Id of anti-PC antibodies where the suppressed Id is expressed by such a vast proportion of the responding cells. At 20 weeks of age as anticipated, new clonotypes begin to emerge and dextran responsiveness was regained in these mice. However, none of them ever expressed the J558 Id. Of course, these experiments were carefully controlled to show that in spite of immunizing across the SJL-BALB/c allotype difference, the suppression was 100% Id specific.

Again, in this system as in the T15 Id system, syngeneically immunized females are difficult to obtain since all BALB/c mice exhibit significant titers of J558 Id-bearing antibody, since these antibodies also represent a naturally occurring response to environmental antigens. This problem was circumvented by obtaining BALB/c mice who were rendered neonatally suppressed for the J558 Id by virtue of being nursed by a J558 immune SJL female, and immunizing them with the J558 myeloma protein to produce a syngeneic anti-id response. Twenty-two percent of the BALB/c progeny of such females also showed a transient dextran unresponsiveness and 59% exhibited a chronic suppression of the J558 Id. These investigators also showed that the progeny of normal BALB/c males and (SJL × BALB/c) F_1 maternally suppressed females, who were immunized with J558 to produce a semisyngeneic anti-J558 Id, also exhibited all the characteristics of maternally induced J558 Id suppression. Interestingly enough, 65 out of 90 of the progeny of the (SJL × BALB/c) F_1 suppressed female showed the transient dextran nonresponsiveness and 85% showed the chronic Id suppression. Perhaps the explanation for this difference between the efficiency with which the suppression is transferred with the BALB/c vs. the (SJL × BALB/c) F_1 females lies in the fact that this latter group of mice was never challenged with dextran. However, the possibility of the difference in specificity between the syngeneic and semisyngeneic anti-J558 Id cannot be excluded.

Finally, Weiler et al.[4] showed that maternal transmission of anti-Id by nursing plays an important role in maintaining the suppression. The maternally suppressed heterozygous offspring of the (SJL × BALB/c) F_1 J558 immune females and BALB/c males were arbitrarily divided such that 1/2 were nursed by a J558 immune SJL female and the other half were nursed by a nonimmune SJL female. Whereas all the mice nursed by the anti-Id-producing female continued exhibiting their maternal suppression, only 40% of the animals nursed by the normal female retained the suppressed phenotype. Even more impressive was the observation that the heterozygous progeny born to a nonimmune SJL female and BALB/c male acquired the suppressed phenotype if they were nursed from J558 immune SJL females.

Experiments in our lab on J558 maternally Id-suppressed mice revealed some interesting features on the cellular expression of this Id during the state of suppression.[47] Females of the A/J (IgC_H^e) strain, which do not express this Id but are known for their vigorous production of anti-Id, were immunized with J558 until anti-Id activity was detected in their sera. At this point they were mated to BALB/c males and the CAF_1 progeny were examined for signs of Id suppression. The animals were followed until 12 weeks of age, at which point no PFC response to dextran could be detected (Table 2), and there were no serum titers of J558 Id-bearing antibodies (<1 $\mu g/m\ell$). It was important to establish that the suppression was completely Id specific by showing that the TNP response was quantitatively and qualitatively (measured by percent of population bearing the minor M460 Id) indistinguishable in the suppressed and normal CAF_1 mice, because this immunization protocol again called for the immunization of a BALB/c (IgC_H^a) immunoglobulin into the allotypically different A/J mice (IgC_H^e). The most exciting results to emerge from these studies were the membrane expression of the J558 Id by the B and T cells of maternally suppressed mice. Utilizing the technique of membrane immunofluorescence, we observed the emergence only in the suppressed mice of a population of splenic T cells displaying a nonimmunoglobulin membrane receptor which specifically stained with the fluoresceinated monoclonal anti-J558 IdI, but not with goat anti-IdX antibodies (Table 2). In other experiments, we showed that these cells were $Lyt2^+$ suppressor cells which could transfer the suppression to naive recipients. More surprising, however, was our observation that in the suppressed animals there was a substantial increase in the number of splenic B cells which bore endogenously synthesized J558 IdI^+ membrane

Table 2
J558 Id SUPPRESSION IN MATERNALLY SUPPRESSED CAF_1 MICE

Animal	Dex[a] PFC/10^6 cells	Percentage inhibition by		TNP[a] PFC/10^6 cells	Percentage inhibition by anti-M460 Id	J558 IdI^+/Ig^{+d} (%)	J558 IdI/Thyl.2^{+e} (%)
		EB3-7-2[b]	GT-anti-IdX[c]				
Normal-CAF_1	565 ± 165	39	78	5120 ± 930	11	0.83 ± 0.13(0.70 ± 0.11)[f]	0
Maternally suppressed CAF_1	0	0	0	4310 ± 300	9	2.95 ± 0.75(2.5 ± 0.23)[f]	3.1 ± 0.6(3.6 ± 0.20)[f]

[a] 12-Week-old mice were immunized with 100 μg Dextran B1355 and 20 μg TNP-Ficoll intraperitoneally. Spleens were removed after immunization for direct PFC determinations.
[b] An A/J allogeneic monoclonal anti-idiotope specific for the J558 IdI.
[c] An affinity-purified xenogeneic reagent specific for the J558 IdX.
[d] Number of cells reacting with the monoclonal anti-J558 IdI antibody, EB3-7-2 among 100 B spleen lymphocytes assessed by membrane immunoglobulin staining.
[e] Number of cells reacting with the monoclonal anti-J558 IdI EB3-7-2 among 100 T spleen cells detected by anti-Thy-1.2 staining.
[f] Value obtained after culturing cells for 24 hr at 37°C.

immunoglobulin (Table 2). There peculiar features of this membrane Ig were that it did not bind dextran and it did not express either the λ light chain or the J558 IdX, two hallmarks of antidextran antibodies. We were subsequently able to immortalize some of these J558 IdI^+ B cells from the suppressed mice as B-cell hybridomas.[48] Detailed immunochemical and molecular analysis reaffirmed our earlier observations that, indeed, these B cells synthesized J558 IdI^+ IdX^-, K $chain^+$ nondextran binding antibody which also derived its V_H from the V_H J558 germline gene family, as, indeed, the antidextran antibodies do. Hence, maternal influence in this system has exerted two almost opposing influences on the immune system. First, all B-cell clones, even the parallel set or nondextran binding ones, were expanded. However, in spite of their increased numbers, these cells remain unresponsive to antigenic stimulation because of the almost simultaneous anti-Id-mediated induction of Id-specific suppressor T cells. These two alleged actions of the anti-Id are separable events, because by administering neonatal BALB/c mice a mere 10 ng of the EB3-7-2 anti-J558 IdI reagent, we can mimic the anti-Id-mediated expansion of J558 IdI^+ B cells (both dextran binding and the parallel set) without recruiting the suppressor T-cell population. Furthermore, even though the J558 IdX is a more widely expressed determinant by antidextran antibodies than the J558 IdI is, it appears that the J558 IdI and not the J558 IdX is a recognized target of regulation by the immune system. Otherwise, the IdX, too, would be obligatorily expressed by the Id-specific suppressor T cells as well as the expanded Id^+ B-cell population.

The study of neonatal and maternally induced Id suppression reveals how the anti-Id antibody can select the immune repertoire of an individual. While no general agreement exists between several of the experimental systems on many of the mechanistic issues of the suppression (e.g., the participation of the suppressor T cells, the variability in the duration of suppression, or the inability to achieve an idiotope-specific suppression with a monoclonal antibody), a general consensus clearly exists on the ability of the anti-Id antibody to irreversibly manipulate the expression of the lymphocytic clones which populate the immune system. This scenario stands in stark contrast to the effect of the anti-Id in the adult or on the mature immune system, where the expression of clones are manipulated, but done in a reversible fashion so as to restore overall equilibrium to the immune system.

B. Enhancing Effects of Anti-Id Antibodies

The anti-Id antibody modulates clonal expression in the immune system through a combination of providing both negative stimuli resulting in Id suppression and positive stimuli resulting in Id enhancement. Jerne's Network theory[1] predicted that the Ab_2, anti-Id antibody, would induce the synthesis of Ab_3, the anti-anti-id antibody. Ab_3 would, in turn, down regulate the production of Ab_2. Thus, if the levels of Ab_2 diminish, so should its suppressive influence on the synthesis of Ab_1, and the levels of Ab_1 should begin to rise. Indeed, the enhancing ability of anti-Id antibodies on Id expression was already seen by investigators studying Id suppression. Eichmann[23] showed that parenteral administration of the IgG fraction of a guinea pig anti-Id reagent, specific for the A5A Id borne by A-CHO antibodies in A/J mice, could significantly enhance expression of these antibodies in adult mice immunized with the bacterium. The IgG_1 anti-Id antibodies were the actual effectors of the enhancement, because if only the IgG_2 antibodies were isolated from this IgG fraction and given to adult mice under the same experimental conditions, then a significant suppression in the expression of these A5A Id^+ antibodies was seen. Kelsoe[15] demonstrated that the dosage of an allogeneic monoclonal anti-idiotope specific for the B1-8 idiotope displayed by anti-NP antibodies in C57BL/6 mice, determined whether or not Id enhancement or suppression was observed. Adult mice receiving 10 ng to 1 μg of anti-AC146 Id antibody showed enhanced levels of AC146 Id^+ anti-NP antibodies following immunization with NP-CGG, while those administered 10 μg showed a profound suppression of this response. Finally, we observed an expansion in the population of J558 Id^+ B cells in (A/J × BALB/c)F_1 mice who were maternally suppressed for expression of the J558 Id.[47]

While the fact that anti-Id antibodies could also stimulate Id expression was consistently demonstrable, several basic questions about this aspect of anti-Id regulation still remained unanswered. According to the Network theory,[1] the Id enhancment observed subsequent to administration of anti-Id antibodies should result from the Ab_2-induced synthesis of Ab_3, a population of antibody specific for the Id borne by the Ab_2 population ($Ab_{3\alpha}$).[59] Therefore, it was interesting to compare the relative incidence of these $Ab_{3\alpha}$ molecules to those ex pressing the Id determinants of Ab_1($Ab_{3\beta}$)[59] in anti-Id-treated animals. Furthermore, within this enhanced Id-bearing $Ab_{3\beta}$ population, what proportion of the antibodies exhibits the Id in question, but not the antigenic specificity which is normally associated with this Id? Such antibodies have been designated as members of the parallel set and are often seen during the course of an unmanipulated immune response.[49] These questions now became the key issues addressed by several researchers studying anti-Id-mediated Id enhancement.

These issues were extensively studied by Bona and colleagues who initiated their studies by analyzing the Id of four members of an Id pathway initiated by A48, a BALB/c β2,6 fructosan binding myeloma protein which protoypically bears the A48 Id.[8] Syngeneic polyclonal antibodies representative of the Ab_2, Ab_3, and Ab_4 populations were generated by immunizing individual BALB/c mice with KLH conjugates of the β2,6 fructosan binding myeloma protein ABPC48 (Ab_1), anti-A48 Id (Ab_2), anti-anti-A48 Id (Ab_3), respectively. Rather surprisingly, the "Ab_3" population must extensively share the A48 Id of Ab_1, because the Ab_4 antibodies recognize not only the Ab_3 population, but also A48 as well. A48 could inhibit 60 to 70% of the binding of radiolabeled Ab_3 to Ab_4 in a radioimmunoassay. Hence, the immunization of syngeneic polyclonal anti-A48 Id antibodies results in the predominance of B-cell clones which express the A48 Id rather than those exhibiting an anti-Id activity for the Ab_2 population.

Rubinstein et al.[50] showed that immunity per se to anti-A48 Id antibodies or the presence of Ab_3 population to neutralize Ab_2 activity was not necessary to achieve A48 Id enhancement. Unmodified anti-A48 Id antibodies administered in saline in a nonimmunogenic form to neonatal BALB/c mice caused a substantial expansion in the B-cell precursors expressing the A48 Id. In constrast to unmanipulated mice where such B cells normally remain silent or unexpressed during the β2, 6-fructosan immune response, in neonatally anti-Id-treated BALB/c animals immunized with bacterial levan (a branched polyfructosan containing a backbone of β2,6-linked-fructose residues), A48 Id-bearing antibodies constituted a major component of the antilevan response. While the anti-Id was shown to specifically enhance the expression of only A48 Id-bearing B cells, it was necessary to immunize with antigen to elicit this response. The anti-Id antibodies seem to directly interact with the B cells through the Id^+ mIg, since T cells did not participate in this expansion. Lethally irradiated BALB/c mice, immunized with bacterial levan following reconstitution with only B cells of anti-Id-treated mice, mounted an A48 Id^+ anti-BL response which was comparable to that observed in the neonatally anti-Id-treated animal. Reconstituting recipients with the T as well as B cells from anti-A48-primed mice did not quantitatively affect the BL response nor the dominant expression of the A48 Id^+ component of that response. On the other hand, mice receiving only T cells from anti-A48 Id-treated mice and normal B cells mounted a respectable anti-BL response which was devoid of A48 Id-bearing antibodies.

By generating hybridomas from the spleen cells of mice treated with anti-A48 Id antibodies, a detailed immunochemical and molecular analysis of those clones expanded by anti-Id treatment in this system was greatly facilitated. Three separate protocols for administration of the anti-Id were devised: (1) BALB/c mice were immunized at birth with 10 ng of polyclonal syngeneic anti-A48 Id antibodies and challenged 1 month later with bacterial levan. This is the original protocol used to show that anti-A48 Id in a nonimmunogenic form could activate the normally silent A48 Id^+ precursor B cells in neonatal mice. Hybridomas derived from these mice were termed Series II antibodies; (2) adult BALB/c mice were hyperimmunized with syngeneic polyclonal anti-A48 Id antibodies covalently conjugated to the KLH carrier protein and challenged 1 month later with bacterial levan. This protocol would optimize $Ab_{3\alpha}$ production, since the anti-Id was being administered in its most immunogenic form. Hybridomas derived from these mice were termed Series III antibodies; (3) adult BALB/c mice were immunized as described for the Series III antibodies, however, covalent KLH conjugates of two syngeneic monoclonal anti-A48 idiotopes rather than polyclonal antibodies were used. This protocol was included in order to explore the possibility that the poor $Ab_{3\alpha}$ response which was observed earlier in the Ab_2-treated neonates was a consequence of Id diversity among the polyclonal population of anti-A48 Id antibodies, with no single Id being present in sufficient quantities to evoke an immune response. Hybridomas deriving from these mice were designated Series AIDA antibodies (kindly donated by Dr. Pierre Legrain, Pasteur Institute, Paris, France).

All hybridomas were initially screened for their ability to inhibit the binding of H^3-A48 protein to syngeneic polyclonal anti-A48-Id antibodies. Those which demonstrated this ability were retained for this study. These hybridomas were compared to the prototypical A48 protein itself in three different areas: expression of the A48 Id, V_H gene origin, and antigen binding specificity.

The expression of the A48 Id by these hybridomas was investigated in a radioimmunoassay using a panel of syngeneic monoclonal anti-A48-Id antibodies (kindly donated by Dr. Pierre Legrain, Pasteur Institute, Paris, France) which all recognized antigen-inhibitable idiotopes on A48. While the various monoclonal anti-A48-Id antibodies bound to most of our monoclonal antibodies, only one, IDA10,[51] was strongly bound by all of them (Table 3). These data make the IDA10 idiotope a good candidate for the target idiotope which may be important in the anti-Id-induced expansion of these clones.

Interestingly enough, at a constant protein concentration, differences were observed in the extent of binding of IDA10 among these monoclonal antibodies. Based on their binding, the antibodies segregate into two groups: Series I and II antibodies which overall bind IDA10 less well than A48, and Series III and AIDA which bind as well or even better than A48 in some cases. These data suggest that the idiotopes being recognized by IDA10 may not be the identical determinant displayed by A48 and may reflect V_H and/or V_L hetrogeneity within this group.

The effects of V_L heterogeneity upon A48 Id expression were evaluated among the monoclonal antibodies by assaying for expression of a K light chain belonging to the V_K10 family. From protein sequence data, it is known that UPC10, another β2,6-fructosan binding myeloma which shares Id[52] and V_H gene origin with A48,[53] uses a V_K10 light chain.[54] The data were obtained from an ELISA assay, in which the direct binding of alkaline phosphatase-labeled A48 Id-positive monoclonal antibodies to affinity-purified rabbit anti-V_K10 antibodies was measured.[55] No correlation was evident between V_K10 light chain expression and the strength of binding to the IDA10 reagent. Hence, these data support the notion of the IDA10 idiotope being associated with V_H determinants, but, of course, does not exclude the trivial possibility of the occurrence of three-dimensional structures associated with the various V_K families sterically interfering with the binding of IDA10 antibodies.

The V_H gene origin of these monoclonal antibodies was more extensively analyzed by Northern blotting techniques. Both A48 and UPC10 derive their rearranged and expressed V_H gene from the V_H^{441-4} germline gene. A V_H^{441-4} germline gene probe (the V_H Gal 39 probe kindly given to us by Dr. S Rudikoff, NCI, Bethesda, Md.) was nick-translated with ^{32}P-labeled deoxynucleotide triphosphates and hybridized to Northern blotted poly A^+ cytoplasmic RNA from each Series II, III, and AIDA hybridoma. With a majority of these A48 Id-positive hybridomas, we observe hybridization of this probe to an mRNA species whose size is consistent with the isotype of the antibody produced by the hybridoma. When the RNA from all those hybridomas not hybridizing with the V_H^{441-4} probe (i.e., Series II

Table 3
A48 IDIOTYPE EXPRESSION AND V_H GENE ORIGIN OF THE MONOCLONAL ANTIBODIES

	Binding to the IDA10 anti-A48 idiotope[a]	Hybridization of H-chain mRNA to V_H441-4 probe[b]	Rearrangement of a V_H X24 germline gene family member[c]
Myeloma			
MOPC460 (α^d,k)	184 ± 17[e]	−	−
A48 (α,k)	5183 ± 289	+	+
UPC10 (γ2α,k)	1492 ± 141	+	+
MOPC173 (γ2β,k)	519 ± 233	+	ND
Series II			
2-1-3 (γ3,k)	679 ± 228	+	+
2-8-2 (μ,k)	804 ± 276	−	−
2-11-1 (μ,k)	728 ± 313	+	+
2-12-10 (μ,k)	1140 ± 136	+	+
2-9-17 (μ,k)	356 ± 257	−	−
2-28-9 (γ3,k)	795 ± 181	+	+
Series III and AIDA			
3-76-4 (μ,k)	1548 ± 128	ND	ND
3-14-9 (μ,k)	3745 ± 152	+	+
3-27-6 (γ1,k)	6030 ± 369	+	+
3-9-9 (γ1,k)	3078 ± 111	+	+
3-101-14 (γ1,k)	2093 ± 41	+	+
AIDA 10-16 (γ1,k)	1616 ± 457	+	+
AIDA 10-21 (γ1,k)	3197 ± 674	+	+
AIDA 23-2 (γ1,k)	9619 ± 107	+	+
AIDA 23-2 (γ,k)	9578 ± 553	+	+

[a] Microtiter plates were coated with the monoclonal test antibodies at 5 μg/mℓ and then incubated with IDA10 anti-A48-Id antibodies. Following extensive washing, the plates were then incubated with ^{125}I-labeled A48.

[b] 200 ng of oligo dT selected RNA was electrophoresed through an 0.8% formaldehyde-containing agarose gel, Northern blotted, and hybridized to a ^{32}P nick-translated V_H441-4 probe.

[c] 10 μg of ECO RI-digested genomic DNA was electrophoresed through a 0.7% agarose gel and Southern blotted. Duplicate filters were hybridized to a ^{32}P nick-translated V_H441-4 and J_H3-J_H4 probe in order to identify any rearrangements to the J_H locus of V_H genes deriving from the V_H X24 germline gene family.

[d] MOPC460 is an IgAk with DNP binding specificity. UPC10 is another β2,6 fructosan binding myeloma, while the binding specificity of MOPC173 is unknown. Both myelomas have been previously shown to share Id and derive their V_H genes from the same V_H gene family as A48 does.[52-58]

[e] Cpm average ± SE after the subtraction of background (3% BSA instead of monoclonal antibodies).

antibodies 2-8-2, 2-11-3, 2-9-17, 2-12-9, and Series III antibodies 3-76-4 and 3-76-42) was hybridized to the appropriate heavy chain isotype probe, only 3-76-4 and 3-76-42 failed to hybridize. These two hybridomas are currently being recloned.

In all those hybridomas where we observed hybridization of heavy chain mRNA to the V_H^{441-4} probe by Southern blotting analysis, we observed a rearrangement to the J_H cluster of a V_H gene belonging to the X24 V_H family. Genomic DNA was digested with Eco RI and Southern blotted. Duplicate blots were hybridized with the V_H^{441-4} probe as well as a J_{H3}-J_{H4} probe to confirm the identity of the rearranged band. Interestingly, all the Series II hybridomas show hybridization of the V_H^{441-4} probe to the same rearranged Eco RI fragment at 2.91 kb, which is different from the A48 type of rearrangement. Among the Series III and AIDA hybridomas, we see five different sizes of rearranged bands (2.95, 2.55, 2.4, 2.2, and 1.65 kb), including the one observed in A48 (2.2 kb). These sizes are consistent with the rearrangement of the V_H^{441-4} or V_H X24 germline gene to each of the four different J_H sequences.

Using a radioimmunoassay, the antigen binding specificities of these monoclonal antibodies was investigated by testing their ability to bind grass levan (100% β2, 6-fructosan linkages), bacterial levan (β2,6-fructosan linkages with β2,1-fructosan-fructosan linkages at the branch points), and inulin (100% β2,1-fructosan linkages). As has been previously reported, A48 and UPC10 are specific for the β2,6-fructosan linkage. Hence, they bind to both grass and bacterial levan, but not to inulin. On the other hand, J606, which is specific for the β2,1-fructosan linkage, will bind to inulin and bacterial levan, but not to grass levan. Therefore, by studying the pattern of binding of these antibodies to each of these polyfructosans, their precise linkage specificity, if any, can be determined. The results of this experiment are summarized in Table 4. All nine of the Series II antibodies bound to bacterial levan quite well. However, only two of them (2-8-2, 2-11-1) showed the β2,6-fructosan linkage specificity by binding to rye levan as well. Four antibodies (2-1-10, 2-11-3, 2-12-10, 2-28-9) bound only to bacterial levan, implying that these antibodies are specific for a conformational determinant present only in bacterial levan. Two antibodies (2-1-3, 2-12-19) bound to all three polysaccharides. However, it should be mentioned that the binding of these two antibodies to bacterial levan was not inhibited with either inulin or grass levan. These data suggest that although the combining site of these antibodies could accommodate either the isolated β2,6- or β2,1-fructosan linkage, they recognize with a much higher affinity a conformational determinant present only in the bacterial levan polysaccharide. One antibody (2-9-17) clearly showed β2,1 linkage specificity by binding to both bacterial levan and inulin.

Among the Series III and AIDA antibodies, only two out of ten antibodies (3-14-9, AIDA 10-16) showed any affinity for bacterial levan. Antibody 3-14-9 bound to all three polysaccharides, while AIDA 10-16 bound only to bacterial levan. These data indicate that they are probably both specific for a conformational determinant in the bacterial levan polysaccharide for the reasons already explained above. Only three other Series III antibodies (3-76-42, 3-27-6, 3-101-4) showed any specificity for a fructosan determinant by respectively binding to grass levan and inulin. Recent sequencing data have shown that the β1,6-D-galactan binding myeloma proteins also derive their rearranged V_H genes from the $V_H^{441\text{-}4}$, as well as the V_H X24 germline V_H genes.[56] In fact, these two genes differ only by seven nucleotide substitutions.[56] This observation prompted us to assay for β2,6-D-galactan binding activity, those Series III and AIDA antibodies which exhibit the A48 Id, but display no specificity for any fructosan determinants. An RIA was used to compare the binding of these A48 Id-positive antibodies, A48 itself, and XRPC 24 (a β1,6-D-galactan binding myeloma protein) to the β1,6-D-galactan determinants in galactan-BSA and in two naturally occurring heteropolysaccharides, arabinogalactan and gum ghatti (Table 4). One series AIDA antibody (AIDA 23-2) clearly showed a specificity for β1,6-D-galactan determinants. Two others (AIDA 10-21 and AIDA 23-3) exhibited much lower galactan binding activities, but ones which, nevertheless, were well above negative control values. This intriguing demonstration of A48 Id expression by galactan binding antibodies was further strengthened by our observation that among four galactan binding myeloma proteins studied (XRPC24, XRPC44, TEPC601, and J539), we showed that XRPC44 could competitively inhibit the binding of syngeneic polyclonal anti-UPC10 Id antibodies to UPC10.[55] As previously men tioned, UPC10 extensively shares Id with A48[52] as well as the β2,6-fructosan antigen specificity and $V_H^{441\text{-}4}$ germline gene origin of its expressed V_H.[53]

Thus, only 1 Series III antibody (3-9-9) out of the entire 20 antibodies analyzed in this study has turned out to be a true $Ab_{3\alpha}$ by the criterion of it not binding to any fructosan or galactan determinants.

These studies in the A48 Id system demonstrate that the anti-Id antibody, even when administered in its most immunogenic form, will preferentially activate and expand B cells synthesizing A48 Id^+ antibody rather than elicit an anti-Id response to its own Id. Since

Table 4
ANTIGEN BINDING SPECIFICITY OF MONOCLONAL ANTIBODIES[a]

Designation	Rye levan (20 μg/mℓ)	Bacterial levan (20 μg/mℓ)	Inulin (5 μg/mℓ)	Arabinogalactan (20 μg/mℓ)	Galactan-BSA (5 μg/mℓ)	Gum ghatti (20 μg/mℓ)
Myeloma						
MOPC460	225 ± 79[b]	376 ± 115	44 ± 2	—	—	—
A48	5,659 ± 275	12,819 ± 945	91 ± 5	299 ± 199	357 ± 105	191 ± 07
UPC10	1,353 ± 95	19,233 ± 723	188 ± 30	—	—	—
MOPC173	194 ± 32	234 ± 45	67 ± 21	—	—	—
J606	360 ± 87	4,265 ± 833	5,875 ± 419	—	—	—
XRPC24	—	—	—	872 ± 13	5,272 ± 161	3,537 ± 51
Series II						
2-1-3	4,013 ± 328	12,570 ± 903	8,347 ± 1,024	—	—	—
2-1-10	802 ± 222	8,503 ± 1,516	249 ± 147	—	—	—
2-8-2	1,057 ± 161	16,232 ± 1,418	98 ± 47	—	—	—
2-11-1	1,592 ± 206	13,286 ± 805	186 ± 40	—	—	—
2-11-3	102 ± 3	12,354 ± 697	151 ± 26	—	—	—
2-12-10	113 ± 76	11,230 ± 1,650	40 ± 13	—	—	—
2-12-19	2,528 ± 408	15,028 ± 1,095	1,453 ± 527	—	—	—
2-9-17	62 ± 15	13,434 ± 2,915	2,228 ± 645	—	—	—
2-28-9	666 ± 294	5,232 ± 1,421	61 ± 21	—	—	—
Series III AND AIDA						
3-76-4	550 ± 69	127 ± 1	77 ± 12	—	—	—
3-76-42	1,544 ± 352	190 ± 41	1,171 ± 271	—	—	—
3-14-9	5,623 ± 947	1,413 ± 263	3,583 ± 777	—	—	—
3-27-6	1,693 ± 293	96 ± 11	177 ± 88	—	—	—
3-9-9	118 ± 30	126 ± 14	105 ± 19	273 ± 45	183 ± 21	189 ± 15
3-101-14	103 ± 19	152 ± 12	1,482 ± 275	—	—	—
AIDA10-16	179 ± 119	2,888 ± 291	125 ± 89	—	—	—
AIDA10-21	143 ± 76	294 ± 145	486 ± 235	730 ± 352	575 ± 64	465 ± 107
AIDA23-2	311 ± 87	151 ± 125	149 ± 34	1,709 ± 324	1,832 ± 300	1,376 ± 54
AIDA23-3	164 ± 44	405 ± 127	851 ± 180	296 ± 112	709 ± 110	483 ± 96

[a] Microtiter plates were coated with rye levan, bacterial levan, arabinogalactan, or gum ghatti at 20 μg/mℓ and inulin-BSA or galactan-BSA conjugates at 5 μg/mℓ. Monoclonal antibodies binding to these antigens were detected by binding to a ^{125}I-rat antimouse C_κ (kappa constant region monoclonal antibody).

[b] Cpm ± SE of triplicates.

monoclonal anti-A48 idiotopes behave in the same fashion as the polyconal anti-A48 Id antibodies, it seems that the inability of the Id of the Ab_2 population to elicit an anti-Id response is not a consequence of Id diversity, with no single Id present at immunogenic concentrations. More likely is the explanation that the Id determinants displayed by syngeneic anti-Id antibodies are simply not efficiently recognized as immunogenic moieties by the immune system. Hence, the regulatory Id (RI) concept was proposed. According to this concept, in a syngeneic system not all idiotopes are recognized by the immune system and, thus, used to mediate immunoregulation. Therefore, the anti-A48 Id antibodies, which can be considered as primarily antiregulatory Id antibodies because of their syngeneic nature, do not seem to bear any regulatory Id themselves; otherwise, their immunization would elicit an anti-anti-Id response. Consequently, the only way such antibodies participate in immunoregulation is by interacting through their paratopes with their regulatory Id-bearing lymphocytic clones and, in this case, expanding those B-cell clones bearing the A48 regulatory Id (RI). The A48 Id^+ hybridomas which were presumably generated from these expanded A48 RI-bearing B clones in anti-A48 Id-treated mice indicate that the IDA10 idiotope may be representative of such a regulatory idiotope, since it was expressed by all of the A48 Id^+ monoclonal antibodies.

Our molecular analysis of these A48 Id^+ hybridomas revealed that the majority, together with A48 and UPC10, derived their V_H regions from one of two highly homologous germline V_H genes (93% nucleotide homology) belonging to the V_H X24 germline gene family. Therefore, it is conceivable that the regulatory idiotope may represent a germline marker of V_H genes. Hence, the diversity in antigen specificities manifested by these monoclonal antibodies may be explained in terms of their expressing highly related V_H genes which, nevertheless, may encode very different hypervariable regions, which may also be free to pair with different types of L chains.

Based on the observations presented in this section as well as those obtained from subsequent experiments, three requirements can be established which an Id must meet in order for it to function as a "regulatory Id". They are

1. The Id must be immunogenic in a syngeneic system.
2. The Id must be borne by antibodies displaying different antigenic specificities.
3. The Idiotype must be recognized by a regulatory T-cell population, which will aid in its dominant expression by different clones.[45]

Takemori[58] showed very interesting differences between the responses of animals who were immunized with KLH conjugates of AC38 and AC146, two monoclonal allogeneic anti-idiotopes generated against the C57BL/6 monoclonal anti-NP antibody, B1-8. AC38 recognizes an idiotope which is not located within, but is near the B1-8 combining site. AC146 recognizes a combining site-associated idiotope of B1-8. AC38 Id^+/AC146 Id^+ and AC38 Id^+/AC146 Id^- antibodies consistently occur at equal frequencies and constitute a large proportion of the anti-NP antibodies in C57BL/6 mice. These antibodies invariantly bear the infrequently expressed lambda (λ) light chain. Adult C57BL/6 mice immunized only with AC38-KLH and not with any NP-bearing antigen show a significant induction of λ-bearing antibodies binding to the AC38 reagent in their sera, which already appeared only 1 week after immunization and remained at this level for the duration of the experiment (8 weeks). However, in contrast to what is observed after immunization with NP, only 5% of this antibody also bound to AC146 and 16% was NP specific. The situation was even more unexpected in the AC146-KLH immunized mice who were also never immunized with any NP-bearing antigen. Again, this treatment induced the appearance of AC146 binding antibodies which peaked 2 to 3 weeks after immunization and achieved a plateau level which persisted for the duration of the experiment (6 weeks). While all the λ-bearing AC146 binding antibodies also bound to AC38 and were specific for NP, they only constituted 5% of the response. In fact, 95% of the AC146 binding antibodies induced by this treatment bore the kappa (κ) light chain and were not NP specific. The possibility that these molecules may represent AC146 Id^+ antibodies bearing κ light chains cannot be excluded, because AC146 will react to some extent with the isolated IgD heavy chains of a B1-8 switch variant, although attempts to fully restore this reactivity by reassociation with various K chain preparations were unsuccessful.

Therefore, in the complete absence of any antigenic challenge by NP-containing antigens, immunization with the AC38-KLH conjugate by itself can preferentially elicit the production of what the authors have termed the $Ab_{3\beta}$ type of antibody[59] by the criteria that 90 to 95% of these antibodies are AC38 Id^+ and bear the λ light chain. Subsequent molecular and sequencing studies on AC38 Id^+, λ^+ monoclonal antibodies derived from AC38-KLH immunized animals have shown them to bear V_H sequences which are very closely related to the germline V_H B1-8 sequence. The production of $Ab_{3\alpha}$, antibodies specific for idiotopes expressed by AC38,[59] are minimal.

In spite of the Id and molecular relatedness of the AC38-induced $Ab_{3\beta}$ population to B1-8, the fact that relatively few of these antibodies are NP specific and coexpress the AC146 idiotope attests to the difference between the AC38 Id^+ B-cell clones which are expanded subsequent to antigenic and anti-Id stimulation. Nevertheless, it is not surprising to find AC38 Id^+, λ^+ non-NP binding antibodies, because expression of this idiotope seems to be determined for the most part by the λ light chain, with a lesser contribution by the heavy chain. This notion is supported by the observation that several AC38 Id^+ hybridomas, which incidentally happen not to be NP specific or AC146 Id^+, express the λ light chain but different D_H sequences and V_H genes which are clearly related to the B1-8 V_H genes, but are not identical to it.

In contrast to the types of clones which were activated by the AC38 antibody, immunization with an AC146-KLH conjugate in the absence of any further antigenic stimulation appears to have resulted only in a very minor production of $Ab_{3\beta}$ antibodies which did, however, share many similarities with the $AC146^+$ antibodies observed after NP immunization. They all bore λ light chains, coexpressed the AC38 idiotope, and bound NP. The vast majority (95%) of the clones activated by the AC146 antibody bore κ light chains and it is unclear whether this entire population represents an $Ab_{3\beta}$ response or is a mixture of $Ab_{3\alpha}$ and $Ab_{3\beta}$ type antibodies.

The participation of a helper T-cell population in the anti-Id-mediated activation of Id-bearing B-cell clones was independently demonstrated in several model Id systems. Bluestone et al.[60] observed this phenomenon in their studies on the anti-Id-mediated induction of anti-H-$2K^k$ antibodies bearing the complementary Id. Adult BALB/c mice were immunized with unmodified, pig or rabbit anti-Id antibodies which were generated against the private idiotopes borne by 3-83P or 11-4.1, two BALB/c monoclonal anti-H-2^k antibodies.

For a period beginning 17 days post anti-Id immunization and lasting for approximately 2 months, antibodies bearing the 3-83P Id or 11-4.1 Id appeared in the sera of these animals. However, only 20% of this Id-bearing antibody showed the anti-H-$2K^k$ specificity. Isoelectric focusing experiments provided further evidence that these xenogeneic anti-Id antibodies had activated a clonotypically different population of Id-bearing B-cell clones from those observed during an alloantigenic immune response. But, that is not to say that those few Id-bearing anti-H-2-K^k B-cell clones which were activated represent an inconsequential action by the anti-Id antibodies. On the contrary, these anti-Id antibodies actually preselected the anti-H2-K^k B-cell repertoire in these animals prior to any antigenic exposure. When C3H(H-$2K^k$) tail skin was grafted onto BALB/c mice (H-$2K^d$), the 3-83P or 11-4.1 Id-bearing antibodies constituted 40 to 60% of the alloantigenic antibody response in the anti-Id immunized animal, but was never consistently detected in untreated mice. Interestingly enough, the titer of the non-H-$2K^k$ binding Id-bearing antibody increases substantially after H-$2K^k$ skin grafting in the pig anti-11-4.1 Id immunized mice. Presumably, this Id in spite of it being defined by xenogeneic antibodies, probably does participate under physiological circumstances in immunoregulation, otherwise it is difficult to explain how an antigenic challenge can increase the levels of nonantigen binding Id-bearing antibody.[61] Auchincloss et al.[62] noticed that pig anti-11-4.1 Id will induce the appearance of Id-bearing antibodies in only one out of every ten nude mice immunized with the anti-Id. The inability of the nude to respond was clearly due to its T-cell deficit, because all nude animals who were reconsituted with syngeneic T cells showed the typical anti-Id-mediated induction of 11-4.1 Id^+ antibodies. Because of the xenogeneic nature of the anti-Id, a series of adoptive transfer experiments was designed to address the possibility that the T-cell participation observed in this system was, indeed, an Id-specific T_H cell and not a carrier-specific T_H elicited by the xenogeneic Fc portion of the anti-Id antibody. Mildly irradiated BALB/c mice who received T cells from anti-Id-treated animals, but themselves never received the anti-Id antibody, mounted a predominantly 11-4.1 Id^+ anti-H-2^k antibody response after being grafted with C3H (H-$2K^k$) tail skin. Since the expression of this Id is absolutely contingent on previous clonal expansion with the anti-Id antibody, these results are consistent with the participation of a 11-4.1 Id-specific T_H cell in this anti-Id-mediated induction system. Furthermore, while a genetic restriction did exist for the expression of this Id within the B-cell compartment, no such restriction was observed for the presence of T_H cells which mediated the expansion of 11-4.1 Id-bearing clones. The production of 11-4.1 Id^+ antibodies was observed only in those strains of mice such as BALB/c or BAB14 which exhibit the $IgV_H{}^a$ genotype. On the other hand, nude mice reconstituted with T cells obtained from BALB/c or CB20 ($IgV_H{}^B$) mice showed an equivalent expression of 11-4.1 Id^+ antibodies following anti-Id treatment, despite the fact that the CB20 congenic strain cannot itself express 11-4.1 Id-bearing antibodies. In a series of experiments where allogeneic bone marrow chimeras were produced between BALB/c and B10.D2 ($IgV_H{}^b$) mice, Auchincloss asked if any differences in the response to anti-11-4.1 antibodies could be observed if the genetic environment in which both the T and B cells matured were altered. B10.D2 and BALB/c mice were irradiated and reconstituted with BALB/c and B10.D2 bone marrow, respectively. Again, B10.D2 do not express the 11-4.1 Id because of their inappropriate IgVh genotype. Following administration of the pig anti-11-4.1 Id antibodies, only the B10.D2 animal receiving BALB/c bone marrow showed the induction of Id-bearing antibodies by the anti-Id. These experiments showed that the ability to respond to these anti-Id antibodies is a genetically determined property of the lymphoid cells which is not subject to alteration by environmental influences. Nevertheless, in this system, the V_H repertoire of the B cells do not influence to any measurable extent the repertoire of Id-enhancing T_H cells.

Similar observations were made by Miller and colleagues while studying the Id expression by staphylococcal nuclease (S. nuclease)-specific antibodies in BALB/c mice.[63] Adult BALB/c mice (2 to 6 months) treated with pig anti-(polyclonal BALB/c anti-S. nuclease antibody) Id, in the absence of any antigenic challenge, showed a significant induction in the expression of antibodies bearing this Id, which, again, for the most part, did not bind to S. nuclease. T_H cells which bear this Id and are nuclease specific are seen in nuclease-primed or anti-Id-treated BALB/c mice and probably participate in the anti-Id-mediated induction of Id-bearing antibodies, since this induction cannot be elicited in nude BALB/c mice. The expression of this Id appears to be IgVh restricted, because it is only infrequently observed at minimal levels in B10.D2 ($IgCh^b$) mice. As expected, nuclease priming of B10.D2 mice does activate nuclease-specific T_H cells which, of course, do not express the BALB/c Id. Moreover, administration of pig anti-BALB/c nuclease Id antibodies to B10.D2 mice will not induce synthesis of Id-bearing antibodies, but it does activate a population of Id-bearing nuclease-specific T_H cells.[64] Again, we see a real difference between the Id expression of the antigen receptors of T and B cells, with neither one exerting an influence over the expression of the other.

Experiments performed in the Id system associated with antibodies binding the synthetic polypeptide (T,G)-A-L showed that anti-Id-mediated enhancement could be achieved in both a T-dependent, as well as a T-independent fashion under different experimental conditions. Weissberger et al.[65] showed that lymph node cells primed in vivo with (T,G)-A-L could be stimulated in vitro to yield a (T,G)-A-L-specific response if they were cocultured only with a rat anti-(C57BL/10 polyclonal anti [T,G]-A-L) Id antibody. The response was quantitatively indistinguishable from cultures containing the (T,G)-A-L antigen itself. This effect was restricted to in vivo primed cells and was observed only for the IgM response, because these in vivo primed lymph nodes spontaneously secreted IgG anti-(T,G)-A-L antibody in vitro which was unaffected by any antigenic or anti-Id stimulus. The mechanism of the anti-Id-mediated induction of the IgM response seemed to involve a direct priming of an $Lyt1^+$ helper population by the anti-Id. This was shown in cultures where the anti-Id alone could induce an IgM anti(T,G)-A-L response when only the T cells were derived from (T,G)-A-L-primed mice and the B cells were obtained from naive animals. Furthermore, the supernatant obtained from cultures containing only the anti-Id antibody and in vivo (T,G)-A-L-primed T cells was sufficient to elicit an IgM anti-(T,G)-A-L response from naive B cells. During the course of these studies, these authors were able to demonstrate that the basis for the I-R gene control which this immune response was subject to seemed to be in the T-cell compartment. An IgM anti-(T,G)-A-L response could be elicited from cultures containing nonresponder strain B cells when they were cocultured with anti-Id primed T cells obtained from responder or (responder × nonresponder) F_1 animals.

The anti-Id antibody can also evoke the expression of Id-bearing antibody molecules under conditions where expression of this Id upon conventional immunization with antigen is linked to the expression of certain immunoglobulin heavy chain allotypes, and the individual receiving the anti-Id does not possess any of the heavy chain allotypes compatible with Id expression. This phenomenon was demonstrated by Leguern et al.,[66] Pene et al.,[67] and Moser et al.,[68] who were studying Id expression by anti-TNP, antidextran, and antiarsonate antibodies, respectively.

Leguern et al.[66] first observed that DBA/2 mice, who normally do not express the M460 Id on their anti-TNP antibodies, could be made to do so if they were first hyperimmunized with a syngeneic anti-M460 Id KLH conjugate.

Pene's[67] experimental system was studying the expression of the J558 MOPC104E IdX borne by antibodies specific for the α1,3 glycosidic linkage. Only mice bearing the $IgCh^a$ allotype (i.e., BALB/c) can mount a J558-MOPC104E IdX^+ response. However, these investigators observed that C57BL/6 or CB20 mice who bear the $IgCh^b$ allotype could synthesize a population of antibodies which could competitively inhibit the interaction of MOPC104E with rabbit anti-J558 IdX antibodies in an RIA if they were previously immunized with rabbit anti-J558-IdX antibodies. Only 10% of these "J558 IdX^+" antibodies bound to dextran; however, in the CB20 animals, immunization with a bacterial dextran B1355-Con A conjugate could raise this proportion upwards to 50% of the entire J558 IdX^+ response. Nevertheless, these dextran-binding J558 IdX^+ antibodies which were induced in these $IgCh^b$ mice are distinct from those observed in BALB/c mice. This conclusion is based on different binding affinities manifested by these two groups of antibodies to a variety of bacterial dextrans possessing an assortment of glycosidic linkages.

Moser et al.[68] studied the expression of antibodies specific for the ars hapten and bearing the ars CRI_A Id. This Id is a cross-reactive Id produced upon immunization with ars only in mice bearing the $IgCh^e$ and $IgCh^d$ allotypes. However, BALB/c mice ($IgCh^a$), who are previously treated with a rabbit anti-ars CRI_A reagent which was generated against a polyclonal population of pooled A/J ($IgCh^e$) CRI_A^+ ars-specific antibodies, can themselves produce a population of antibodies, even without arsonate immunization, which are sound competitive inhibitors in a radioimmunoassay for CRI_A expression. Many of these CRI_A^+ antibodies in BALB/c do manifest the ars specificity, because several hybridomas have been generated from ars-immunized, Id-treated BALB/c mice which secrete ars-binding CRI_A^+ antibodies. Interestingly, the CRI_A^+ antibodies in A/J mice appear to be encoded by a very limited number of germline V_H genes which are clearly absent from the BALB/c repertoire. Hence, in this instance, it is clear that the basis for this shared Id expression between these two genetically distinct strains of mice must be either: (1) a conserved nucleotide sequence shared by at least two otherwise different groups of germline V_H genes which encode the structural correlates for this Id; (2) different nucleotide sequences in the BALB/c V_H genes which encode amino acids giving rise to three-dimensional Id structures on these antibodies which are serologically indistinguishable from those present on the A/J antibody. Further molecular analysis should distinguish between these two possibilities.

Along these same lines of thought, Urbain[70] and colleagues showed that an anti-Id antibody could evoke the expression of Id-bearing antibody molecules in an individual of another species where that Id is not normally expressed in that species. Their studies began with their observations on the Id expression of antibodies specific, either for tobacco mosaic virus (TMV) or micrococcus lysodeikticus carbohydrate (ML), in the rabbit. Since their rabbits were not from an inbred colony, it was not surprising to find that no cross-reactive Id expression could be detected between the TMV- or ML-specific antibodies of different rabbits. However, this situation could be drastically altered if rabbits were immunized with an anti-Id generated against the Ab_1 anti-TMV or anti-ML population of an individual rabbit. Rabbits immunized in this fashion could now mount a TMV or ML response which shared Id between themselves and, of course, with the animal whose Ab_1 antibody was used to generate the anti-Id.[69] These workers extended their observations by treating BALB/c mice with the same anti-Id preparations used to immunize the rabbits described above.[70] Even across species lines, these anti-Id antibodies could induce in these mice a population of antibodies which not only shared a cross reaction with the individual rabbit's Ab_1 population used as the immunogen for the anti-Id, but even more astoundingly shared either its TMV or ML specificity. Extensive experimentation ruled out the trivial possibility that these anti-Id used to treat the mice bore the internal image of the antigen; hence, they were stereochemically mimicking the antigen which could explain how they could evoke these responses even across species barriers. Therefore, the authors conclude that these results are attributable to the sharing of an interspecies germline-encoded regulatory Id.

The experiments presented in this section collectively demonstrate that anti-Id-mediated enhancement of Id expression can proceed by the direct interaction of the anti-Id molecule with the Id-bearing B cell or helper T cell. At this point, it is important to emphasize that this enhancement is purely the result of Id-anti-Id interactions and is not attributable to the anti-Id antibody bearing the internal image of the antigen. This is evident by the fact that this enhancement often results in the appearance of clones which do express the complimentary Id, but not necessarily the antigen-binding activity associated with expression of that Id. In these experiments, the term enhancement has been shown to encompass a very broad range. Indeed, in the A48 Id and anti-H-$2K^k$ Id systems, silent clones are expanded by treatment with anti-Id until they comprise a major part of the immune response. In the MOPC460 Id, ars CRI_A, and MOPC104E-J558 IdX systems, anti-Id evokes the expression of clones in individuals who are thought not to possess the prototypical V_H and/or V_L structural genes necessary for expansion of the respective Id. In the TMV and ML Id systems, anti-Id can evoke the expression of an Id across a species barrier. Finally, it is worthwhile commenting at this point on the lack of parallelism between Id expression by the B- and T-cell repertoire. In several instances, we see Id expression by the T-cell repertoire, but not the B-cell repertoire. The basis for this dichotomy will undoubtedly emerge as we increase our knowledge of the structural basis for Id expression, particularly by the T-cell receptor.

IV. EFFECTS OF ANTI-ID ANTIBODIES ON EFFECTOR T-CELL FUNCTIONS

A fundamental assumption in believing that Id interactions form a basic communications network among the clones of the immune system is that clones deriving from both the B- and T-cell lineages participate. Supporting this point of view is the fact that numerous investigators have demonstrated that despite the fact that T cells do not possess endogenously synthesized membrane immunoglobulin, they do display stereochemical structures on their membranes which react very specifically with anti-Id antibodies generated against immunoglobulin Id. Furthermore, as was presented in the previous two sections, anti-Id-mediated modulation of humoral immune response, in many instances, involved the recruitment of Id specific regulatory T cells. Anti-Id antibodies can also influence the activities of effector-type T cells, such as those mediating mixed lymphocyte reactions (MLC, MLR) delayed-type hypersensitivity responses (DTH), and cell-mediated lysis which are Id specific.

Binz and Wigzell[71] demonstrated that they could generate an anti-Id reagent by injecting DBA/2 mice with DBA anti-C3H alloreactive blast cells generated in in vitro MLR reactions, which would react with DBA anti-C3H alloantibodies. Andersson et al.[72] observed that anti-Id sera generated in this fashion could inhibit the MLC-induced proliferation as well as the subsequent generation of cytotoxic DBA/2 cells when the stimulator cells in the culture expressed the same alloantigens as those which were used to originally generate the DBA/2 blasts used for the production of the anti-Id. Furthermore, pretreating the DBA/2 responder population with the anti-Id plus complement precluded any type of response in the above-described culture situation. Binz et al.[73,74] succeeded in demonstrating that prolonged in vitro incubation of the cells with anti-Id will induce proliferation and the subsequent generation of cytotoxic T cells in the absence of any alloantigenic stimulation which were absolutely specific for the alloantigen expressed on the stimulator population used to generate the Id-bearing alloreactive blasts.

These types of observations have been repeated in rat and guinea pig systems by Andersson et al.[72]

Strassman et al.[75] showed that allogeneic anti-poly(L Tyr, L Glu)-poly (DL Ala)- - poly(L Lys) (T,G)-A--L) Id serum could elicit a DTH response in naive recipients infused with (T,G)-A--L-educated T cells. The anti-Id seemed to be directly stimulating the educated T cells, because a response could not be elicited from T cells deriving from a strain of mouse which does not synthesize anti-(T,G)-A--L antibodies bearing that Id.

Arnold et al.[76] also showed that a PC-specific DTH response could be elicited in PC-sensitized BALB/c mice either with the antigen or with a mixture of monoclonal anti-T15 idiotopes. The individual anti-idiotopes could not elicit this response. Furthermore, the anti-Id-induced elicitation of this DTH response, in contrast to the antigen-induced response, did not show any H-2 restriction. Only the anti-Id antibody and not antigen could induce a DTH response from PC-sensitized BALB/c (H-2^d) lymph node cells which were transferred in BALB/k (H-2^k) mice.

In addition to eliciting a DTH response from an antigen-primed T-cell population, Sy et al.[77] and Jayaraman et al.[78] showed that anti-Id could also prime naive T cells for an antigen-specific DTH response. Sy et al.'s model system is the CRI Id system of ars-specific antibodies produced by A/J mice. This group showed that an ars-specific DTH could be elicited in mice who were administered rabbit anti-CRI Id antibody subcutaneously. This response could be abrogated by treatment with anti-CRI and complement. Furthermore, only in mice bearing the $IgCh^e$ allotype, the only strains synthesizing ars-specific antibody bearing this Id, could these anti-CRI antibodies elicit this response. Working in the same CRI Id system, Thomas et al.[79] could use an allogeneic monoclonal anti-idiotope to prime naive T cells for an ars-specific DTH response. The anti-idiotope, 14A was gene rated in a (SJL ×

BALB/c)F_1 animal against 7.1.3, an A/J CRI^+ ars-specific monoclonal antibody. The 14A idiotope is located within or near the antibody combining site and is considered a minor idiotope among ars-specific antibodies. Again, the DTH-mediating T cells primed by this anti-idiotope bore the 14A idiotope on their membranes, since the DTH response was abrogated by treatment with 14A and complement, and also showed the H-2 restriction associated with T DTH.

Jayaraman et al.[78] showed that A/J mice injected subcutaneously with rabbit antiphenyltrimethyl ammonium (TMA) Id antibodies will be sensitized for a TMA-specific DTH reaction. Again, the ability of mice to produce this Id is linked to the $IgCh^e$ locus, as is the ability of these anti-Id antibodies to prime the TMA-specific T_{DTH} cells. These T_{DTH} cells do bear TMA Id determinants, as anti-TMA Id antibodies will block the DTH reaction sensitized by the anti-Id.

Anti-Id antibodies can also suppress a DTH reaction elicited by antigen in an Id-specific fashion. Sy et al.[80] and Yamamoto et al.,[81] respectively, showed that the DTH response induced by sensitization with ars-coupled spleen cells or PC-coupled peritoneal exudate cells could be inhibited by passive administration of anti-ars CRI or anti-T15 Id antiserum. In both instances, the suppression was mediated by suppressor T cells which were induced by the anti-Id reagents. Sy et al.[80] clearly showed that the anti-CRI Id-induced suppression showed the same genetic restriction as the ability to produce CRI Id^+ anti-ars antibodies. Namely, only A/J mice who can produce this type of antibody are susceptible to anti-CRI Id-induced suppression of the ars-specific DTH response, while BALB/c who do not produce this Id are not susceptible to this suppression.

In conclusion, these results show that anti-Id antibodies can influence effector T-cell functions in an Id-specific fashion. In contrast to what was observed in the previous section, the expression of Id by these T cells did parallel the same genetically determined pattern of expression which was observed by the B cells. Since the T cells described in the previous section which did not parallel the B-cell Id expression were helper T cells, it is possible that it is only this class of T cell which represents the exception to this rule.

REFERENCES

1. **Jerne, N. K.,** Towards a network theory of the immune system, *Ann. Immunol.*, 125C, 373, 1974.
2. **Eichmann, K.,** Expression and function of idiotypes on lymphocytes, *Adv. Immunol.*, 26, 195, 1978.
3. **Bona, C.,** Idiotype suppression in adults, in *Lymphocytic Regulation by Antibodies*, Bona, C. and Cazenave, P. A., Eds., John Wiley & Sons, New York, 1981, chap. 12.
4. **Weiler, I. J.,** Neonatally and maternally induced idiotypic suppression, in *Lymphocytic Regulation by Antibodies*, Bona, C. and Cazenave, P. A., Eds., John Wiley & Sons, New York, 1981, chap. 13.
5. **Cosenza, H.,** Detection of anti-idiotype reactive cells in the response to phosphorylcholine, *Eur. J. Immunol.*, 6, 114, 1976.
6. **Bona, C., Lieberman, R., Chien, C. C., Mond, J., House, S., Green, I., and Paul, W. E.,** Immune response to levan. I. Kinetics and ontogeny of anti-levan and anti-inulin antibody response and of expression of cross-reactive idiotype, *J. Immunol.*, 120, 1436, 1978.
7. **Schrater, A. F., Goidl, E. A., Siskind, G. W., and Thorbecke, G. J.,** Regulation of the immune response by autoanti-idiotypic antibody, *J. Supramol. Struct.*, Suppl. 3, 294, 1979.
8. **Bona, C. A., Heber-Katz, E., and Paul, W. E.,** Idiotype-anti-idiotype regulation. I. Immunization with a levan-binding myeloma protein leads to the appearance of auto-anti(anti-idiotype) antibodies and to the activation of silent clones, *J. Exp. Med.*, 153, 951, 1981.
9. **Cosenza, H. and Kohler, H.,** Specific suppression by antibodies to receptors, *Proc. Natl. Acad. Sci. U.S.A.*, 69, 2701, 1972.
10. **Cosenza, H. and Kohler, H.,** Specific inhibition of plaque formation to phosphorylcholine by antibody against antibody, *Science*, 176, 1027, 1972.

11. **Kohler, H.**, The response to phosphorylcholine, *Transplant. Rev.*, 27, 24, 1975.
12. **Strayer, D. S., Cosenza, H., Lee, W. M. F., Rowley, D. A., and Kohler, M.**, Neonatal tolerance induced by antibody against antigen-specific receptor, *Science*, 186, 640, 1974.
13. **Strayer, D. S., Lee, W. M. F., Rowley, D. A., and Kohler, H.**, Anti-receptory antibody. II. Induction of long term unresponsiveness in neonatal mice, *J. Immunol.*, 114, 728, 1975.
14. **Kearney, J. F., Barletta, R., Quan, Z. S., and Quintans, J.**, Monoclonal vs. heterogeneous anti-H8 antibodies in the analyses of the anti-phosphorylcholine response in BALB/c mice, *Eur. J. Immunol.*, 11, 877, 1981.
15. **Kelsoe, G., Reth, M., and Rajewsky, K.**, Control of idiotope expression by monoclonal anti-idiotope and idiotope bearing antibody, *Eur. J. Immunol.*, 11, 418, 1981.
16. **Bona, C., Stein, K. E., Lieberman, R., and Paul, W. E.**, Direct and indirect suppression induced by anti-idiotype antibody in the inulin-bacterial levan antigenic system, *Mol. Immunol.*, 16, 1093, 1979.
17. **Hart, D. A., Wang, A. L., Pawlak, L. S., and Nisonoff, A.**, Suppression of idiotypic specificities in adult mice by administration of antiidiotypic antibody, *J. Exp. Med.*, 135, 1293, 1972.
18. **Nisonoff, A., Shyr, T. J., and Owen, F. L.**, Studies of structure and immunosuppression of a cross-reactive idiotype in strain A mice, *Immunol. Rev.*, 34, 89, 1977.
19. **Ward, K., Cantor, H., and Nisonoff, A.**, Analysis of the cellular basis of idiotype-specific suppression, *J. Immunol.*, 120, 2016, 1978.
20. **Hirai, Y. and Nisonoff, A.**, Selective suppression of the major idiotypic component of an antihapten response by soluble T cell-derived factors with idiotypic or anti-idiotypic receptors, *J. Exp. Med.*, 151, 1213, 1980.
21. **Rothstein, R. L., Miller, R. A., Parker, D. J., Kelly, E., Vastola, P. A., and Marshak-Rothstein, A.**, Induction of idiotope suppression in the azophenylarsonate response of T depleted A/J mice, *J. Exp. Med.*, 159, 1283, 1984.
22. **Hornbeck, P. V. and Lewis, G. K.**, Idiotype connectance in the immune system. I. Expression of a cross-reactive idiotype on induced anti-p-azophenylarsonate antibodies and on endogenous antibodies not specific for arsonate, *J. Exp. Med.*, 157, 1116, 1983.
23. **Eichmann, K.**, Idiotype suppression. I. Influence of the dose and of the effector functions of anti idiotypic antibody on the production of an idiotype, *Eur. J. Immunol.*, 4, 296, 1974.
24. **Hetzelberger, D. and Eichmann, K.**, Idiotype suppression. III. Induction of unresponsiveness to sensitization with anti-idiotypic antibody: identification of the cell types tolerized in high zone and in low zone, suppressor cell mediated, idiotype suppression, *Eur. J. Immunol.*, 8, 839, 1978.
25. **Kohler, H., Richardson, B. C., Rowley, D. A., and Smyk, S.**, Immune response to phosphorylcholine. III. Requirement of the Fc portion and equal effectiveness of IgG subclasses in anti-receptor antibody-induced suppression, *J. Immunol.*, 119, 1979, 1977.
26. **Müller, C. E. and Rajewsky, K.**, Idiotope regulation by isotype switch variants of two monoclonal antiidiotope antibodies, *J. Exp. Med.*, 159, 758, 1984.
27. **Bordenave, G. R.**, A study of idiotypic suppression in adult rabbits immunized with Salmonella aborties-equi, *Immunology*, 28, 635, 1975.
28. **Getlen, D. and Morphis, L.**, Systems of materno-foetal transport of γ-gamma immunoglobulin in the mouse, *Nature (London)*, 223, 195, 1969.
29. **Culbertson, J. T.**, The natural transmission of immunity against *Trypanasoma duttoni* from mother mice to their young, *J. Immunol.*, 38, 51, 1940.
30. **Halliday, R.**, Prenatal and postnatal transmission of passive immunity to young rats, *Proc. R. Soc. London*, 144, 427, 1955.
31. **Halliday, R.**, The termination of the capacity of young rats to absorb antibody from the milk, *Proc. R. Soc. London*, 145, 179, 1955.
32. **Augustin, A. and Cosenza, H.**, Expression of new idiotypes following neonatal idiotypic suppression of a dominant clone, *Eur. J. Immunol.*, 6, 497, 1976.
33. **Berek, C., Schreier, M., Sidman, C. L., Jaton, J. C., Kocher, H. P., and Cosenza, H.**, Phosphorylcholine binding hybridoma proteins of normal and idiotypically suppressed BALB/c mice. I. Characterization and idiotypic analysis, *Eur. J. Immunol.*, 10, 258, 1980.
34. **Cosenza, H., Augustin, A. A., and Julius, M. H.**, Idiotypes and anti-idiotypes as probes in analysis of immunoregulation, *Cold Spring Harbor Symp. Quant. Biol.*, 41, 709, 1976.
35. **Du Clos, T. and Kim, B.**, Suppressor T cells presence in mice rendered tolerant by neonatal treatment with anti-receptor antibody or antigen, *J. Immunol.*, 119, 1769, 1977.
36. **Kim, B. and Greenberg, J.**, Mechanisms of idiotype suppression. IV. Functional neutralization in mixtures of idiotype-specific suppressor and hapten-specific suppressor T cells, *J. Exp. Med.*, 154, 809, 1981.
37. **Fung, J. and Kohler, H.**, Mechanism of neonatal idiotype suppression. II. Alterations in the T cell compartment suppress the maturation of B cell precursor, *J. Immunol.*, 125, 2489, 1980.
38. **Fung, J. and Kohler, H.**, Mechanism of neonatal idiotypic suppression. I. State of the suppressed B cells, *J. Immunol.*, 125, 1998, 1980.

39. **Berek, C.,** Antibodies specific for different T15 idiotopes induce neonatal suppression of T15 idiotype, *Eur. J. Immunol.,* 13, 766, 1983.
40. **Takemori, T. and Rajewsky, K.,** Specificity, duration and mechanism of idiotype suppression induced by neonatal injection of monoclonal antiidiotope antibodies into mice, *Eur. J. Immunol.,* 14, 656, 1984.
41. **Rothstein, T. L. and Vastola, P.,** Homologous monoclonal antibodies induce idiotope specific suppression in neonates through maternal influence and in adult exposed during fetal and neonatal life, *J. Immunol.,* 133, 1151, 1984.
42. **Bona, C., Lieberman, R., Chien, C. C., Mond, J., House, S., Green, I., and Paul, W. E.,** Immune response to levan. I. Kinetics and ontogeny of anti-levan and anti-inulin antibody response and of expression of cross-reactive idiotype, *J. Immunol.,* 120, 1436, 1978.
43. **Lieberman, R., Potter, M., Humphrey, W., and Chien, C. C.,** Idiotypes of inulin-binding antibodies and myeloma proteins controlled by genes linked to the allotype locus of the mouse, *J. Immunol.,* 117, 2105, 1976.
44. **Cosenza, H., Julius, M. H., and Augustin, A. A.,** Idiotypes as variable region markers: analogies between receptors on phosphorylcholine-specific T and B lymphocytes, *Immunol. Rev.,* 34, 3, 1977.
45. **Kresina, T. F. and Nisonoff, A.,** Properties of suppressive cells and soluble suppressive factors in idiotypically suppressed, hyperimmunized mice. I. Passive transfer of the idiotypically suppressed state by serum and transfer of suppression from mothers to offspring, *J. Exp. Med.,* 157, 15, 1983.
46. **Weiler, I. J., Weiler, E., Sprenger, R., and Cosenza, H.,** Idiotype suppression by maternal influence, *Eur. J. Immunol.,* 7, 591, 1977.
47. **Victor, C., Bona, C., and Pernis, B.,** Idiotype determined circuits in maternally suppressed mice, in *Immune Networks,* Bona, C. A. and Kohler, M., Eds., The New York Academy of Sciences, New York, 1983, 220.
48. **Victor-Kobrin, C., Bona, C., and Pernis, B.,** Expansion of idiotype positive B cells in maternally idiotype suppressed mice, *J. Mol. Cell Immunol.,* 1, 331, 1984.
49. **Oudin, J. and Cazenave, P. A.,** Similar idiotypic specificities in immunoglobulin fractions with different antibody functions or even without detectable antibody function, *Proc. Natl. Acad. Sci. U.S.A.,* 68, 2616, 1971.
50. **Rubinstein, L. J., Goldberg, B., Hiernaux, J., Stein, K. E., and Bona, C.,** Idiotype anti-idiotype regulation. V. The requirement for immunization with antigen or monoclonal anti-idiotypic antibodies for the activation of $\beta 2 \rightarrow 6$ and $\beta 2 \rightarrow 1$ polyfructosan-reactive clones in BALB/c mice treated at birth with minute amounts of anti-A48 idiotype antibodies, *J. Exp. Med.,* 158, 1129, 1983.
51. **Legrain, P., Voegle, D., Buttin, G., and Cazenave, P. A.,** Idiotype-anti-idiotype interactions and the control of the anti-$\beta(2 \rightarrow 6)$ polyfructosan response in the mouse: specificity and idiotype of anti-ABPC48 anti-idiotypic monoclonal antibodies, *Eur. J. Immunol.,* 11, 678, 1981.
52. **Goldberg, B., Paul, W. E., and Bona, C.,** Idiotype-anti-idiotype regulation. IV. Characterization of regulatory idiotopes on $\beta 2,6$ fructosan binding monoclonal antibodies and monoclonal proteins with different antigen specificities, *J. Exp. Med.,* 158, 515, 1983.
53. **Auffrey, C., Skeorav, J. L., Ollo, R., and Rougeon, F.,** Correlation between D region structure and antigen binding specificity from the comparison of closely related immunoglobulin V_H sequence, *Ann. Immunol.,* 132, 77, 1977.
54. **Kabat, E. A., Wu, T. T., and Belofsky, H.,** Sequences of Immunoglobulin Chains, Publ. No. 80-2008, National Institutes of Health, Bethesda, Md., 1983, 37.
55. **Victor-Kobrin, C., Bonilla, F. A., Bellon, B., and Bona, C.,** Immunochemical and molecular characterization of regulatory idiotopes expressed by monoclonal antibodies exhibiting or lacking $\beta 2 \rightarrow 6$ fructosan binding activity, *J. Exp. Med.,* 162, 647, 1985.
56. **Hartman, A. and Rudekoff, S.,** V_H genes encoding the immune response to $\beta(1,6)$ galactan: somatic mutation in IgM molecules, *EMBO J.,* 3, 3023, 1984.
57. **Rubinstein, L. J., Yeh, M., and Bona, C.,** Idiotype anti-idiotype network. II. Activation of silent clones by treatment at birth with idiotypes is associated with the expansion of idiotype specific helper T cells, *J. Exp. Med.,* 156, 506, 1982.
58. **Takemori, T., Tesch, M., Reth, M., and Rajewsky, K.,** The immune response against anti-idiotope antibodies. I. Induction of idiotope-bearing antibodies and analysis of the idiotope repertoire, *Eur. J. Immunol.,* 12, 1040, 1982.
59. **Tesch, H., Takemori, T., and Rajewsky, K.,** The immune response against antiidiotope antibodies. II. The induction of antibodies bearing the target idiotope ($Ab_{3\beta}$) depends on the frequency of the corresponding B cells, *Eur. J. Immunol.,* 13, 726, 1983.
60. **Bluestone, J. A., Epstein, S. L., Ozato, K., Sharrow, S. O., and Sachs, D. M.,** Anti-idiotypes to monoclonal anti-H-2 antibodies. II. Expression of anti-H-$2K^k$ idiotypes on antibodies induced by anti-idiotype or H-$2K^k$ antigen, *J. Exp. Med.,* 154, 1305, 1981.
61. **Rabinowitz, R., Bluestone, J. A., and Sachs, D. M.,** Evidence for a regulatory idiotypic network in the in vivo response to H-2 antigens, *J. Exp. Med.,* 162, 745, 1985.

62. **Auchincloss, H., Jr., Bluestone, J. A., and Sachs, D. M.,** Antiidiotypes against anti-H-2 monoclonal antibodies. V. In vivo anti-idiotype treatment induces idiotype specific helper T cells, *J. Exp. Med.*, 157, 1273, 1983.
63. **Miller, G. G., Nadler, P. I., Asano, Y., Hodes, R. J., and Sachs, D. M.,** Induction of idiotype bearing, nuclease specific helper T cells by in vivo treatment with anti-idiotype, *J. Exp. Med.*, 154, 24, 1981.
64. **Miller, G. G. P., Nadler, P. I., Hodes, R. J., and Sachs, D. M.,** Modification of T cell antinuclease idiotype expression by in vivo administration of anti-idiotype, *J. Exp. Med.*, 155, 190, 1982.
65. **Weissberger, M. Z., Shenk, R. R., and Rickler, H. B.,** Antiidiotype stimulation of antigen-specific antigen-independent antibody responses in vitro. I. Evidence for stimulation of helper T lymphocyte function, *J. Exp. Med.*, 158, 465, 1983.
66. **Leguern, C., Ben Aissa, F., Juy, D., Mariamé, B., Buttin, G., and Cazenave, P. A.,** Expression and induction of MOPC460 idiotopes in different strains of mice, *Ann. Immunol. (Inst. Pasteur)*, 130C, 293, 1979.
67. **Pene, J., Bekkhoucha, F., Desmayard, C., Zaghouani, H., and Stanislavski, M.,** Induction of a cross-reactive idiotype dextran positive antibody response in two Igh-C^b mouse strains treated with anti-J558 cross-reactive idiotype antibodies, *J. Exp. Med.*, 157, 1573, 1983.
68. **Moser, M., Leo, O., Hiernaux, J., and Urbain, J.,** Idiotypic manipulation in mice: BALB/c can express the cross-reactive idiotype of A/J mice, *Proc. Natl. Acad. Sci. U.S.A.*, 80, 4474, 1983.
69. **Wikler, M., Franseen, J. D., Collignon, C., Leo, O., Mariame, B., Van de Walle, P., De Groote, D., and Urbain, J.,** Idiotypic regulation of the immune system. I. Common idiotypic specificities between idiotypes and antibodies raised against anti-idiotypic antibodies in rabbits, *J. Exp. Med.*, 150, 184, 1979.
70. **Francotte, M. and Urbain, J.,** Induction of anti-tobacco mosaic virus antibodies in mice by rabbit antiidiotypic antibodies, *J. Exp. Med.*, 160, 1485, 1984.
71. **Binz, H. and Wigzell, M.,** Shared idiotypic determinants, on B and T lymphocytes reactive against the same antigenic determinants. I. Demonstration of similar or identical idiotypes on IgG molecules and T cell receptors with specificity for the same alloantigens, *J. Exp. Med.*, 142, 197, 1975.
72. **Andersson, L. C., Aguet, M., Wight, E., Andersson, R., Binz, M., and Wigzell, M.,** Induction of specific immune unresponsiveness using purified mixed leukocyte culture activated T lymphoblasts as autoimmunogen. I. Demonstration of a general validity as to species and histocompatibility barriers, *J. Exp. Med.*, 146, 1124, 1977.
73. **Binz, M., Frisckknecht, M., and Wigzell, M.,** Some studies on idiotypes and anti-idiotypic reactions and receptors in anti-allo-MHC T cell immunity, *Ann. Immunol. (Inst. Pasteur)*, 130C, 273, 1979.
74. **Binz, M., Frisckknecht, M., Shen,, F. W., and Wigzell, M.,** Idiotypic determinants on T cell subpopulations, *J. Exp. Med.*, 149, 910, 1979.
75. **Strassman, G., Lefshitz, R., and Mozes, E.,** Elicitation of delayed type hypersensitivity responses to poly(L Tyr, L Glu)-poly (DL Ala)— poly (L Lys) by anti-idiotypic antibodies, *J. Exp. Med.*, 152, 1448, 1980.
76. **Arnold, B., Wallech, R., and Hammerling, G. J.,** Elicitation of delayed-type hypersensitivity to phosphorylcholine by monoclonal anti-idiotypic antibodies in an allogeneic environment, *J. Exp. Med.*, 156, 670, 1982.
77. **Sy, M. S., Brown, A. R., Benacerraf, B., and Greene, M. I.,** Antigen and receptor driven regulatory mechanisms. III. Induction of delayed type hypersensitivity to azobenzenearsonate with anti-cross-reactive idiotypic antibodies, *J. Exp. Med.*, 151, 896, 1980.
78. **Jayaraman, S. and Bellone, C. J.,** Hapten specific responses to the phenyltrimethylamino hapten. I. Evidence for idiotype-anti-idiotype interactions in delayed-type hypersensitivity in mice, *Eur. J. Immunol.*, 12, 272, 1982.
79. **Thomas, W. R., Morahan, G., Walker, J. D., and Miller, J. F. A. P.,** Induction of delayed type hypersensitivity to azobenzene arsonate by a monoclonal antiidiotype antibody, *J. Exp. Med.*, 153, 743, 1981.
80. **Sy, M. S., Bach, B. A., Dohi, Y., Nisonoff, A., Benacerraf, B., and Greene, M. I.,** Antigen and receptor driven regulatory mechanisms. I. Induction of suppressor T cells with anti-idiotypic antibodies, *J. Exp. Med.*, 150, 1216, 1979.
81. **Yamamoto, H., Nonaka, M., and Katz, D. H.,** Suppression of hapten specific delayed type hypersensitivity responses in mice by idiotype specific suppressor T cells after administration of anti-idiotypic antibodies, *J. Exp. Med.*, 150, 818, 1979.

Chapter 9

ANTIBODIES SPECIFIC FOR THE T-CELL RECEPTOR

F. W. Fitch

TABLE OF CONTENTS

I. INTRODUCTION

The idea, first proposed by Jerne,[1,2] that idiotypes (Id) and complementary anti-idiotypes (anti-Id) constitute a network of interactions that plays a major role in the regulation of immune responses now is generally accepted. Id are the antigenic specificities of antibodies produced by an individual or a group of individuals in response to a given antigen.[3] Any given Id is the set of epitopes displayed by the variable regions of a set of antibody molecules.[1] An Id is identified on the basis of reactivity with an anti-Id antibody. Since the number of different antibody specificities is large, the number of Id (and corresponding anti-Id) is large. Unique amino acid sequences in the variable regions of antibody light and heavy chains seem to provide the structural basis for both antibody specificity and Id. Information regarding the structural basis for some idiotopes is accumulating, and particular amino acid sequences have been correlated with expression of specific Id.[4] However, as is true for many immunological terms, Id and idiotopes can be defined at present only in operational ways. In spite of the somewhat unsatisfactory working definition of immunoglobulin (Ig) Id and differing opinions with respect to the "completeness" of the Id network, involvement of an Id network in the regulation of B-lymphocyte responses presents no conceptual problems.[5,6]

However, an Id network involving T lymphocytes is a more complicated issue. T-lymphocyte Id have been dealt with in two quite different contexts. In the first, T and B lymphocytes have been considered to share Id. However, in spite of extensive supporting data,[7-12] this concept presents a number of problems. Information interpreted as showing expression of Ig Id by T lymphocytes usually was provided by observations made with incompletely characterized antigens and with heterogeneous populations of antibodies and lymphoid cells. The complexity inherent in such model systems made it difficult to be certain that the observed phenomena were uniquely the result of sharing of Id by the T-cell receptor (TCR) for antigen and antibodies. In addition, T and B cells appear to recognize antigens in fundamentally different ways. B lymphocytes react with antigens directly via the variable regions of their surface Ig. Recognition of antigen by T lymphocytes is restricted by molecules of the major histocompatibility complex (MHC).[13] Thus, the basic recognition mechanisms employed by B and T lymphocytes appeared to differ. Finally, it now is clear that genes encoding the α, β, and γ chains of the TCR are distinct and separate from those encoding the heavy and light chains of Ig peptides, although there are similarities in structure, organization, and mechanisms of rearrangement of genes for TCR and genes for Ig.[14-16] Therefore, if T lymphocytes and Ig do share Id, this cannot be based on utilization of shared genes.

In the second context, T cells have been considered to express Id that are analogous to, but distinct from, those of antibodies. Unique amino acid sequences in the variable domains TCR peptide chains seem to provide the structural basis for T-cell specificity. The gene segments encoding the variable, diversity, and joining regions of the α, β, and γ chains of the TCR are homologous to, but quite separate from, those encoding comparable regions of Ig peptide chains.[14-16] By analogy to Ig Id, T-cell Id can be defined as the antigenic specificities of T cells produced by an individual or a group of individuals in response to a given antigen. A T-cell Id, by this definition, is a set of epitopes displayed by the variable regions of a set of TCR. In this context, T-cell and Ig Id should be quite distinct. An antiserum reactive with an Ig Id would not be expected to react with a T-lymphocyte Id, although cross reactivity might occur by chance.

In the following discussion, anti-Id antibodies reactive with the TCR will be considered in both contexts. Emphasis will be placed on studies which have utilized monoclonal antibodies (mAb) and clonal populations of T cells, since results obtained with such systems usually are less ambiguous. T-cell Id analogous to, but distinct from, Ig Id will be discussed first. Evidence interpreted as indicating the sharing of Id by Ig and T cells then will be considered rather briefly, and an attempt will be made to reconcile the two differing concepts concerning T-cell Id. Portions of this material have been presented elsewhere.[17]

II. ANTIBODIES REACTIVE WITH THE T-CELL RECEPTOR FOR ANTIGEN

The definition of Ig Id was greatly facilitated by the availability of large quantities of homogeneous Ig. Initially, this was provided by myeloma proteins. Later, hybridoma antibodies reactive with specific antigens were used. The identification of the TCR and the characterization of T-cell Id also were facilitated by the availability of large numbers of homogeneous T cells.

A. Clonal Populations of T Lymphocytes

Several different approaches have been used to obtain clonal populations of T cells. T-cell lymphomas can be cloned and grown readily in culture. However, an independent identification of the antigen receptor on lymphoma cells may prove to be difficult. T-cell lymphomas that retain inducible immunologic functions apparently occur infrequently;[18] T-cell lymphomas having a particular function have been induced occasionally.[9-21] In spite of these difficulties, a T-cell lymphoma was used in one of the earliest studies that demonstrated the TCR biochemically.[22]

Construction of T-cell hybridomas, using modifications of the fusion method that has been applied so successfully for obtaining antibody-producing B-cell hybridomas,[23] has been a successful alternative approach for obtaining clonal populations of T cells. However, T-cell hybridomas are inherently unstable because of chromosome loss, and repetitive cloning at frequent intervals is necessary to maintain phenotypic and genetic homogeneity. Identification of particular hybrid cells as the fusion product of two T cells may not always be direct; some hybridomas formed by fusion of B and T tumor cell lines express the Thy-1 antigen of each parent cell.[24] Also, the tumor cell partner may contribute to the observed functions in ways that may be difficult to recognize.[25-27]

A third source of homogeneous functional T lymphocytes is cloned "normal" T cells. The discovery of T-cell growth factor, later called interleukin 2 (IL-2), made this approach feasible.[28] Although it may be possible to grow activated T cells in IL-2 alone, the frequency of cells capable of growing under these conditions appears to be low.[29] Often, activated T cells cultured in IL-2 alone grow well for about 2 months and then undergo a "crisis" with slowing of the growth rate. Cells then either die or suddenly begin to grow better. The characteristics of uncloned lymphocytes that survive after passage in IL-2 alone for several months often suggest that they are clonally derived,[29] but such cells also may be functionally unstable.[30] Most, if not all, cells grown in IL-2 alone for extended periods have chromosomal abnormalities, probably reflecting the selective growth of variant cells.[31]

Cloned cytolytic T lymphocytes (CTL) and helper T lymphocytes (HTL) that retain normal phenotypic characteristics can be maintained by repetitive stimulation at about weekly intervals with the appropriate antigen in the presence of accessory cells and relatively small amounts of IL-2.[32-35] For T cells reactive with conventional soluble antigens, irradiated syngeneic spleen cells usually are employed as a source of accessory cells, but clonal populations of B-lymphoma cells may be used.[36] The accessory cells serve as antigen-presenting cells, but they may also carry out other functions as well. Interleukin 1, secreted by or bound to accessory cells, appears to be required for the growth of at least some cloned murine T lymphocytes.[37,38] For alloreactive T lymphocytes, irradiated allogeneic murine spleen cells or transformed human peripheral blood B lymphocytes usually are used as a source of alloantigen; these cells meet other accessory cell requirements as well. Cloned T cells maintained in this manner usually are functionally stable and appear to be normal in phenotype and karyotype.

Maintaining cloned cells with antigen and small amounts of IL-2 appears to provide a strong selective pressure for T cells that respond to specific antigenic stimulation. Exposure to antigen increases expression of IL-2 receptors, thus, favoring the growth of specifically reactive T cells.[39] Passage at intervals of at least 7 days was found empirically to be optimal.[33] This rather lengthy culture cycle seems to be required for HTL, because this type of cell becomes unresponsive to restimulation following antigenic stimulation,[40] apparently as a result of exposure to IL-2 secreted in response to the initial antigenic stimulus.[41]

Each of these methods for obtaining homogeneous populations of T lymphocytes has advantages and disadvantages. Each type of cell has provided important information about T-cell Id and about the molecules that are involved in the recognition of antigen by T lymphocytes.

III. ANTI-ID ANTIBODIES REACTIVE WITH THE T-CELL ANTIGEN RECEPTOR

The first anti-Id antibody reactive with the TCR was identified indirectly. A tumor-specific mAb, obtained by immunizing with a murine T-cell lymphoma, precipitated a cell surface molecule that was composed of disulfide-linked 39- and 41-kdalton peptide subunits.[22] Although this mAb did not react with normal splenic lymphocytes, a similar heterodimeric structure could be identified when lysates of surface-labeled splenic T cells and thymocytes, but not B cells, were examined using the technique of two-dimensional electrophoresis.[22] In this procedure, cell extracts are separated first by electophoresis under nonreducing conditions. The gel containing the separated peptides is then treated with a reducing agent, and electrophoresis carried out in the second dimension at right angles to the first. Disulfide-linked structures are located ''off-diagonal'' in such gels. A set of peptides from normal T lymphocytes which appeared in an off-diagonal location in two-dimensional gels was located in the same positions as the peptides precipitated by the ''tumor-specific'' mAb.

The characteristics of this structure indicated that it was not one of the previously identified molecules that was specific for T cells. The fact that normal cells expressed a molecular complex biochemically similar to, but immunologically distinct from, that of a T-cell lymphoma suggested that this structure was a likely candidate for the long sought-after TCR. Subsequently, a xenoantiserum was obtained by immunizing rabbits with immune precipitates prepared from the T-cell lymphoma with the clonotypic mAb. Immunoprecipitates prepared with this antiserum showed that molecules from different T-cell populations had homologous structure. Two-dimensional tryptic peptide maps indicated that both peptides had regions of constant and variable structure, properties expected for the TCR.[42] Because an antigen-specific function for this T-cell lymphoma-specific cell surface molecule could not be demonstrated, the initial antiserum could not be identified with certainty as an anti-Id antibody reactive with a TCR.

IV. FUNCTIONAL EFFECTS OF ANTI-ID ANTIBODIES REACTIVE WITH THE T-CELL ANTIGEN RECEPTOR

The first candidates for anti-Id antibodies were identified on the basis of their ability to react uniquely with cloned T lymphocytes, and it seemed likely that such clonotypic mAb reacted with the TCR. Additional evidence that these clonotypic mAb were reactive with the TCR was provided by the finding that they inhibited antigen-specific responses of the appropriate T-cell clone. The size of the T-cell repertoire, at least for CTL, is rather large.[43] This is true even when T-cell responses are limited to the differences associated with substitution of a single amino acid in the α chain of the H-$2K^b$ molecule.[44] Given this extensive repertoire for antigen recognition, the prospect of developing antibodies reactive with the antigen receptor of individual T cells became realistic only when functional T-cell clones were developed for use as immunogen and for screening the mAb that were generated. This approach for generating anti-Id antibodies was based on the reasonable assumption that the TCR would be the most likely structure to be distributed clonally.

A number of antibodies reactive with specific T-cell clones have been obtained, but the general experience has been that their frequency is very low. A striking exception has been the experience with one particular cloned HTL that appears to stimulate the production of anti-TCR antibodies, perhaps by directly activating B cells bearing complementary receptors.[45] Two mAb reactive with an allotypic determinant of the TCR have been derived independently.[46,47] They seem to have the same specificity and react with about 20% of T cells from many common mouse strains, although the determinant appears to be absent in several strains. One of these mAb has been shown to react with epitopes encoded by a limited subset of V_β genes.[48] Monoclonal antibodies reactive with a variable proportion (up to 6%) of normal human T cells have been prepared by immunizing mice with human T-cell leukemic cells.[49,50] It is of some interest that T cells in cultures activated by one of these mAb contain both HTL and CTL cells bearing the idiotope.[50] It is somewhat surprising that immunization with cloned T cells has yielded mainly clonotypic antibodies which presumably are reactive with the variable domains of TCR.[37] Antisera which react with the constant region of denatured α or β TCR subunits in T-cell extracts have been prepared, but these antisera appear not to react with intact T cells.[51]

A. Inhibitory Effects of Anti-Id Antibodies Reactive with the T-Cell Antigen Receptor

The first reported clonotypic mAb was found to bind specifically with, and to block the cytolytic activity of, the cloned CTL used for immunization; it did not react with other cloned CTL.[52] Based on the amount of antibody bound, it was estimated that there were about 10,000 receptor molecules per cell.[53] Additional clonotypic mAb having similar properties soon were described.[37,54-58] It seems certain that these antibodies reacted with idiotopes on the TCR because they were clone-specific, and they specifically precipitated from these T-cell clones similar, but not identical, structures that had both variable and constant peptide regions.

Reinherz and colleagues provided the first extensive information about the functional effects of anti-Id mAb reactive with the TCR. They developed alloreactive human CTL clones and showed that such clones bearing the CD4 surface structure[59] reacted with Class II MHC antigens; clones bearing the T8 surface structure reacted with Class I MHC antigens.[34] They then derived clonotypic mAb reactive with clones of each phenotype and demonstrated that these mAb blocked antigen-specific cytolytic activity and antigen-induced proliferation of the appropriate clones.[55,56] These inhibitory effects were not due simply to an inactivation of the cloned cells as a result of antibody treatment, since the same mAb caused an augmentation of proliferation induced by IL-2.[60] About 30,000 sites were present per T cell,[55] and peptides of 43 and 49 to 51 kdalton were identified in immunoprecipitates prepared with these mAb.[55,56] Similar mAb, reactive with human inducer T lymphocytes, were also produced.[61]

Clonotypic antibodies reactive with the TCR of murine HTL hybridomas were identified on the basis of inhibition of antigen-induced lymphokine secretion.[54,57] There were from 15,000 to 25,000 receptor sites per cell, and two distinct peptides of 40,000 to 44,000 kdalton and 45,000 to 50,000 kdalton were found in immunoprecipitates.[62,63] Although most of the clonotypic mAb reacted only with the immunizing murine clone, one was found to react with a small proportion of cells enriched for T cells reacting with the same alloantigen.[52] Also, Marrack et al. screened about 400 T-cell hybridomas for reactivity with one of their clonotypic mAb and found one hybrid that reacted strongly.[64] This cross-reactive hybridoma was shown to have a fine specificity pattern of antigen recognition identical to that of the original hybridoma, both in terms of nominal antigen and MHC restriction. In addition, the maps of tryptic digests prepared from receptor peptides of the two cloned hybridomas were identical, suggesting that these two independently derived hybridomas had identical TCR.[64] Recently, a third hybridoma sharing these properties has been identified.[27] These findings would be expected if the TCR is clonally distributed and if the clonotypic mAb react with Id determinants on the TCR.

B. Stimulatory Effects of Anti-Id Antibodies Reactive with the T-Cell Antigen Receptor

Soluble clonotypic antibodies generally have been found to inhibit the functional activities of the cloned T cells with which they react. However, some of the first reported anti-Id antisera reactive with T cells stimulated proliferation of the appropriate T-cell clone but not other clones.[65] Thus, these sera appeared to contain both anti-Id antibodies reactive with the TCR as well as antibodies having other specificities.

In contrast to the inhibitory effects observed with soluble forms of antibody, anti-Id mAb reactive with the TCR induced proliferation and IL-2 secretion by the appropriate cloned T cells when linked to a solid support.[66] This effect was observed with human CTL clones reactive with Class I or Class II MHC antigens[66] as well as an antigen-reactive, Class II MHC antigen-restructed HTL.[61] Comparable effects have been observed with murine CTL and HTL cultured with immobilized mAb reactive with Id or allotypic determinants on the TCR.[67] Apparently, multimeric interaction between anti-Id mAb and the TCR is required for T-cell activation, since neither mAb not linked to surfaces[60] nor monovalent Fab fragments of anti-Id mAb activate.[68] This interpretation is not inconsistent with reports that clonotypic antisera can stimulate proliferation of cloned T cells.[65],[69] Such antisera have been found to stimulate better in the presence of irradiated syngeneic accessory cells.[69] Binding of anti-Id antibodies to Fc receptors on accessory cells may provide an appropriate array of antibody. In addition, binding of different soluble antibodies specific for separate epitopes on the TCR may result in multimeric interactions sufficient to activate T cells.

Proliferation of HTL and some CTL induced by immobilized anti-Id mAb appears to be due to induction of endogenous IL-2 secretion which, in turn, interacts with IL-2 receptors to cause T-cell division.[70] This autocrine pathway does not operate in those CTL which do not produce IL-2. However, an IL-2-independent pathway for proliferation can be activated in such CTL by immobilized anti-Id or anti-allotypic mAb.[67]

V. OTHER T-CELL SURFACE MOLECULES INVOLVED IN ANTIGEN RECOGNITION

Based on the evidence reviewed above, it seems clear that the α/β heterodimeric structure of the TCR constitutes the antigen-recognition unit of T lymphocytes and that anti-Id mAb reactive with idiotopes on this structure can modulate T-cell responses. However, there are other T-cell surface components which are involved in T-cell activation. The α/β heterodimeric structure is closely associated with, but not covalently linked to, the CD3 molecular complex. The involvement of CD3 in antigen recognition was first suggested by the observation that mAb reactive with CD3 blocked both the induction of CTL as well as the lytic activity of CTL and also inhibited antigen-induced T-cell proliferation.[61,71] Anti-CD3 mAb can be mitogenic for T cells.[72] Modulation of the CD3 complex by mAb also modulates the expression of cell surface TCR.[56] Immunoprecipitates obtained with anti-CD3 mAb frequently include antigen-receptor peptides.[73,74] There appears to be an obligatory requirement for the coexpression of the TCR and CD3. Mutants of the T-cell tumor line Jurkat which lacked either CD3 or the TCR failed to express both of these structures on the cell surface.[75] Several mutants were shown not to express a full-length mRNA for the β chain of the TCR. Transfection of one of these mutants with β chain cDNA induced led to expression of a functional CD3-TCR complex on the cell surface.[76]

The CD3 complex may be involved in transduction of the signal initiated by interaction of the TCR with antigen. TCR peptides themselves are not phosphorylated during activation.[77] However, 20- and 25-kdalton peptides, precipitated along with the α and β chain peptides by anti-Id mAb, are phosphorylated in response to activation of a murine T-cell hybridoma by antigen or by concanavalin A.[77,78] Although evidence that these phosphorylated peptides are part of the CD3 complex is indirect, the size and characteristics of these and other peptides found in the immunoprecipitation strongly suggest that this is the case.

CD4 and CD8 cell surface antigens are expressed on mutually exclusive subsets of T lymphocytes. The involvement of these structures in T-cell activation is indicated by the finding that mAb reactive with CD4 and CD8 inhibits antigen-specific functions of T cells.[34,79-81] T lymphocytes that react with or are restricted by Class I MHC antigens express CD8; most T lymphocytes that react with or are restricted by Class II MHC antigens expressed CD4. This is true both with human[34,82] and murine[81] lymphocytes. The genes encoding human CD4[83] and CD8[84,85] have been cloned. The protein structures for these two molecules, deduced from cDNA, reveal that both are integral membrane proteins which share significant amino acid and structural homologies with members of the Ig supergene family. The CD8 gene does not seem to be rearranged in cells which express the protein.[86] The CD4 and CD8 structures appear to serve as associative recognition structures, contributing to the overall avidity of interaction between the responding T cell and the antigen-presenting cell. It seems likely that nonpolymorphic determinants on MHC molecules are the target structures for CD4 and CD8, although this has not been demonstrated directly.

The LFA-1 molecular complex, one member of a family of related surface recognition molecules,[87] also seems to have an associative recognition function. LFA-1 consists of two peptide chains, an α subunit of approximately 170 kdalton and a β subunit of 95 kdalton.[88] Another member of this family, identified by several mAb (Mo1/MAC-1/OKM1) and found on granulocytes, monocytes, and some bone marrow cells,[89] shares a β subunit with LFA-1, but has a distinctive α subunit of 165 kdalton. A third member of this polypeptide family sharing the β subunit has been identified, but the function of this structure is not known. In addition, mAb reactive with CD2[90] and against a T-cell-specific peptide of 44 kdalton[91] can induce human T cells to release IL-2 and to proliferate.

VI. IMMUNOGLOBULIN ID AND T LYMPHOCYTES

Until it became clear that distinct sets of genes encoded Ig and TCR peptides, the hypothesis that B and T lymphocytes shared at least some variable region gene segments and, therefore, Id was quite attractive.[10,92,93] Such a mechanism would provide an efficient means for functionally distinct cells to utilize a common recognition process. Several different approaches yielded results which were consistent with the postulated sharing of Id by Ig and T lymphocytes. The rather large amount of data in this area will not be reviewed. Rather, results obtained with different model systems will be summarized briefly with reference mainly to review articles which contain extensive bibliographies.

The first evidence suggesting that T cells expressed Id determinants was provided by Ramseier and Lindenmann.[94,95] Their experiments were based on the concept that F_1 hybrid animals derived from inbred parental strains should express most, if not all, of the genetic information including MHC antigens from each parent. However, F_1 animals should not express the Id determinants present on the TCR encoded by genes from one parent and reactive with the MHC antigens of the other parent. T cells bearing such TCR would be self-reactive in the F_1 animal and, according to the clonal selection hypothesis, should have been deleted. To test this concept, lymphoid cells from one parental strain were injected into F_1 hybrid animals, and the resulting antisera were tested for effects on mixed leukocyte culture (MLC). These "antireceptor" antibodies inhibited T-cell reactivity in a highly specific way, although a complicated bioassay was used to measure the "product of antigen recognition".[96]

Similar approaches were used by Binz and Wigzell.[10,97] They found that anti-Id antisera raised by immunizing (Lewis × DA) F_1 hybrid rats with Lewis rat T cells could be used together with complement to deplete Lewis rat spleen cells capable of mediating specific Lewis anti-DA graft-vs.-host reactivity and Lewis anti-DA reactivity in MLC. Evidence for sharing of Ig and T-cell Id was provided by their observation that Lewis anti-DA antibody could absorb the activity of anti-Id antisera for Lewis rat T cells reactive with DA antigen. Heavy chains, but not light chains, of Lewis anti-DA antibody were capable of absorbing the anti-Id activity, suggesting that the relevant T-cell Id bore a V_H-like structure. Isolated monomeric 140-kdalton molecules produced by normal Lewis T cells were found to bind to anti-Idiotypic antibody and to DA alloantigen. Collectively, these data suggested that the antigen-binding portion of the TCR bore a V_H region.

Similar conclusions were reached by Eichmann and Rajewsky who used anti-Id antibody raised in guinea pigs against mouse antibody.[8,92] They studied the effects of such anti-Id antisera on the activity of T cells having the same specificity as the antibody used to immunize the guinea pigs. Small amounts of IgG1 antibody reactive with antistreptococcal A polysaccharide antibody primed helper T cells to respond to streptococcal A polysaccharide antigen. Anti-V_H-Id antibodies had similar effects, while anti-Id antibody reactive mainly with V_L did not prime T cells.[98] Several other kinds of evidence have suggested a relationship between Ig and TCR. A genetic linkage between T-cell Id and Ig heavy chain genes has been reported,[99,100] and Ig[101] and Ig-related[12,102] have been identified on the surface of T cells. Id-bearing, antigen-binding molecules have been isolated from T lymphocytes.[102]

It is difficult to explain these findings in light of the current evidence regarding the genetic basis for Ig and TCR structure. The modulation of immune responses attributed to anti-Id antibodies appears to be specific in each of these models. However, in the allograft models, a coordinated and nearly complete inhibition of both antibody and cell-mediated responses to multiple histocompatibility epitopes apparently occurs. The molecular nature of antigen-binding, Id-bearing molecules from T cells also is unclear. Conventional CTL and HTL appear not to secrete soluble TCR molecules. Perhaps, situations involving modulation of T-cell responses by anti-Id antibody are dominated by suppressor T cells. Although suppressor T-cell hybridomas have been constructed, most of them have shown no rearrangements of the β-chain gene of the TCR.[103,104]

Recently, data linking Ig and TCR Id have been provided with two reasonably well-defined model systems. The first involved synthetic peptides corresponding to an entire $J_{\beta 1}$ region and part of the D_β region predicted from the sequence of a human β-chain gene.[105] Antisera were prepared against these peptides, and affinity-purified anti-TCR peptides bound to intact IG and to light and heavy chains from Ig.[103] This result was expected based on significant homology between this peptide and J regions of several Ig heavy and light chains.[106] These results suggest that sufficient structural homology exists in isolated regions of Ig and TCR peptides to lead to immunologic cross reactivity in spite of the fact that genes are not directly shared.

The other model system involves a murine virus, several mAb, and murine CTL cell lines. The murine CTL response to reovirus type 3 is predominantly directed against the viral hemagglutinin (HA).[107] The antibody response to the HA of this virus is of limited heterogeneity,[108] and it was possible to generate a mAb which reacted with the HA and neutralized virus infection.[109] The anti-HA mAb was used, in turn, to generate an anti-Id mAb designated 87.92.6 which reacted with the mAb used for immunization and also with a receptor for the viral HA present on somatic cells.[110] This anti-Id mAb also reacted with reovirus-specific CTL clones obtained by limiting dilution.[111] The reactivity of anti-Id mAb 87.92.6 has been explored further using reovirus-specific CTL lines. The lytic activity of

CTL lines for virally infected target cells could be inhibited by monoclonal anti-Id antibody, by the anti-reovirus mAb used to generate the anti-Id mAb, and by anti-MHC antibodies.[112] The Id expressed by this CTL line seemed to represent a dominant Id, since 25% of reovirus type 3-specific CTL recognized a specific anti-Id determinant.[110,111] The monoclonal anti-Idiotypic antibody was capable of inducing T-cell-mediated immune responses when administered to mice in vivo.[113,114] This immunity was mapped to the neutralizing domain of the viral hemagglutinin, the region of the virus with which the mAb used for generating the anti-Id mAb reacted.[110] Thus, in this well-characterized model system, the TCR of a murine CTL line and a mAb reactive with the hemagglutinin of reovirus type 3 shared an Id identified by a monoclonal anti-Id antibody generated by immunization with the anti-viral mAb. The anti-Id antibody could induce immune responses in vivo and, therefore, provides a means for regulating both antibody and T-cell-mediated immune responses.

However, the situation is actually more complicated. It appears that anti-Id mAb 87.92.6, in addition to its anti-Id characteristics, also bears an "internal image" of the cell surface binding site of the reovirus type 3 hemagglutinin.[115] When the β sheet structures of the complementary-determining regions (CDR) of the anti-Id mAb 87.92.6 were compared with β sheet structures in the hemagglutinin globular region of reovirus type 3, homologies were detected. A high level of homology was evident between a region within and just adjacent to the second CDR of the light chain polypeptide and a portion of the globular region of the viral hemagglutinin thought to be involved in reovirus infectivity.[115] In addition to the anti-Id properties of mAb 87.92.6, this molecule acts as an internal image of the cell surface binding site of reovirus type 3 and, as a consequence of this property, is able to bind to the cellular receptor for reovirus and act as an autoimmune antibody.[115] It is not yet known how common this sort of mimicry is; a number of other examples have been identified.[116] Sharing of primary sequences by idiotopes and external ligands provides another mechanism for generating interacting regulatory immune networks. These considerations may relate to the relative immunogenicity of idiotopes. This type of antigen mimicry may account for sharing of T- and B-cell Id in other situations where more direct explanations seem unlikely.

VII. A SUMMING UP

Recent information obtained using clonal populations of T lymphocytes indicates that the α/β chains of the TCR are encoded by genes that are distinct from those encoding Ig peptides. However, the structure, organization, and patterns of rearrangements of these genes are quite similar to those of Ig genes. Genes for the γ chain also are distinct from those of Ig, but the relationship of this chain to the functional TCR on mature T lymphocytes is not clear. Evidence that the α/β heterodimeric structure constitutes the antigen-specific recognition component of the TCR is largely indirect, but is rather compelling. In addition to the α/β heterodimeric structure of the TCR, the functional receptor unit includes the CD3 molecular complex. Other T-cell surface molecules including CD4, CD8, LFA-1, and CD2 are involved in T-cell activation by antigen. However, assuming that the α/β subunit of the TCR is the antigen recognition unit, T lymphocytes do seem to express unique Id determinants analogous to, but distinct from, Ig Id.

It is less clear how T lymphocytes widely share Id with B lymphocytes. Several years ago, this question was addressed provocatively in a series of short editorials dealing specifically with Ig gene expression by T cells.[117-123] The summarizing editorial concluded that if TCR and Ig genes were related, the postulated homology between the TCR and Ig is sufficiently remote to obliterate detectable cross-hybridization with gene probes.[117] More recent results suggest that such homologies may exist, but that they are not extensive.[106] Some of the in vivo and in vitro effects of anti-Id antibody may be mediated by B-cell and antibody-Id targets intrinsic to the assays rather than by T cells.[124] However, these explanations seem to be insufficient to account for all instances of Id sharing. "Antigen mimicry", such as that observed in the primary sequence identity of reovirus type 3 and anti-Id mAb, provides another mechanism for generating immunoregulatory Id networks. It seems likely that other mechanisms will be discovered to explain why T and B lymphocytes may share Id in situations where Id networks appear to play dominant roles in the regulation of immune responses. Exclusion of gene sharing by T and B lymphocytes does not rule out other mechanisms that may result in sharing of immunologically defined Id.

REFERENCES

1. **Jerne, N.,** Towards a network theory of the immune system, *Ann. Immunol. (Inst. Pasteur),* 125, 373, 1974.
2. **Jerne, N.,** The generative grammar of the immune system, *EMBO J.,* 4, 847, 1985.
3. **Oudin, J.,** L'idiotypie des anticorps, *Ann. Immunol. (Inst. Pasteur),* 125C, 309, 1974.
4. **Davie, J., Seiden, M., Greenspan, N., Lutz, C., Bartholow, T., and Clevinger, B.,** Structural correlates of idiotopes, *Annu. Rev. Immunol.,* 4, 147, 1986.
5. **Coutinho, A.,** The self-nonself discrimination and the nature and acquisition of the antibody repertoire, *Ann. Immunol. (Inst. Pasteur),* 131D, 235, 1980.
6. **Langman, R. and Cohn, M.,** The 'complete' idiotypic network is an absurd immune system, *Immunol. Today,* 7, 100, 1986.
7. **Ramseier, H. and Lindenmann, J.,** Aliotypic antibodies, *Transplant. Rev.,* 10, 57, 1972.
8. **Eichmann, K. and Rajewsky, K.,** Induction of T and B cell immunity by anti-idiotypic antibody, *Eur. J. Immunol.,* 5, 661, 1975.
9. **Cosenza, H., Julius, M., and Augustin, A.,** Idiotypes as variable region markers: analogies between receptors on phosphorylcholine-specific T and B lymphocytes, *Immunol. Rev.,* 34, 3, 1977.
10. **Binz, H. and Wigzell, H.,** Antigen-binding, idiotypic T-lymphocyte receptors, *Contemp. Top. Immunobiol.,* 7, 113, 1977.
11. **Janeway, C.,** Idiotypes, T-cell receptors, and T-B cooperation, *Contemp. Top. Immunobiol.,* 9, 171, 1980.
12. **Cone, R.,** Molecular basis for T lymphocyte recognition of antigens, *Prog. Allergy,* 29, 182, 1981.
13. **Zinkernagel, R. and Doherty, P.,** MHC-restricted cytotoxic T cells: studies on the biological role of polymorphic major transplantation antigens determining T-cell restriction-specificity, function, and responsiveness, *Adv. Immunol.,* 27, 51, 1979.
14. **Davis, M.,** Molecular genetics of the T cell-receptor beta chain, *Annu. Rev. Immunol.,* 3, 537, 1985.
15. **Hood, L., Kronenberg, M., and Hunkapiller, T.,** T cell antigen receptors and the immunoglobulin supergene family, *Cell,* 40, 225, 1985.
16. **Mak, T. and Yanagi, Y.,** Genes encoding the human T cell antigen receptor, *Immunol. Rev.,* 81, 221, 1984.
17. **Fitch, F.,** T cell clones and T cell receptors, *Microbiol. Rev.,* 50, 50, 1986.
18. **Gillis, S., Scheid, M., and Watson, J.,** Biochemical and biologic characterization of lymphocyte regulatory molecules. III. The isolation and phenotypic characterization of interleukin-2 producing T cell lymphomas, *J. Immunol.,* 125, 2570, 1980.
19. **Fathman, C. and Weissman, I.,** Production of alloreactive T-cell lymphomas, *Nature (London),* 283, 404, 1980.
20. **Finn, O., Boniver, J., and Kaplan, H.,** Induction, establishment in vitro and characterization of functional antigen-specific, carrier-primed murine T-cell lymphomas, *Proc. Natl. Acad. Sci. U.S.A.,* 76, 4033, 1979.
21. **Ricciardi-Castagnoli, P., Doria, G., and Adorini, L.,** Production of antigen-specific suppressive T cell factor by radiation leukemia virus-transformed suppressor T cells, *Proc. Natl. Acad. Sci. U.S.A.,* 78, 3804, 1981.
22. **Allison, J., McIntyre, B., and Bloch, D.,** Tumor-specific antigen of murine T-lymphoma defined with monoclonal antibody, *J. Immunol.,* 129, 2293, 1982.
23. **Kohler, G. and Milstein, C.,** Continuous cultures of fused cells secreting antibodies of predefined specificities, *Nature (London),* 256, 495, 1975.
24. **Taussig, M., Holliman, A., and Wright, L.,** Hybridization between T and B lymphoma cell lines, *Immunology,* 39, 57, 1980.
25. **Clark, A. and Capra, J.,** Ubiquitous nonimmunoglobulin p-azobenzene-arsonate-binding molecules from lymphoid cells, *J. Exp. Med.,* 155, 611, 1982.

26. **Pacifico, A. and Capra, J.,** T cell hybrids with arsonate specificity. I. Initial characterization of antigen-specific T cell products that bear a cross-reactive idiotype and determinants encoded by the murine major histocompatibility complex, *J. Exp. Med.*, 152, 1289, 1980.
27. **Yague, J., White, J., Coleclough, C., Kappler, J., Palmer, E., and Marrack, P.,** The T cell receptor: the α and β chains define idiotype, and antigen and MHC specificity, *Cell,* 42, 81, 1985.
28. **Morgan, D., Ruscetti, F., and Gallo, R.,** Selective in vitro growth of T lymphocytes from normal human bone marrows, *Science,* 193, 1007, 1976.
29. **Haas, W., Mathur-Rochat, J., Pohlit, H., Nabholz, M., and Von Boehmer, H.,** Cytotoxic T cell responses to haptenated cells. III. Isolation and specificity analysis of continuously growing clones, *Eur. J. Immunol.*, 10, 828, 1980.
30. **Nabholz, M., Engers, H., Collavo, D., and North, M.,** Cloned T cell lines with specific cytolytic activity, *Curr. Top. Microbiol. Immunol.*, 81, 176, 1978.
31. **Johnson, J., Cianfriglia, M., Glasebrook, A., and Nabholz, M.,** Karyotype evolution of cytolytic T cell lines, in *Isolation, Characterization, and Utilization of T Lymphocyte Clones,* Fathman, C. G. and Fitch, F. W., Eds., Academic Press, New York, 1982, 183.
32. **Fathman, C. and Hengartner, H.,** Clones of alloreactive T-cells, *Nature (London),* 272, 617, 1978.
33. **Glasebrook, A., Sarmiento, M., Loken, M., Dialynas, D., Quintans, J., Eisenberg, L., Lutz, C., Wilde, D., and Fitch, F.,** Murine T lymphocyte clones with distinct immunological functions, *Immunol. Rev.*, 54, 225, 1981.
34. **Meuer, S., Schlossman, S., and Reinherz, E.,** Clonal analysis of human cytotoxic T lymphocytes: T4+ and T8+ effector T cells recognize products of different major histocompatibility complex regions, *Proc. Natl. Acad. Sci. U.S.A.*, 79, 4395, 1982.
35. **Reiss, C., Hemler, M., Englehard, V., Mier, J., Strominger, J., and Burakoff, S.,** Development and characterization of allospecific long-term human cytolytic T-cell lines, *Proc. Natl. Acad. Sci. U.S.A.*, 77, 5432, 1980.
36. **Glimcher, L., Kim, K.-J., Green, I., and Paul, W.,** Ia antigen-bearing B cell tumor lines can present protein antigen and alloantigen in a major histocompatibility complex-restricted fashion to antigen-reactive T cells, *J. Exp. Med.*, 155, 445, 1982.
37. **Kaye, J., Porcelli, S., Tite, J., Jones, B., and Janeway, C. J.,** Both a monoclonal antibody and antisera specific for determinants unique to individual cloned helper T cell lines can substitute for antigen and antigen-presenting cells in the activation of T cells, *J. Exp. Med.*, 158, 836, 1983.
38. **Kurt-Jones, E., Beller, D., Mizel, S., and Unanue, E.,** Identification of a membrane-associated interleukin 1 in macrophages, *Proc. Natl. Acad. Sci. U.S.A.*, 82, 1204, 1985.
39. **Hemler, M., Brenner, M., McLean, J., and Strominger, J.,** Antigenic stimulation regulates the level of expression of interleukin 2 receptor on human T cells, *Proc. Natl. Acad. Sci. U.S.A.*, 81, 2172, 1984.
40. **Wilde, D. and Fitch, F.,** Antigen-reactive cloned helper T cells. I. Unresponsiveness to antigenic restimulation develops after stimulation of cloned helper T cells, *J. Immunol.*, 132, 1632, 1984.
41. **Wilde, D., Prystowsky, M., Ely, J., Vogel, S., Dialynas, D., and Fitch, F.,** Antigen-reactive cloned helper T cells. II. Exposure of murine cloned helper T cells to IL 2-containing supernatant induces unresponsiveness to antigenic restimulation and inhibits lymphokine production after antigenic stimulation, *J. Immunol.*, 133, 636, 1984.
42. **McIntyre, B. and Allison, J.,** Biosynthesis and processing of murine T-cell antigen receptor, *Cell,* 38, 659, 1984.
43. **Sherman, L.,** The specificity repertoire of cytolytic T lymphocytes, in *Isolation, Characterization and Utilization of T Lymphocyte Clones,* Fathman, C. G. and Fitch, F. W., Eds., Academic Press, New York, 1982, 313.
44. **Sherman, L.,** Recognition of conformational determinants on H-2 by cytolytic T lymphocytes, *Nature (London),* 297, 511, 1982.
45. **Tite, J., Kaye, J., Saizawa, K., Ming, J., Katz, M., Smith, L., and Janeway, C., Jr.,** Direct interactions between B and T lymphocytes bearing complementary receptors, *J. Exp. Med.*, 163, 189, 1986.
46. **Haskins, K., Hannum, C., White, J., Roehm, N., Kubo, R., Kappler, J., and Marrack, P.,** The antigen-specific major histocompatibility complex-restricted receptor on T cells. VI. An antibody to a receptor allotype, *J. Exp. Med.*, 160, 452, 1984.
47. **Staerz, U., Rammensee, H.-G., Benedetto, J., and Bevan, M.,** Characterization of a murine monoclonal antibody specific for an allotypic determinant on T cell antigen receptor, *J. Immunol.*, 134, 3994, 1985.
48. **Sim, G. and Augustin, A.,** V_β gene polymorphism and a major polyclonal T cell receptor idiotype, *Cell,* 42, 89, 1985.
49. **Bigler, R., Posnett, D., and Chiorazzi, N.,** Stimulation of a subset of normal resting T lymphocytes by a monoclonal antibody to a crossreactive determinant of the human T cell antigen receptor, *J. Exp. Med.*, 161, 1450, 1985.
50. **Boylston, A. and Cosford, P.,** Growth of normal human T lymphocytes induced by monoclonal antibody to the T cell antigen receptor, *Eur. J. Immunol.*, 15, 738, 1985.

51. **Fabbi, M., Acuto, O., Bensussan, A., Poole, C., and Reinherz, E.,** Production and characterization of antibody probes directed at constant regions of the α and β subunit of the human T cell receptor, *Eur. J. Immunol.*, 15, 821, 1985.
52. **Lancki, D., Lorber, M., Loken, M., and Fitch, F.,** A clone-specific monoclonal antibody that inhibits cytolysis of a cytolytic T cell clone, *J. Exp. Med.*, 157, 921, 1983.
53. **Sarmiento, M., Dialynas, D., Lancki, D., Wall, K., Lorber, M., Loken, M., and Fitch, F.,** Cloned T lymphocytes and monoclonal antibodies as probes for cell surface molecules active in T cell-mediated cytolysis, *Immunol. Rev.*, 68, 135, 1982.
54. **Haskins, K., Kubo, R., White, J., Pigeon, M., Kappler, J., and Marrack, P.,** The major histocompatibility complex-restricted antigen receptor on T cells. I. Isolation with a monoclonal antibody, *J. Exp. Med.*, 157, 1149, 1983.
55. **Meuer, S., Acuto, O., Hussey, R., Hodgdon, J., Fitzgerald, K., Schlossman, S., and Reinherz, E.,** Evidence for the T-3 associated 90K heterodimer as the T-cell antigen receptor, *Nature (London)*, 303, 808, 1983.
56. **Meuer, S., Fitzgerald, K., Hussey, R., Hodgdon, J., Schlossman, S., and Reinherz, E.,** Clonotypic structures involved in antigen-specific human T cell function. Relationship to the T3 molecular complex, *J. Exp. Med.*, 157, 705, 1983.
57. **Samelson, L., Germain, R., and Schwartz, R.,** Monoclonal antibodies against the antigen receptor on a cloned T-cell hybrid, *Proc. Natl. Acad. Sci. U.S.A.*, 80, 6972, 1983.
58. **Staerz, U., Pasternack, M., Klein, J., Benedetto, J., and Bevan, M.,** Monoclonal antibodies specific for a murine cytotoxic T-lymphocyte clone, *Proc. Natl. Acad. Sci. U.S.A.*, 81, 1799, 1984.
59. IUIS-WHO Nomenclature Subcommittee, Nomenclature for clusters of differentiation (CD) of antigens defined on human leukocyte populations, *Bull. W.H.O.*, 62, 809, 1984.
60. **Reinherz, E., Acuto, O., Fabbi, M., Bensussan, A., Milanese, C., Royer, H., Meuer, S., and Schlossman, S.,** Clonotypic surface structure on human T lymphocytes: functional and biochemical analysis of the antigen receptor complex, *Immunol. Rev.*, 81, 93, 1984.
61. **Meuer, S., Cooper, D., Hodgdon, J., Hussey, R., Fitzgerald, K., Schlossman, S., and Reinherz, E.,** Identification of the receptor for antigen and major histocompatibility complex on human inducer T lymphocytes, *Science*, 222, 1239, 1983.
62. **Kappler, J., Kubo, R., Haskins, K., White, J., and Marrack, P.,** The mouse T cell receptor: comparision of MHC-restricted receptors on two T cell hybridomas, *Cell*, 34, 727, 1983.
63. **Samelson, L.,** An analysis of the structure of the antigen receptor on a pigeon cytochrome c-specific T cell hybrid, *J. Immunol.*, 134, 2529, 1985.
64. **Marrack, P., Shimonkevitz, R., Hannum, C., Haskins, K., and Kappler, J.,** The major histocompatibility complex-restricted antigen receptor on T cells. IV. An antiidiotypic antibody predicts both antigen and I-specificity, *J. Exp. Med.*, 158, 1635, 1983.
65. **Infante, A., Infante, P., Gillis, S., and Fathman, C.,** Definition of T cell idiotypes using anti-idiotypic antisera produced by immunization with T cell clones, *J. Exp. Med.*, 155, 1100, 1982.
66. **Meuer, S., Hodgdon, J., Hussey, R., Protentis, J., Schlossman, S., and Reinherz, E.,** Antigen-like effects of monoclonal antibodies directed at receptors on human T cell clones, *J. Exp. Med.*, 158, 988, 1983.
67. **Moldwin, R., Lancki, D., Herold, K., and Fitch, F.,** An antigen-receptor-driven, IL-2 independent pathway for proliferation of murine CTL clones, *J. Exp. Med.*, 163, 1566, 1986.
68. **Kaye, J. and Janeway, C. J.,** The Fab fragment of a directly activating monoclonal antibody that precipitates a disulfide-linked heterodimer from a helper T cell clone blocks activation by either allogeneic Ia or antigen and self-Ia, *J. Exp. Med.*, 159, 1397, 1984.
69. **Frelinger, J., Sing, A., Infante, A., and Fathman, C.,** Clonotypic antibodies which stimulate T cell clone proliferation, *Immunol. Rev.*, 81, 21, 1984.
70. **Meuer, S., Hussey, R., Cantrell, D., Hodgdon, J., Schlossman, S., Smith, K., and Reinherz, E.,** Triggering of the T3-Ti antigen-receptor complex results in clonal T-cell proliferation through an interleukin 2-dependent autocrine pathway, *Proc. Natl. Acad. Sci. U.S.A.*, 81, 1509, 1984.
71. **Reinherz, E., Hussey, R., and Schlossman, S.,** A monoclonal antibody blocking human T cell function, *Eur. J. Immunol.*, 10, 758, 1980.
72. **Van Wauwe, J., De Mey, J., and Goossens, J.,** OKT3: a monoclonal antihuman T lymphocyte antibody with potent mitogenic properties, *J. Immunol.*, 124, 2708, 1980.
73. **Borst, J., Prendiville, M., and Terhorst, C.,** Complexity of the human T lymphocyte-specific cell surface antigen T3, *J. Immunol.*, 128, 1560, 1982.
74. **Reinherz, E., Meuer, S., Fitzgerald, K., Hussey, R., Hodgdon, J., Acuto, O., and Schlossman, S.,** Comparison of T3-associated 49- and 43-kilodalton cell surface molecules on individual human T-cell clones: evidence for peptide variability in T-cell receptor structures, *Proc. Natl. Acad. Sci. U.S.A.*, 80, 4104, 1983.

75. **Weiss, A. and Stobo, J. B.,** Requirement for the coexpression of T3 and the T cell antigen receptor on a malignant human T cell line, *J. Exp. Med.,* 160, 1284, 1984.
76. **Ohashi, P., Mak, T., Van Den Elsen, P., Yanagi, Y., Yoshikai, Y., Calman, A., Terhorst, C., Stobo, J., and Weiss, A.,** Reconstitution of an active surface T3/T-cell antigen receptor by DNA transfer, *Nature (London),* 316, 606, 1985.
77. **Samelson, L., Harford, J., Schwartz, R., and Klausner, R.,** A 20-kDa protein associated with the murine T-cell antigen receptor is phosphorylated in response to activation by antigen or concanavalin A, *Proc. Natl. Acad. Sci. U.S.A.,* 82, 1969, 1985.
78. **Samelson, L. Harford, J., and Klausner, R.,** Identification of the components of the murine T cell antigen receptor complex, *Cell,* 43, 223, 1985.
79. **Engleman, E., Benike, C., Glickman, E., and Evans, R.,** Antibodies to membrane structures that distinguish suppressor/cytotoxic and helper T lymphocyte sub-populations block the mixed leukocyte reaction in man, *J. Exp. Med.,* 154, 193, 1981.
80. **Ledbetter, J. and Seaman, W.,** The Lyt-2, Lyt-3 macromolecules; structural and functional studies, *Immunol. Rev.,* 68, 197, 1982.
81. **Dialynas, D., Wilde, D., Marrack, P., Pierres, A., Wall, K., Havran, W., Otten, G., Loken, M., Pierres, M., Kappler, J., and Fitch, F.,** Characterization of the murine antigenic determinant, designated L3T4a, recognized by monoclonal antibody GK1.5: expression of L3T4a by functional T cell clones appears to correlate primarily with class II MHC antigen-reactivity, *Immunol. Rev.,* 74, 29, 1983.
82. **Engleman, E., Benike, C., Grumet, F., and Evans, R.,** Activation of human T lymphocyte subsets: helper and suppressor/cytotoxic T cells recognize and respond to distinct histocompatibility antigens, *J. Immunol.,* 127, 2124, 1981.
83. **Maddon, P., Littman, D., Godfrey, M., Maddon, D., Chess, L., and Axel, R.,** The isolation and nucleotide sequence of a cDNA encoding the T cell surface protein T4: a new member of the immunoglobulin gene family, *Cell,* 42, 93, 1985.
84. **Kavathas, P., Sukhatme, V., Herzenberg, L., and Parnes, J.,** Isolation of the gene encoding the human T-lymphocyte differentiation antigen Leu-2 (T8) by gene transfer and cDNA subtraction, *Proc. Natl. Acad. Sci. U.S.A.,* 81, 7688, 1984.
85. **Littman, D., Thomas, Y., Maddon, P., Chess, L., and Axel, R.,** The isolation and sequence of the gene encoding T8: a molecule defining functional classes of T lymphocytes, *Cell,* 40, 237, 1985.
86. **Sukhatme, V., Sizer, K., Vollmer, A., Hunkapiller, T., and Parnes, J.,** The T cell differentiation antigen Leu-2/T8 is homologous to immunoglobulin and T cell receptor variable regions, *Cell,* 40, 591, 1985.
87. **Springer, T.,** The LFA-1, Mac-1 glycoprotein family and its deficiency in an inherited disease, *Fed. Proc. Fed. Am. Soc. Exp. Biol.,* 44, 2660, 1985.
88. **Sanchez-Madrid, F., Nagy, J., Robbins, E., Simon, P., and Springer, T.,** A human leukocyte differentiation antigen family with distinct α-subunits and a common β-subunit: the lymphocyte function-associated antigen (LFA-1), the C3bi complement receptor (OKM1/Mac-1), and the p150,95 molecule, *J. Exp. Med.,* 158, 1785, 1983.
89. **Springer, T., Galfre, G., Secher, D., and Milstein, C.,** Mac-1: a macrophage differentiation antigen identified by monoclonal antibody, *Eur. J. Immunol.,* 9, 301, 1979.
90. **Meuer, S., Hussey, R., Fabbi, M., Fox, D., Acuto, O., Fitzgerald, K., Hodgdon, J., Protentis, J., Schlossman, S., and Reinherz, E.,** An alternative pathway of T-cell activation: a functional role for the 50 kd T11 sheep erythrocyte receptor protein, *Cell,* 36, 897, 1984.
91. **Hara, T., Fu, S., and Hansen, J.,** Human T cell activation. II. A new activation pathway used by a major T cell population via a disulfide-bonded dimer of a 44 kilodalton polypeptide (9.3 antigen), *J. Exp. Med.,* 161, 1513, 1985.
92. **Rajewsky, K. and Eichmann, K.,** Antigen receptors of T helper cells, *Contemp. Top. Immunobiol.,* 7, 69, 1977.
93. **Eichmann, K.,** Expression and function of idiotypes on lymphocytes, *Adv. Immunol.,* 26, 195, 1978.
94. **Ramseier, H. and Lindenmann, J.,** Aliotypic antibodies, *Transplant. Rev.,* 10, 57, 1972.
95. **Ramseier, H., Aguet, M., and Lindenmann, J.,** Similarity of idiotypic determinants of T- and B-lymphocyte receptors for alloantigens, *Immunol. Rev.,* 34, 50, 1977.
96. **Ramseier, H.,** Spontaneous release of T-cell receptors for alloantigens. I. Recognition of alloantigens and receptor release dynamics, *J. Exp. Med.,* 140, 603, 1974.
97. **Binz, H. and Wigzell, H.,** Antigen-binding, idiotypic receptors from T lymphocytes: an analysis of their biochemistry, genetics, and use as immunogens to produce specific immune tolerance, *Cold Spring Harbor Symp. Quant. Biol.,* 41, 275, 1976.
98. **Krawinkel, U., Cramer, M., Berek, C., Hammerling, G., Black, S. J., Rajewsky, K., and Eichmann, K.,** On the structure of the T-cell receptor for antigen, *Cold Spring Harbor Symp. Quant. Biol.,* 41, 285, 1976.

99. **Krammer, P. and Eichmann, K.,** T cell receptor idiotypes are controlled by genes in the heavy chain linkage group and the major histocompatibility complex, *Nature (London),* 270, 733, 1977.
100. **Rubin, B., Hertel-Wulff, B., and Kimura, A.,** Alloantigen-specific idiotype-bearing receptors on mouse T lymphocytes. I. Specificity characterization and genetic association with the heavy-chain IgG allotype, *J. Exp. Med.,* 150, 307, 1979.
101. **Warner, N.,** Membrane immunoglobulins and antigen receptors on B and T lymphocytes, *Adv. Immunol.,* 19, 67, 1974.
102. **Marchalonis, J.,** Antigen-binding molecules of T cells: distinction from MHC-restricted molecules and segmental homology to immunoglobulin V_H and T-cell receptor genes, *Scand. J. Immunol.,* 24, 99, 1985.
103. **Blanckmeister, C., Yamamoto, K., Davis, M., and Hammerling, G.,** Antigen-specific, I-A-restricted suppressor hybridomas with spontaneous cytolytic activity. Functional properties and lack of rearrangement of the T cell receptor β chain genes, *J. Exp. Med.,* 162, 851, 1985.
104. **Hedrick, S., Germain, R., Bevan, M., Dorf, M., Engel, I., Fink, P., Gascoigne, N., Heber-Katz, E., Kapp, J., Kaufmann, Y., Kaye, J., Melchers, F., Pierce, C., Schwartz, R., Sorensen, C., Taniguchi, M., and Davis, M.,** Rearrangement and transcription of a T-cell receptor β-chain gene in different T-cell subsets, *Proc. Natl. Acad. Sci. U.S.A.,* 82, 531, 1985.
105. **Yanagi, Y., Yoshikai, Y., Leggett, K., Clark, S., Aleksander, I., and Mak, T.,** A human T cell-specific cDNA clone encodes a protein having extensive homology to immunoglobulin chains, *Nature (London),* 308, 145, 1984.
106. **Schluter, S. and Marchalonis, J.,** Antibodies to synthetic joining segment peptide of the T-cell receptor β-chain: serological cross-reaction between products of T-cell receptor genes, antigen binding T-cell receptors and immunoglobulins, *Proc. Natl. Acad. Sci. U.S.A.,* 83, 1872, 1986.
107. **Finberg, R., Weiner, H., Fields, B., Benacerraf, B., and Burakoff, S.,** Generation of cytolytic T lymphocytes after reovirus infection: role of S1 gene, *Proc. Natl. Acad. Sci. U.S.A.,* 76, 442, 1979.
108. **Nepom, J., Weiner, H., Dichter, M., Tardieu, M., Spriggs, D., Gramm, C., Powers, M., Fields, B., and Greene, M.,** Identification of a hemagglutinin-specific idiotype associated with reovirus recognition shared by lymphoid and neural cells, *J. Exp. Med.,* 155, 155, 1982.
109. **Burstin, S., Spriggs, D., and Fields, B.,** Evidence for functional domains on the reovirus Type 3 hemagglutinin, *Virology,* 117, 146, 1982.
110. **Noseworthy, J., Fields, B., Dichter, M., Sobotka, C., Pizer, E., Perry, L., Nepom, J., and Greene, M.,** Cell receptors for the mammalian reovirus. I. Syngeneic monoclonal anti-idiotypic antibody identifies a cell surface receptor for reovirus, *J. Immunol.,* 131, 2533, 1983.
111. **Ertl, H., Greene, M., Noseworthy, J., Fields, B., Nepom, J., Spriggs, D., and Finberg, R.,** Identification of idiotypic receptors on reovirus-specific cytolytic T cells, *Proc. Natl. Acad. Sci. U.S.A.,* 79, 7479, 1982.
112. **Sharpe, A., Gaulton, G., Ertl, H., Fineberg, R., McDade, K., Fields, B., and Greene, M.,** Cell receptors for the mammalian reovirus. IV. Reovirus-specific cytolytic T cell lines that have idiotypic receptors recognize anti-idiotypic B cell hybridomas, *J. Immunol.,* 134, 2702, 1985.
113. **Sharpe, A., Gaulton, G., McDade, K., Fields, B., and Greene, M.,** Syngeneic monoclonal antiidiotype can induce cellular immunity to reovirus, *J. Exp. Med.,* 160, 1195, 1984.
114. **Ertl, H., Homans, E., Tournas, S., and Finberg, R.,** Sendai virus-specific T cell clones. V. Induction of a virus-specific response by antiidiotypic antibodies directed against a T helper cell clone, *J. Exp. Med.,* 159, 1778, 1984.
115. **Bruck, C., Co, M., Slaoui, M., Gaulton, G., Smith, T., Mullins, J., and Greene, M.,** Nucleic acid sequence of an internal image-bearing monoclonal anti-idiotype and its comparison to that of the external image, *Proc. Natl. Acad. Sci. U.S.A.,* 83, 6578, 1986.
116. **Gaulton, G. and Greene, M.,** Idiotypic mimicry of biological receptors, *Annu. Rev. Immunol.,* 4, 253, 1980.
117. **Coutinho, A. and Meo, T.,** Immunoglobulin gene expression by T lymphocytes, *Scand. J. Immunol.,* 18, 79, 1983.
118. **Honjo, T.,** The T-lymphocyte antigen receptor — an imaginary monster?, *Scand. J. Immunol.,* 18, 83, 1983.
119. **Cone, R.,** On the expression of immunoglobulin genes by T lymphocytes, *Scand. J. Immunol.,* 18, 86, 1983.
120. **Goding, J. and Nossal, G.,** The T-cell receptor for antigen: past, present and future, *Scand. J. Immunol.,* 18, 89, 1983.
121. **Julius, M.,** Antigen recognition structures on T cells: involvement of immunoglobulin gene expression, *Scand. J. Immunol.,* 18, 93, 1983.
122. **Rajewsky, K.,** Cross-reacting idiotypes on antibodies and T-cell receptors: how can the data be interpreted?, *Scand. J. Immunol.,* 18, 95, 1983.

123. **Rubin, B.,** On the genes responsible for expression of antigen-specific T-cell recognition and function, *Scand. J. Immunol.,* 18, 97, 1983.
124. **Miller, J., Morahan, G., and Walker, I.,** T-cell antigen receptors: fact and artefact, *Immunol. Today,* 4, 141, 1983.

Chapter 10

THE IDIOTYPE-SPECIFIC REPERTOIRE IS DETERMINED BY IDIOTYPE PREVALENCE *

K. Bottomly

TABLE OF CONTENTS

* Supported by National Institutes of Health grant CA-38350.

I. INTRODUCTION

The study of idiotypes (Id) and the regulation of their expression has attracted a good deal of attention since Jerne enunciated the Id network hypothesis in 1973;[1] indeed, it makes up the theme of the present volume. In this chapter the following questions will be addressed: what is an Id? Is the expression of Id regulated independently of the expression of antibody levels? What is the function of such regulation in the immune response? What is the nature of the regulatory apparatus? And how do such regulatory elements specific for Id arise?

Strictly speaking, an Id is an antigenic determinant on the variable domain of an antibody molecule, as detected by a specific antibody. When different antibody molecules expressing a shared Id are analyzed structurally, it is found that they share structural elements in the variable region. Thus, probing an antibody response with an anti-idiotypic (anti-Id) antibody allows one to determine the contribution of the structural element so detected to the response as a whole. The totality of Id expressed in an individual is said to comprise that individual's repertoire of Id or antibody structures.

Thus, anti-Id antibodies serve to allow the rapid structural definition of antibody repertoires, avoiding the necessity of determining the structure of each contributing antibody.

Why should the characterization of repertoires be of interest? There are several answers to this question. First, in the early stages of analyzing the variability of immunoglobulins, Kunkel and others used the frequency of occurrence of Id immunoglobulins in normal sera to determine the number of individual structures in the immunoglobulin repertoire, and concluded that a given individual could make at least 10^8 different antibody molecules.[2] Second, the use of anti-Id antibodies also revealed that certain structures are expressed as a major component of certain immune responses in inbred strains of mice. These so-called recurrent Id could then be used to analyze the regulation of Id expression and to determine whether or not independent regulation of Id-bearing antibody occurred. Third, specific dysfunctions in the immune response, such as may occur in autoimmunity or in the failure to respond to a particular pathogen, could reflect the presence or absence of immunoglobulin structures critical for the particular response. Thus, the actual structure of Id repertoires will clearly have medical importance.

In this chapter, the evidence for and nature of Id-specific regulation will be the central focus. In particular, evidence for the existence and function of Id-specific helper T cells will be summarized. It will be emphasized that the *quantity* of Id present in an individual has a decisive influence on the development of Id-specific helper T cells. This, in turn, will be interpreted to mean that only certain Id are normally under the control of such Id-specific helper T-cell influences, and that these are the Id present at the highest frequency in the repertoire.

II. ID-SPECIFIC REGULATION IN ANTIBODY RESPONSES

There have been numerous reports of Id-specific regulation occurring as part of the antibody response. In particular, the role of anti-Id antibody, of Id-specific helper T cells, and of Id-specific suppressor T cells has been studied. Most studies of regulation of Id expression by anti-Id antibody[3-10] have involved the injection of such antibodies into an animal during immunization; analysis of the production of autologous anti-Id antibody has not been extensively studied, and its importance in Id-specific regulation is not presently clear. Likewise, Id-specific suppressor cells have largely been characterized in mice immunized not only with antigen, but also with anti-Id antibody;[11-19] their definition as part of the normal immune response has not been characterized to any degree. Nevertheless, Rajewsky and colleagues[20] have described an Id-specific suppressor cell that arises following neonatal injection of antigen rather than anti-Id, and such cells could obviously play an important role in the determination of Id repertoires.

By contrast, several laboratories have reported the presence of helper T cells specific for Id which selectively augment the production of antibody bearing that Id.[21-29] Such cells arise during normal immunization of unmanipulated mice and, thus, are quite likely to play a role in the regulation of Id expression during antibody responses to antigen immunization. In this chapter, the findings in the TEPC15/antiphosphorylcholine (PC) antibody system will be the focus.

The response to phosphorylcholine in BALB/c mice is dominated by the antibodies bearing the T15 Id, first characterized on the BALB/c PC-binding myeloma TEPC15.[30] This Id dominance is seen in both thymus-independent and thymus-dependent responses.[31,32] In analyzing the helper T-cell contribution to the thymus-dependent form of PC, it was noted that helper T cells derived from mice that lacked expression of the Id, either genetically or due to experimental B-cell depletion,[23,24] would not induce Id-dominated anti-PC antibody responses. That this deficiency was due to the lack of a subset of helper T cells was subsequently demonstrated by restoring the response with Lyt-2$^-$ T cells derived from normal donor mice primed with an irrelevant antigen. An unusual feature of this activity was the requirement that such cells be restimulated with their immunizing antigen at the time of assay. Thus, such Id-specific helper T cells appear to be specific for two distinct entities, antigen and Id. Subsequent studies in other Id systems have revealed identical behavior.[27,28] Such cells are termed ThId.

As will be pointed out subsequently, ThId cells actually bind to native Id.[33] They are present in Id-positive mice and absent from Id-negative mice.[23,24] ThId cells cannot activate B cells in the absence of other conventional, MHC-restricted, antigen-specific helper T cells (ThMHC). A completely distinct type of helper T cell, also specific for Id, can be detected in mice immunized with Id,[34-37] such as TEPC 15 protein,[36] in strong adjuvants. Such helper T cells are conventionally detected by their ability to help for responses to haptens physically coupled to the Id immunoglobulin. These cells appear to be conventional, MHC-restricted helper T cells whose antigen is simply an Id determinant.[34-37] Interestingly, such cells specific for T15 cannot be elicited in normal mice by immunization with TEPC 15 protein;[38] however, they are readily detectable in mice lacking expression of TEPC 15 in normal serum. Thus, their development appears to be the reciprocal of that of the ThId. Such cells are, thus, termed anti-IdTh.

In some studies, it has been shown that anti-IdTh can actually directly activate B cells bearing complementary Id; indeed, this process can be observed in in vitro cultures using a cloned line of helper T cells of this type.[39] However, it is not clear whether such cells arise spontaneously in vivo, whether they regulate responses to antigen, and how they contribute to repertoire formation. It is possible that during antibody responses to bacteria and other particulate antigens, antibody molecules complexed to the bacteria might be processed and presented to anti-IdTh, leading to their activation. This natural form of immunization might play an important role in inducing this form of Id-specific regulatory cell. Data from several studies suggest that such cells are specific for fragments of Id molecules and would, thus, tend to select for sequence-specific Id, while ThId are specific for native Id and would, thus, tend to select for conformational Id determinants.

From this analysis of the specificity of ThId and anti-ThId, one might expect that their requirements for self-MHC recognition might also differ. Thus, ThId, which interact with native Id, might be expected to recognize Id independent of the MHC expressed on the B cell, while anti-IdTh, which recognize sequential Id determinants, might be expected to be MHC restricted in their recognition of Id. This is, indeed, the case, with one notable exception. Thus, ThId not only bind to native Id on plastic surfaces,[21,33] but also interact with Id-bearing B cells independent of the MHC genotype of the B cell.[40,41] By contrast, anti-IdTh are MHC restricted in their interaction with B cells. In one case in which anti-IdTh interact with Id-bearing B cells directly, antigen is required, apparently to induce the processing of the Id determinants by the B cell.[34,37] As noted above, there is one reported exception to this overall picture, and its importance is not yet clear. Cloned helper T cells can directly induce the production of idiotypically restricted anti-T-cell receptor antibody by MHC disparate B cells.[39] While such Th cells are MHC restricted in their recognition of nominal antigen, they are MHC independent in their recognition of anti-T-cell receptor antibody. Whether ThId are, in fact, typical MHC-restricted T cells simply observed as interacting with complementary receptors on B cells is not known.

III. THE DEVELOPMENT AND ACTIVATION OF ID-SPECIFIC HELPER T CELLS

Implicit in the observation that ThId cells selectively expand production of antibody of a particular structure, as detected by the production of a particular Id, is the notion that such cells exist only for certain Id. Should ThId exist for all Id in equal numbers, then this Id preference in ThId function could not be detected. Thus, one has to ask what determines the specificity of ThId for Id. Several possibilities exist. First, it could reflect the available genetic repertoire of the still-to-be-defined ThId receptor for Id. Second, it could reflect interactions of these receptors with antigen and/or MHC, which are known to affect the repertoires of T-cell receptors. Third, it could reflect the encounter of ThId cells with their natural target, Id-bearing B cells. It will be argued that it is this latter interaction that determines the prevalence of ThId cells of various types in the total ThId repertoire.

In analyzing the ontogeny of ThId in the T15 system, several observations point directly to a critical role for Id in the development of ThId cells. First, in mice bearing the X-linked immune deficiency marker and, thus, lacking B cells that produce T15, one finds few, if any, T15-specific ThId cells.[23] While this observation is controversial, it has now been reported in several studies[29,42] and, thus, is likely to be correct. Second, in mice lacking B cells altogether, one fails to observe ThId cell function.[24] Third, in mice lacking the genetic capability to make a T15-dominated anti-PC antibody response and expressing little or no T15 in normal serum, one also does not observe ThId cell function. Thus, all of these studies point to a central role for Id in the development of ThId cells bearing complementary receptors. This conclusion is difficult to prove, although recent studies in mice expressing rearranged Igh genes as transgenes strongly support it (see below).[43] It should also be pointed out that B-cell-deprived mice lack ThId or helper cells that are phenotypically indistinguishable from ThId in several different experimental systems studied in several laboratories.

While the above analysis points to Id as playing a central role in the development of ThId, much as MHC is thought to play a role in expanding self-MHC-recognizing T cells, the analysis does not explain why ThId in the anti-PC response are seen primarily for T15. As pointed out in an earlier review,[44] the most likely explanation for this dominance of T15-specific ThId is the very high level of T15 expression found normally as reflected in a high titer of Id in normal serum. A similar situation appears to exist for several of the Id systems analyzed to date, such as Id-460, Ars-CRI, and others.

This analysis leads directly to two conclusions. First, not all Id will be regulated within the network. Rather, those present at high frequency will induce regulatory cells, while those present at low levels will not. Thus, some Id will fall within the definition of regulatory Id or idiotopes,[45] and others will not. This is, of course, a necessity in any case, as one could not envision an immune system in which there were complementary cells for every Id, since this would lead to an endless expansion of specificities. The regulatory idiotopes will be those present at high levels which, thus, induce high levels of regulatory cells. As a simplifying assumption, this hypothesis also contains the notion that regulatory idiotopes will not be distinguishable from other Id on structural grounds alone, but will be distinguishable on the basis of their level of expression. Some Id occur recurrently at high levels in normal serum, and it is easy to detect ThId cells specific for these idiotopes. Interestingly, these normal serum Id appear to be germline-encoded antibacterial (fungal, worm, etc.) antibodies. Second, this analysis suggests that analyzing Id with anti-idiotope antibodies may be highly misleading, since the idiotope that is regulated may be the one recognized by ThId cells, for example, and not the one measured with the anti-idiotope antibody. Nevertheless, since it is clear that multiple idiotopes are expressed on single antibody molecules, generally appearing as a group since they are reflections of different portions of a particular VH and/or VL gene, one may see a pattern of regulation that appears to be specific for a nonregulatory idiotope. Two practical considerations derive from this analysis. First, anti-idiotopes that react with normal serum immunoglobulin, such as anti-T15 antibodies, are more likely to reflect the regulatory effects of ThId cells than are anti-idiotopes directed at idiotopes not found in normal serum, and second, the critical parameter in Id regulation is that idiotope is recognized by the regulatory cell itself, rather than detected serologically.

What role does antigen play in the establishment and functioning of ThId cells? It seems likely that antigen will play a role in the expansion of B cells expressing germline-encoded antibacterial antibodies which, as noted above, frequently appear to bear regulatory idiotopes that induce ThId. Nevertheless, it should be noted that studies of germ-free animals have not been notably informative in studying the ontogeny of ThId cells. However, antigen does play a decisive role in the activation and functioning of ThId. The basis for this antigen effect is, as noted above, both unknown and highly unusual. Thus, in the T15 system and several others, one finds that ThId must be derived from antigen-immune mice and must be restimulated with that antigen in order to function.[23,24,40,41] Unlike the antigen requirements of MHC-restricted, classical Th cells, ThId cell antigen stimulation does not require physical linkage of the antigen to a ligand for which the Id B cell is specific, nor does it require that the antigen in question induce production of the Id. Indeed, as discussed in the next section, the antigen appears to be recognized in an MHC independent fashion. Clearly, this aspect of ThId function in highly intriguing and needs a great deal more work. One might speculate that it imposes an important control step in the process of ThId cell activation, as ThId cell function independent of antigen might lead to uncontrolled proliferation of the ThId and its complementary B cells. It can also be argued that the interaction with antigen has to be independent of Id, because a linkage of these two forms of recognition would lead to a highly restricted response, a situation that would compound the difficulty of generating cells that regulate a large number of distinct Id.

Conventional, MHC-restricted Th (ThMHC) will interact only with B cells bearing self-Ia molecules, and are under MHC-linked Ir gene control in their response to antigen. By contrast, ThId cells do not show this behavior. Thus, Th cells derived from F_1 into parent chimeric mice will show two different patterns of interaction with B cells derived from the two parental strains.[41] ThMHC will only collaborate with B cells from the parent that is Ia identical with the recipient in the chimera, while ThId will collaborate with B cells of both parental genotypes. Indeed, using cloned ThId cells, it can be shown that collaboration is identical with syngeneic and fully allogeneic B cells. As might be expected from these results, ThId can also be activated by antigen in Ir gene nonresponder mice.[40] Thus, mice primed with antigen to which they fail to generate T-cell proliferative or antibody responses due to MHC-linked Ir genes, also fail to generate ThMHC; however, T cells from the same mouse make normal ThId cell responses, and the ThId cells need to be restimulated with the same genetically controlled antigen to which the donor animal was primed in order to function. Thus, antigen recognition in this system is apparently completely distinct from antigen recognition in the conventional, MHC-restricted set of mice.

While these studies suggest that ThId cells do not recognize antigen in the context of self-MHC, and do not interact with B cells via self-MHC recognition, they do not rule out the possibility that ThId are, in fact, MHC-restricted Th which cross react with particular idiotopes. Implicit in the finding of clonotypic monoclonal anti-T-cell receptor antibodies directed as such receptors is the notion that such interactions can occur. Indeed, in one system it has been shown that a conventional, antigen plus self-MHC-specific cloned helper T cell line can interact directly with B cells bearing complementary receptors, and that this interaction is independent of the MHC genotype of the B cell. Indeed, this cloned ThMHC can induce an idiotypically restricted B-cell response directed at its own receptor. One might, thus, conclude that ThId cells are actually ThMHC that cross react with certain Id, and that ThMHC cells having this cross-reactive specificity would be selectively expanded by contact with Id B cells. That this is unlikely to be the case is suggested by one experiment in the PC-T15 system. T-cell-depleted mice were repopulated with the activated cells derived from the early stages of a primary mixed lymphocyte reaction (MLR).[46] After some time, these mice were immunized with antigen and their ThMHC and ThId cell function analyzed. As might be predicted from the finding that the same receptor accounts for both self-MHC plus antigen and nonself MHC recognition, ThMHC function was normal in these mice. That the majority of the T cells in the recipient were, in fact, responsive to the selecting alloantigen was shown by a repeat MLR. However, these mice lacked ThId or ThId-like cells in both systems assayed. Thus, this experiment suggests that ThId and ThMHC derive from different lineages of cells. However, it must be admitted that the receptors on cells responding to the selecting alloantigen could have lacked structures that could be complementary to the T15 Id analyzed. A clear resolution to the question of whether ThId are simply a different form of ThMHC or a different lineage of cells having unique receptor structures will await a molecular definition of the receptors on cloned ThId cell lines.

IV. WHAT IS THE FUNCTION OF ThId?

While ThId are interesting objects of study for a cellular immunologist interested in the structure of lymphocyte repertoires, one would like to know whether they play an important functional role in the protective immune response, or whether they are simply an intellectual curiosity. One might have argued similarly about H-2 antigens or about differentiation antigens in the past; both are now known to have essential roles in the physiology of the immune response now. Likewise, it seems unlikely that ThId cells would exist and yet not have an important functional role. However, it must be admitted that a critical test of the significance of ThId has not yet been performed and awaits a technique for the selective in vivo depletion of such cells.

Despite these limitations, one can infer what might be the biological importance of ThId from studies of their effect on the immune response to PC. First, they clearly augment the T15-bearing component of the anti-PC antibody response. This increase has now been analyzed by B-cell-limiting dilution experiments and has been shown to be due to the ability of the ThId cells to render B-cell precursors susceptible to activation by conventional, ThMHC cells.[47] In addition, single B-cell precursors activated in the presence of ThId cells produce larger numbers of antibody-forming cells than do the same cells activated in the absence of ThId. The net effect is that while the percent of antibody-forming cells expressing the T15 Id rises from 30 to 90%, the number of anti-PC antibody-forming cells of the T15 Id produced increases by nearly 20-fold. This is a remarkable increase in an antibody response. It should be noted that the increase is entirely restricted to T15-positive anti-PC B cells. Thus, not only do ThId cells bind T15, they act only on T15-bearing B cells.

It has been shown in the anti-PC antibody response that the T15-bearing B cell has, on average, lower surface density of Ia antigens than does the T15-negative precursor B cell.[48] The reason for the association of Ia antigen density with Id is not known. However, it does suggest a possible mechanism of action for ThId cells. ThId may, on encounter with an

Idiotype-bearing B cell, and upon appropriate stimulation with the antigen for which the ThId is also specific, induce a marked increase in Ia antigen density on the T15-bearing B cell. This increase in Ia antigen density would, in turn, render that B cell able to present antigen to an antigen-specific, Ia-restricted ThMHC, leading to activation of the B cell and the production of antibody. This should be testable using cloned lines of ThId cells. If they produce Ia-inducing factors upon appropriate stimulation by antigen and/or Id, then it seems likely that the proposed mechanism of action is correct.

A second action of the ThId and ThId-like cells that has been less well characterized is their ability to accelerate antibody responses. Thus, in adoptive transfer experiments in the antibody response to DNP, two different helper types, analogous to ThId and ThMHC, were observed as contributing to the early phases of the secondary adoptive antibody response, but only the ThMHC contributed significantly to its later phases.[49]

The increased production of antibody bearing a regulatory idiotope, as well as the acceleration in the antibody response induced by ThId cells, would obviously increase the protective efficiency of an antibody response. It should be reemphasized that for many ThId, the regulatory idiotope appears in normal serum as an antibacterial antibody. Indeed, in the T15 system it has been shown that among anti-PC antibodies tested, those bearing the T15 Id are best at protecting against infection with *Streptococcus pneumoniae*.[50,51] Thus, the relationship of ThId to germlike-encoded antibacterial antibodies may also say something about the biological relevance of such helper cells.

V. EVIDENCE FOR ThId IN OTHER EXPERIMENTAL SYSTEMS

In addition to the T15-PC system, studies in several other systems support the findings outlined here. Because different approaches have been used in the studies in other laboratories, these studies are worth summarizing here and comparing with the conclusions reached based on the T15 system. However, for detailed analysis of the findings in each system, the reader is referred to the other chapters in this volume as well as the original reports of the findings in these systems.

First, it should be pointed out that several other investigators have found cells similar to ThId in a variety of experimental systems. These are the Ars-CRI system,[21] the anti-DNP antibody response,[49] the Tyr-TMA system,[27] the MOPC 315 system,[28] and the A5A system.[22] Indeed, the initial description of Ig-specific helper T cells[52] appears to reflect a cell similar to ThId but specific for an immunoglobulin allotype. Recently, Kohler has also detected ThId-like cells in the PC-T15 system,[29] and Teale reported findings in the splenic focus assay consistent with a role for ThId in this analytical read-out as well.[42,53] Thus, the case for the existence of T cells with ThId-like function appears to be solid, and failures to demonstrate such cells are the exception rather than the rule. As might be expected for cells that alter the nature of an antibody response, but are clearly not necessary for its occurrence, ThId are not observable in every published report. Likewise, nude mice do not have hair or T cells, but can live; this does not mean that hair and T cells are not important for survival.

Are all Id-specific helper effects due to ThId cells? This question is more difficult to answer. In particular, the distinction between ThId and anti-IdTh needs to be kept clearly in mind in interpreting data. However, many reports on Id-specific helper effects are not sufficiently clear to allow such a distinction. This distinction is not just intellectually interesting, but of great importance in determining the role of these two cell types, and possible other cell types, in the immune response. Particularly difficult to categorize are Id-specific cells that are present normally[27,54] or that are recovered from antigen immunizations, but not further characterized.[55-57]

argument that Thld cells arise in response to exposure to Id, and that regulatory idiotopes are those present in the system which, in turn, induce Thld. The first is the finding that Thld for the Id-dominated secondary response to hen egg lysozyme only arise after immunization with lysozyme which induces Id production.[58] This suggests that not all Thld are present prior to antigen immunization, and that altering the repertoire of B cells causes a corresponding change in the repertoire of complementary Thld cells. These studies do not analyze the Thld cells in sufficient detail to determine whether they are in all ways similar to the Thld in the T15 system, nor do they clearly demonstrate that it is Id, and not exposure of the Thld themselves to antigen, that is critical for their induction. The second is the observation by Bona and co-workers[59] of Thld-like cells induced by passive injection of soluble A48 protein into neonatal mice. This injection allows the mice to make A48 Id, which they would normally not do, in response to bacterial levan. In addition, it could be shown that the effect was transferrable with T cells. Again, it was not determined whether these cells were fully analogous to Thld described in the T15 system. However, in this case, it can be seen clearly that Id alone is sufficient to induce a complementary set of Th cells specific for Id. Finally, in recent experiments of Weaver et al.[43] mice were generated which carry a rearranged Igh-V gene. This rearranged Igh-V gene is expressed in a large percentage of B cells in the transgenic mice. However, some B cells express rearranged endogenous VH and VL genes. What is remarkable about these mice is that hybridomas derived from their B cells frequently express an Id not normally found on any B cells from the recipient mouse, but expressed by the hybridoma that donated the rearranged VH gene, and do not express the rearranged transgene at all. Although it is possible that the expression of Id by the rearranged endogenous genes reflects DNA/DNA interactions during B-cell development, the finding that many of the Id-positive B cells rearrange nonhomologous genes that, nevertheless, allow expression of Id more strongly suggests that such expression reflects network interactions. Whether these findings are due to the activation of Thld cells by expression of Id immunoglobulin derived from the rearranged transgene, or to some other effect, is being determined. If the former is true, then these studies will provide strong support for the model proposed in this review, namely, that the repertoire of Thld is determined by the level of particular Id in the normal serum or B-cell pool of immunoglobulin molecules or receptors.

VI. ARE REGULATORY IDIOTOPES SPECIAL?

Based on the present analysis, one can conclude that regulatory idiotopes are both special and not special. They are special in that they represent those antibodies present at the highest levels in an immune system. In unmanipulated mice, these appear to be mainly germline-encoded antibacterial antibodies; however, this conclusion is based on a very small sample size, and exceptions to it seem likely to appear. Based on studies in manipulated mice, it would appear that any Id can be a regulatory Id, provided its level is increased during B-cell development. This, in turn, implies that the repertoire of potential Thld receptors is open, consistent with the openness of B-cell and MHC-restricted T-cell receptor repertoire potentials, and that, like MHC-restricted T-cell receptor repertoires, exposure to complementary structures during ontogeny imposes limitations on the expression of this potential repertoire. These limitations or restrictions, in turn, appear as Id-selective effects mediated by the Thld cells. Thus, one would predict that Thld cells in unmanipulated mice would be specific for prevalent idiotopes, but that Thld cells not found in this normal repertoire could readily be induced by increasing the level of expression of an idiotope. This, in turn, implies that the immune system is, indeed, a network, and that any Id can be regulated within this network; however, in normal mice, only those Id that are prevalent to begin with are likely to be regulated, and, thus, one observes selective regulation of particular idiotopes within such responses. The challenge now would, therefore, appear to be to purify, clone, and fully characterize ThId cells, and to use them as reagents to measure Id responses. Since it is the ThId cells that probably regulate Id expression, it is the idiotopes recognized by such cells that one expects to find most predictably regulated.

REFERENCES

1. **Jerne, N. K.,** Toward a network theory of the immune system, *Ann. Immunol. (Paris),* 125C, 373, 1974.
2. **Kunkel, H. G., Mannik, M., and Williams, R. C.,** Individual antigenic specificity of isolate antibodies, *Science,* 140, 1218, 1963.
3. **Hart, D. A., Wang, A. C., Pawlak, L., and Nisonoff, A.,** Suppression of idiotypic specificities in adult mice by administration of anti-idiotypic antibody, *J. Exp. Med.,* 135, 1293, 1972.
4. **Strayer, D. S., Consenza, H., Lee, W. M. F., Rowley, D. A., and Kohler, H.,** Neonatal tolerance induced by antibody against antigen-specific receptor, *Science,* 186, 640, 1974.
5. **Eichmann, K. and Rajewsky, K.,** Induction of T and B cell immunity by anti-idiotypic antibodies, *Eur. J. Immunol.,* 5, 661, 1975.
6. **Bona, C., Stein, K. E., Lieberman, R., and Paul, W. E.,** Direct and indirect suppression induced by anti-idiotype antibody in the inulin-bacterial levan antigenic system, *Mol. Immunol.,* 16, 1093, 1979.
7. **Kelsoe, G., Reth, M., and Rajewsky, K.,** Control of idiotype expression by monoclonal anti-idotypic antibodies, *Immunol. Rev.,* 52, 75, 1980.
8. **Rajewsky, K. and Takemori, T.,** Genetic, expression and function of idiotypes, *Annu. Rev. Immunol.,* 1, 569, 1983.
9. **Cerny, J., Cronkhite, R., and Heussen, C.,** Antibody response of mice following neonatal treatment with a monoclonal anti-receptor antibody. Evidence for B cell tolerance and T suppressor cells specific for different idiotypic determinants, *Eur. J. Immunol.,* 13, 244, 1983.
10. **Berek, C.,** Antibodies specific for different T15 idiotopes induce neonatal suppression of the T15 idiotype, *Eur. J. Immunol.,* 13, 766, 1983.
11. **Ward, K., Cantor, H., and Boyse, E. A.,** Clonally-restricted interactions among T and B cell subclasses, in *Immune System: Genetics and Regulation,* Sercarz, E., Herzenberg, L. A., and Fox, C. F., Eds., Academic Press, New York, 1977, 397.
12. **Owen, F. L. and Nisonoff, A.,** Effect of idiotype-specific suppressor T cells on primary and secondary responses, *J. Exp. Med.,* 148, 182, 1978.
13. **Hetzelberger, D. and Eichmann, K.,** Idiotypic suppression. III. Induction of unresponsiveness to sensitization with anti-idiotypic antibody: identification of the cell types tolerized in high zone and in low zone, suppressor cell-medicated, idiotype suppression, *Eur. J. Immunol.,* 8, 839, 1978.
14. **Bottomly, K., Mathieson, B. J., and Mosier, D. E.,** Anti-idiotype induced regulation of helper cell function for the response to phosphorylcholine in adult BALB/c mice, *J. Exp. Med.,* 148, 1216, 1978.
15. **Bona, C. and Paul, W. E.,** Cellular basis of regulation of expression of idiotype. I. Suppressor cells specific for MOPC 460 idiotype regulate the expression of cells secreting anti-TNP antibodies bearing 460 idiotypes, *J. Exp. Med.,* 149, 592, 1979.
16. **Rohrer, J. W., Odermatt, B. O., and Lynch, R. G.,** Immunoregulation of murine myelomas: isologous immunization with M315 induces idiotype-specific T cells that supress IgA secretion by MOPC 315 cells in vivo, *J. Immunol.,* 122, 2011, 1979.
17. **Abbas, A. K., Perry, L. C., Bach, B. A., and Green, M. I.,** Idiotype-specific T cell immunity. I. Generation of effector and suppressor T lymphocytes reactive with myeloma idiotypic determinants, *J. Immunol.,* 8, 839, 1978.
18. **Kelsoe, G., Takemore, T., Reth, M., and Rajewsky, K.,** Generation of specific regulatory T cells with monoclonal anti-idiotype antibody: induction of suppressor T cells, in *Lymphocytes in the Immune Response: Functional, Developmental and Interactive Properties,* Klinman, N. R., Mosier, D. E., Sher, I., and Vitetta, E. S., Eds., Elsevier/North-Holland, New York, 1981, 423.
19. **Kim, B. S. and Greenberg, P.,** Mechanisms of idiotype suppression. IV. Functional neutralization in mixtures of idiotype-specific suppressor and hapten-specific suppressor T cells, *J. Exp. Med.,* 154, 809, 1982.
20. **Tokuhisa, T. and Rajewsky, K.,** Antigen induces chronic idiotype suppression, *Proc. Natl. Acad. Sci. U.S.A.,* 82, 4217, 1985.
21. **Woodland, R. and Cantor, H.,** Idiotype-specific T cells are required to induce idiotype-positive B memory cells to secrete antibody, *Eur. J. Immunol.,* 7, 600, 1978.

22. **Hetzelberger, P. and Eichmann, K.,** Recognition of idiotypes in lymphocyte interactions. I. Idiotypic selectivity in the cooperation between T and B lymphocytes, *Eur. J. Immunol.,* 8, 846, 1978.
23. **Bottomly, E. and Mosier, D. E.,** Mice whose B cells cannot produce the T15 idiotype also lack an antigen-specific T cell required for T15 expression, *J. Exp. Med.,* 150, 1399, 1979.
24. **Bottomly, K., Janeway, C. A., Jr., Mathieson, B. J., and Mosier, D. E.,** Absence of an antigen-specific helper T cell required for the expression of the T15 idiotype in mice treated with anti-μ antibody, *Eur. J. Immunol.,* 10, 159, 1980.
25. **Adorini, L. M., Harvey, H., and Sercarz, E. E.,** The fine specificity of regulatory T cells. IV. Idiotypic complementarity and antigen bridging interactions, *Eur. J. Immunol.,* 9, 906, 1979.
26. **Bottomly, K.,** Activation of the idiotypic network. Environmental and regulatory influences, in *Immunoglobulin Idiotypes,* Janeway, C. A., Jr., Sercarz, E. E., and Wigzell, H., Eds., Academic Press, New York, 1981, 517.
27. **Jayaraman, S., Swierkosz, J. E., and Bellone, C. J.,** T cell replacing factor substitutes for an I-J$^+$ idiotype-specific T helper cell, *J. Exp. Med.,* 155, 641, 1982.
28. **Rohrer, J. W., Gershon, R. K., Lynch, R. G., and Kemp, J.,** The enhancement of B lymphocyte secretory differentiation by an Ly1$^+$2$^-$, 2a-1$^+$ helper T cell subset that sees both antigen and determinants on immunoglobulin, *J. Mol. Cell. Immunol.,* 1, 50, 1983.
29. **Smyk, S. K., McNamara, M. K., Gleason, K. S., and Kohler, H.,** Differences in T15 expression of primary and secondary anti-PC responses with T cells from T15$^+$ and T15$^-$ donors, *J. Immunol.,* 134, 23, 1985.
30. **Sher, A. and Cohn, M.,** Inheritance of an idiotype associated with the immune responses of inbred mice to phosphorylcholine, *Eur. J. Immunol.,* 2, 319, 1972.
31. **Lee, W., Consenza, H., and Kohler, H.,** Clonal restriction of the immune response to phosphorylcholine, *Nature (London),* 247, 55, 1974.
32. **Claflin, J. L. and Cubberley, M.,** Clonal nature of the immune response to phosphorylcholine. VI. Molecular uniformity of a single idiotype among BALB/c mice, *J. Immunol.,* 121, 1410, 1978.
33. **Dunn, E. B. and Bottomly, K.,** T15-specific helper T cells: analysis of idiotype specificity by competitive inhibition analysis, *Eur. J. Immunol.,* 15, 728, 1985.
34. **Jorgenson, T. and Hannestad, K.,** Helper T cell recognition of the variable domains of a mouse myeloma protein (315). Effect of the major histocompatibility complex and domain conformation, *J. Exp. Med.,* 155, 1587, 1982.
35. **Eichmann, K., Falk, I., and Rajewsky, K.,** Recognition of idiotypes in lymphocyte interactions. II. Antigen-independent co-operation between T and B lymphocytes that possess similar and complementary idiotypes, *Eur. J. Immunol.,* 8, 853, 1978.
36. **Gleason, K., Pierce, S., and Kohler, H.,** Generation of idiotype specific T cell help through network perturbation, *J. Exp. Med.,* 153, 924, 1981.
37. **Kawahara, D. J., Marrack, P., and Kappler, J. W.,** H-2-linked Ir gene control of V_H determinant(s)-specific helper T cells, *J. Mol. Cell. Immunol.,* 2, 255, 1986.
38. **Sakato, N., Janeway, C. A., Jr., and Eisen, H. N.,** Immune response of BALB/c mice to the idiotype T15 and other myeloma proteins of BALB/c origin: implications for an immune network and antibody multispecificity, in *Cold Spring Harbor Symp. Quant. Biol.,* 41, 1977, 719.
39. **Janeway, C. A., Jr., Broughton, B., Smith, L. A., Marion, T. N., and Bottomly, K.,** Direct receptor:receptor interactions between T and B lymphocytes: idiotypic restriction in the antibody response to a cloned helper T cell receptor, *J. Mol. Cell Immunol.,* 3, 83, 1987.
40. **Bottomly, K. and Maurer, P. H.,** Antigen-specific helper T cells required for dominant production of an idiotype (ThId) are not under immune response (Ir) gene control, *J. Exp. Med.,* 152, 1571, 1980.
41. **Bottomly, K. and Mosier, D. E.,** Antigen-specific helper T cells required for dominant idiotype expression are not H-2 restricted, *J. Exp. Med.,* 154, 411, 1981.
42. **Teale, J.,** Abnormalities in isotype expression in CBA/N mice due to stimulatory environment rather than a B cell defect, *J. Immunol.,* 130, 72, 1983.
43. **Weaver, D., Reis, M. H., Albanese, C., Costantini, F., Baltimore, D., and Imanishi-Kari, T.,** Altered repertoire of endogenous immunoglobulin gene expression in transgenic mice containing a rearranged mu heavy chain gene, *Cell,* 45, 247, 1986.
44. **Bottomly, K.,** 1984: All idiotypes are equal, but some are more equal than others, *Immunol. Rev.,* 79, 45, 1984.
45. **Paul, W. E. and Bona, C.,** Regulatory idiotopes and immune networks: a hypothesis, *Immunol. Today,* 3, 9, 1982.
46. **Bottomly, K. and Janeway, C. A., Jr.,** Selected populations of alloreactive T cells contain helper T cells but lack ThId, an antigen-specific helper T cell required for dominant production of the T15 idiotype, *Eur. J. Immunol.,* 11, 170, 1981.
47. **Dunn, E. B., Kim, J., and Bottomly, K.,** A cloned T cell line that selectively augments antibody responses of phosphorylcholine-specific B cells bearing the T15 idiotype, *J. Mol. Cell. Immunol.,* 2, 209, 1986.

48. **Bottomly, K., Jones, B., Kaye, J., and Jones, F., III,** Subpopulations of B cells distinguished by cell surface expression of Ia antigens. Correlation of Ia and idiotype during activation by cloned Ia-restricted T cells, *J. Exp. Med.*, 158, 265, 1983.
49. **Janeway, C. A., Jr., Murgita, R. A., Weinbaum, F. I., Asofsky, R., and Wigzell, H.,** Evidence for an immunoglobulin-dependent antigen-specific helper T cell, *Proc. Natl. Acad. Sci. U.S.A.*, 74, 4582, 1977.
50. **Briles, D.E., Nahm, M., Schroer, K., Davie J., Baker, P., Kearney, J., and Barletta, R.,** Anti-phosphorylcholine antibodies found in normal mouse serum are protective against intravenous infection with type 3 *Streptococcus Pneumoniae, J. Exp. Med.*, 153, 694, 1981.
51. **Briles, E.E., Forman, C., Hudak, S., and Claflin, J.L.,** Antiphosphorylcholine antibodies of the T15 idiotype are optimally protective against *Streptococcus pneumoniae, J. Exp. Med.*, 156, 1177, 1982.
52. **Herzenberg, L.A., Okumura, K., Cantor, H., Sato, V.L., Shen, F.W., Boyse, E., and Herzenberg, L.A.,** T cell of alliotype-specific helper T cells and their specific removal by suppressor T cells, *J. Exp. Med.*, 144, 330, 1976.
53. **Teal, J.M. and Janeway, C.A., Jr.,** Influence of immunoglobulin dependent T cells on antibody class switching, manuscript submitted for publication.
54. **Cerny, J. and Caulfield, M.J.** Stimulation of specific antibody-forming cells in antigen-primed nude mice by the adoptive transfer of syngeneic anti-idotypic T cells, *J. Immunol.*, 126, 2262, 1981.
55. **L'Age-Stehr, J., Tuchmann, H., Gershon, R.K., and Cantor, H.,** Stimulation of regulatory T cell circuits by Ia-associated structures on activated B cells, *Eur. J. Immunol.*, 10, 21, 1980.
56. **L'Age-Stehr, J.,** Priming of T helper cells by antigen activated B cells: B cell primed Lyt-1^+; helper cells are restricted to cooperate with B cells expressing the IgV_H phenotype of the priming B cells, *J. Exp. Med.*, 153, 1236, 1981.
57. **Nutt, N., Haber, J., and Wortis, H.H.,** Influence of Igh-linked gene products on the generation of T helper cells in the response to sheep erythrocytes, *J. Exp. Med.*, 153, 1225, 1981.
58. **Adorini, L.M., Harvey, M., and Sercarz, E.E.,** The fine specificity of regulatory T cells. IV. Idiotypic complementarity and antigen bridging interactions, *Eur. J. Immunol.*, 9, 906, 1979.
59. **Bona, C.A., Victor-Kobrin, C., Manheimer, A.J., Bellon, B., and Rubinstein, L.J.,** Regulatory arms of the immune network, *Immunol. Rev.*, 79, 25, 1984.

Chapter 11

IDIOTYPE-SPECIFIC SUPPRESSOR T CELLS

S. Jayaraman and C. J. Bellone

TABLE OF CONTENTS

I. INTRODUCTION

Jerne has proposed that the immune system comprises a network of idiotypes (Id) and anti-idiotypes (anti-Id) which are intimately involved in regulation.[1] The theory implies that each combining site, in addition to binding a number of foreign antigenic determinants, necessarily also combines with a number of Id determinants within the same immune system. This leads to a formation of a large number of Id-anti-Id bonds involving receptors on lymphocytes as well as soluble antigen-recognizing molecules, thus, establishing a "formal" network. This is based on the assumption that Id determinants are highly immunogenic and that they can trigger a chain of complementary anti-Id responses: antibody Ab_1 bearing Id_1 stimulating Ab_2 bearing Id_2 which, in turn, triggers the formation of Ab_3 bearing Id_3 and so on, in the same individual. Experimental findings supporting this notion led to the suggestion of the existence of a "functional" network which is primarily supported by the findings of the occurrence of anti-Id autoantibodies as well as the ability of some anti-Id antibodies to mimic foreign antigens. Such functional networks are of two types: suppressive and enhancing. The existence of enhancing networks is well documented and treated in a number of reviews.[2-9] It has been documented that a functional suppressive network exists at the T-cell level in many antigen systems.[10-17] These interactions occur primarily between the so-called first-order T suppressor (Ts_1), second-order Ts (Ts_2), and the third-order Ts (Ts_3) subsets in antigen systems which are dominated by well-characterized cross-reactive Id (CRI). The understanding of the relationship among Ts subpopulations and between the Ts subsets and immune effector lymphocytes is of immense importance for manipulation of immune responses.

A number of excellent reviews have been written dealing with the characterization of Ts subsets, their factors, and their relevance to the control of a variety of immune responses.[10-14,16,17] In this review we will deal exclusively with the Id-specific Ts subset which appears to play a pivotal role in suppressor pathways characterized by dominant CRI. In particular, we will review what is known about (1) inductive signals required for Id-specific Ts cells; (2) their functional and cellular properties; and (3) physiological significance. We will also document some evidence for the existence of a unique Id-specific Ts cell which has specificity for T-cell and not immunoglobulin-(Ig) associated Id.

II. ID SUPPRESSION

Id structures, at least at the B-cell surface, represent the antibody variable (V) region gene products and, thus, serve as useful markers for the study of development, differentiation, function, and regulation of B-cell clones carrying these Id determinants. The evidence that B-cell Id structures serve as a target for discrete immune modulation comes from the early studies of Hart et al.[18] in the azobenzenearsonate (ABA) system, and Cosenza and Kohler[19] in the phosphorylcholine (PC) system. Subsequent studies in a number of antigen systems substantiated these findings that dominant Id-bearing antibody populations could be suppressed when anti-Id reagents were introduced into the host prior to antigen administration.[20-22] Further studies showed that not only anti-Id, but also a variety of reagents such as monovalent antigen,[21,23] a tolerogenic dose of antigen,[24] antigen plus Id-bearing antibody complexes,[25] anti-Id antibodies plus antigen,[26] tolerogen,[27] and hapten-coupled to isologous gamma globulin[28] all result in Id suppression at the B-cell level.

In contrast to B cells, T cells do not use Ig V_H gene segments related to those found in B cells.[29,30] Nonetheless, T and B cells of the same antigen specificity can bear serologically similar Id structures[31] and, moreover, anti-Id antibodies can induce a wide variety of T-cell activities. These include helper,[32,33] mixed-lymphocyte reactivity,[34] delayed-type hypersensitivity (DTH),[35-39] as well as activation of lymphocytes reactive to a number of pathogens.[40]

In addition, allogeneic anti-Id sera[41-44] and syngeneic monoclonal anti-Id[45] induce antigen-specific immune suppression at the T-cell level. Analysis of modulation at both the T- and B-cell level revealed that no one mechanism accounted for the observed effects. Mechanisms like B-cell tolerance,[46] direct interaction of anti-Id with Id-bearing B cells,[47-49] preemption of virgin CRI-positive B cells by memory B cells,[50-52] lack of Id-specific help,[42,46,53,54] and active suppression by Ts cells,[21,22,41,43,44,53-60] either singly or in combination, may produce unresponsiveness at both the T- and B-cell levels.

Eichmann[41] was the first to demonstrate that anti-Group A streptococcal carbohydrate (A-CHO) antibodies bearing a dominant CRI could be suppressed in mildly irradiated recipients by adoptive transfer of T cells from anti-Id-treated mice. Such an anti-Id-induced Ts has also been shown to mediate suppression in an antigen-specific fashion in the ABA,[44,45] PC,[25,26,42,43,59,60] and phenyltrimethylammonium (TMA)[21] systems. In many of these early studies, it was inferred, but not directly demonstrated, that anti-Id-mediated suppression involved Ts cells specific for the Id involved. Owen et al.[55-57] were the first to demonstrate that Id-specific antibody suppression was mediated by a Ts population that bears surface receptors specific for Id determinants. Bona and Paul[61] subsequently demonstrated naturally occurring Id-specific Ts cells directed to the Id associated with the trinitrophenol (TNP)-binding mouse myeloma protein MOPC 460, suggesting these cells may play a general physiological role in immune regulation. Since these initial studies, Id-recognizing Ts, induced by a variety of experimental manipulations, have been described in several antigen systems. It is clear from all these studies that the Id-specific Ts either act at the induction[54,57,62-68] or efferent phase of the immune response.[66,67,69-73] In some cases they apparently function as final effector Ts populations.[23,74-78] Moreover, the majority of these Ts appear to be analogous to the second-order Ts, the Ts_2,[12] described in the Id-nondominated systems, in that they function in a genetically restricted fashion and require other Ts subset(s) to manifest suppression. These cells will be described in more detail in the following section.

III. ID-SPECIFIC Ts CELLS

A. General Properties

1. Cells

Id-specific Ts cells and factors have now been described in a variety of experimental systems. These include model antigen,[21,25,26,41,46,55,57,59-61,65-71,73,79-89] tumor systems,[64,74-76,90-92] experimental interstitial nephiritis,[78] and schistosomiasis system.[93] Although some differences do exist with respect to function and phenotype, the majority of cells share most of the following properties. Without exception, all bear Thy1.1 and most possess the Lyt 1^-2^+ phenotype[23,52,59,60,65,67,70,76,78,88,92] as well as I-J-encoded determinants.[58,64,67,73,78,82,88] Functionally, with few exceptions,[42,54,57,63-68,88] these cells suppress ongoing immune responses and, hence, are called efferent-phase suppressors. Operationally, these Ts can limit both ongoing antibody and DTH responses even when introduced hours before the time of assay. These efferent-acting cells can be categorized as Ts_2, since most can be shown to be induced by Ts_1/Ts_1-derived factor (TsF_1).[65,66,69,75,78,83,94,95] The induced Ts_2 is genetically restricted,[67,69,78] i.e., the Ts_2 cannot function in adoptive transfer protocols unless the recipients are matched at both the MHC and Igh genetic loci. As will be discussed in a later section in greater detail, the Id-specific Ts in DTH systems, with possibly one exception,[78] require the presence of an antigen-binding Id^+ Ts_3 subset to function. In these cases the anti-Id Ts perform as a transducer population, bridging the Id^+ inducer (Ts_1) and Id^+ effector (Ts_3) subsets.

A common feature of all well-characterized Id-specific Ts is their ability to bind to Id associated with Igs which are either coated onto polystyrene petri dishes,[59-61,64,65,67,69-71,74,75,77,78,88] coupled to red blood cells,[55,56] or Sepharose® 4B.[76] Suppression of both antibody and DTH is mediated by such Id-binding Ts or TsF derived from them. In many systems the Id-specific Ts appear to have specificity for the major CRI found on serum antibodies.[25,55,59,65] In the TMA system, these cells bind to a heterogeneous preparation of CRI^+ anti-TMA antibodies[67,83] as well as the monoclonal (m.c.) anti-TMA antibody B-5.4 which is represented predominantly in serum antibodies.[96] It is interesting that Ts_2 induced by tolerizing doses of nitrophenyl acetyl (NP) coupled to spleen cells (NP-SC) do not recognize the predominant serologically detected NP^b-Id, but rather recognize minor serologically detected Id represented in serum antibodies.[71] On the other hand, in this same system, Ts induced by immunizing doses of NP coupled to keyhole limpet hemocyanin (KLH) readily recognize the predominant Id associated with anti-NP antibodies.[77] However, these cells, designated T_{sid}, differ phenotypically as well as functionally from that of the tolerogen-induced Id-specific Ts_2. Thus, efferent-acting Id-specific Ts do not appear to represent an absolute homogeneous population of Ts, particularly with respect to fine specificity for Ig-associated Id. It would appear that dominant B-cell clones responding to immunizing doses of antigen may, in fact, dictate the fine Id specificity of these cells.

A major unresolved question involves the number and nature of the target idiotopes which play a role in immune suppression. Since IgV regions contain multiple Id determinants, which, if any, are key in the suppressor network system? Do Id-specific Ts and Th cells recognize the same or distinct Id when regulating target lymphocytes? The network hypothesis would predict that Ts would recognize only Id outside of the paratope region on receptors. The use of highly characterized m.c. antibodies with respect to localization of Id, along with binding studies, should aid in answering these questions.

2. Ts_2-Derived Factor(s)

Investigations into the nature of Ts cell interactions have been greatly facilitated by the use of cell extracts, cell-free products, and the secreted factors from monoclonal hybrids. To date, most of the information on the properties of Ts_2-derived TsF_2 is indirect and comes from experiments using various ligands and serological reagents coupled to Sepharose® 4B. The early work of Hirai and Nisonoff demonstrated that the ABA-TsF_2 induced in hyperimmune suppressed mice is sensitive to trypsin, but not to DNase or RNase treatment, and does not possess conventional Ig determinants. The molecular weight estimated by gel filtration is 50,000 to 100,000.[79] Further studies showed that TsF_2, which is involved in both humoral[79] and DTH[66] regulation, bears H-2 determinants and binds to CRI. Similarly, the m.c. hybridoma-derived NP-TsF_2 does not possess mouse Ig as well as NP^b-Id determinants, but does bear I-J region-encoded structures.[80] Moreover, the NP-TsF_2 has binding specificity only for NP^b-Id determinants and not for NP-KLH. Similarly, TsF involved in murine schistosomiasis bears I-J determinants and binds to Id.[93] In the TMA system, physical disruption of antigen-induced Ts_2 cells yields TsF_2 which is composed of two polypeptide chains connected by disulfide bond(s),[83] one of which bears I-J subregion-encoded determinants. The integrity of the two-chain structure is essential for its function, but the role for each is not known. The TMA-TsF_2 can be bound to and eluted from immunoadsorbents coupled with Id^+, but not to Id^- anti-TMA monoclonal antibodies.[84,85] Moreover, the TsF_2 does not bind to TMA-coupled Sepharose® 4B.[96]

Functionally, the TsF_2, like the Ts_2 cells, produce suppression both at induction as well as efferent phases of DTH responses in the ABA[66] and TMA[23] systems. However, the m.c. NP-TsF_2, like the tolerogen-induced Ts_2 cells, suppresses only the efferent phase of NP-specific responses.[80] Nevertheless, all three TsF_2 are functionally restricted by both H-2 and allotype-region-linked gene products,[66-67,80] and all, like Ts_2,[72,82,97,98] depend[84,99-102] upon the Ts_3 subset for function. Thus, despite minor differences between the individual systems studied, the overall properties of both Ts_2 cells and factors derived from them appear similar.

As yet, there are no reports describing the isolation of these factors in sufficient amounts to biochemically characterize them. This is undoubtedly due to the minute amounts produced by Ts and also cloned Ts_2-hybridomas. It is unlikely that the first structure-function information will come from studies at the protein level, but rather deduced from cloned and sequenced Ts_2 genes.

B. Induction

1. General Considerations

The original finding that inoculation of anti-Id and antigen resulted in Id-specific suppression[18] has been reproduced in several antigen systems dominated by well-defined CRI. In addition, other studies have demonstrated that antigen-antibody complexes,[25] anti-Id plus antigen complexes,[26] and Id-bearing antibodies in solution[74,90,91] as well as coupled to syngeneic SC[62,64,75,92,97,103-105] all serve as sufficient inductive signals for the generation of Id-specific Ts_2 cells. All of these studies provided some information about initial inductive signal(s) and further documented the existence of Id-specific Ts in several model systems. However, they provided no insight into the cellular events that occur between the initial signal and the eventual formation of Id-specific Ts.

Significant insight into Ts induction, in general, came from the early studies of Tada in the KLH,[106] Waltenbaugh and associates in the L-glutamic acid[50]-L-tyrosine[50] (GT), and L-glutamic acid[60]-L-alanine[30]-L-tyrosine[10] (GAT) systems[107,108] and Cantor and colleagues in the sheep erythrocyte (SRBC) systems.[109] Soluble suppressor factors (TsF) derived from one population of Ts cells were shown to function by inducing subsequent Ts cell types. Although Ts cells in the KLH, GAT, and SRBC systems are antigen and not Id specific, these findings indicated the existence of amplification loops in suppressor systems. This approach in Id-defined systems also revealed that Id^+-Ts_1/TsF_1 trigger the formation of Id-specific Ts_2. Since all these studies involved experimental manipulation, it was not clear whether these inductive mechanisms reflected physiological events. The question remained whether antigen alone could trigger Ts_2 suppressor cells at some point in an immune response. This was first suggested by Alevy and Bellone who showed that injection of the synthetic antigen L-tyrosine-*p*-azophenyltrimethylammonium (tyr[TMA]) alone in Freund's complete adjuvant (FCA) results in the induction of Id-specific Ts.[21] These cells appeared 6 weeks after a single inoculation of antigen and functioned to selectively suppress the Id^+ component of the anti-TMA antibody response. Weinberger and colleagues demonstrated that i.v. injection of NP-SC stimulated the formation of both induction-phase Ts_1 as well as an Id-specific effector-phase Ts_2 population.[69] They further demonstrated that NP-binding Ts_1 cells can, in the presence of NP-SC, induce a population of effector phase Ts_2 cells, suggesting the sequential induction of Ts_1 and Ts_2 cells. If the stimulation of Ts_2 by Ts_1 has any in vivo relevance, one should be able to detect in the same animal first the Id-bearing Ts_1 followed by the appearance of Id-binding Ts_2 in the course of an immune response to antigen or to tolerization by haptenated SC. Such a possibility was demonstrated in the TMA system. Injection of adult mice with tyr(TMA) in FCA triggered an orderly sequence of nonoverlapping regulatory T-cell populations. Within 1 week, an Id-bearing T helper population was detected in the absence of any Ts activity.[96,110] An antigen-binding, Id-bearing, induction-phase Ts_1 population appeared 1 week later,[23] and between 3 and 7 weeks after antigen administration, an Id-binding Ts_2 population was detected in the same experimental animals.[67,96] These results demonstrated that antigen administered under *nontolerogenic* conditions can induce a wave of regulatory T cells which appear to interact by complementary Id-anti-Id receptor recognition.

Since the above results strongly implicated Ts_1/TsF_1 as a key inductive signal for Ts_2, we and others have studied conditions required for the induction of Id-specific Ts_2 utilizing the Ts_1-derived TsF_1. Three systems have mainly been studied which include the ABA,[13] NP,[16] and TMA[15] systems. These model systems share important similarities which include: (1)

antibody to their respective ligands is dominated by well-characterized Id; (2) these Id are also shared by some Ts populations; and (3) similar Ts_1, Ts_2 (Id-specific), and Ts_3 populations have been identified in the regulation of immune responses. Several questions have been approached regarding Ts_2 induction: what is the role, if any, of major histocompatibility (MHC) gene products? Is TsF_1 a sufficient inductive signal or is antigen also required? If so, what role does antigen play regarding subsequent cellular events?

2. *Role of MHC Products*

In view of the fact that Ts_2 cells are functionally restricted by both MHC and allotype region-linked gene products, it was hypothesized that the induction of Ts_2 by TsF_1 may also be influenced by the products of these same gene complexes. It is important to recall that TsF_1 involved in the ABA[111] and NP[94] systems is not H-2 restricted, but only allotype restricted, whereas in the TMA system,[83] it is neither H-2 nor allotype restricted for function. These observations suggest that at least the H-2 genotype of the inducer Id^+ TsF_1 is not responsible for the MHC restriction of the induced Ts_2 cells. Furthermore, it was observed that the allotype-restricted NP-TsF_1 could generate Ts_2-like cells across an H-2 and allotype barrier, but failed to function due to the lack of an appropriate target in the recipient mice.[94] This phenomenon, termed pseudogenetic restriction, appears to reflect a requirement for homology between anti-Id Ts_2 cells and another cell population which, presumably, bears complementary Id receptors. In the case cited above, only Id determinant(s) on TsF_1 appeared to play a key role in subsequent Ts_2 cell activation and function. In the TMA system, we have observed that A/J (H-2^a; Igh-1^e)-derived TsF_1 acts across both an H-2 and allotype barrier.[83] When A/J TsF_1 was injected into SJL/J (H-2^s; Igh-1^b) mice, the reulting Ts cells produced suppression in the SJL/J mice, but not in the A/J strain.[112] The cells were found to be effector-phase and antigen-specific, but failed to bind Id associated with anti-TMA antibodies produced in A/J mice. These data demonstrated that (1) TMA-TsF_1 can induce Ts_2 in allogeneic mice; (2) the induced Ts_2 cells function in the host strain which produced them and not in the TsF_1 donor, unlike the NP system; (3) the genetic restriction is not imposed by the TsF_1, but rather by the host which produces the Ts_2; and finally, (4) the Ts_2 cells induced across an allotype barrier do not have specificity for Id determinants of the donor strain. Collectively, the data indicate that TsF_1 is processed and re-presented by host factor-presenting cells which appear to play an important role in the subsequent Ts_2 restriction. In the NP system, it was shown that induction of Ts_2 cells across an H-2 barrier requires presentation of m.c. TsF_1 by I-J^+ macrophages/dendritic cells.[95] The I-J phenotype of this factor-presenting population and not the genotype of the TsF_1 controls the H-2 restriction of Ts_2 cells. Similarly, in the ABA system it was observed that when A/J-derived TsF_1 is administered into A.BY (H-2^b; Igh-1^e), the subsequent Ts_2 and its factor are restricted to H-2^b rather than the H-2^a gene products present on A/J-ABA-TsF_1 itself.[99] Thus, it appears that Ts_1-mediated induction of Ts_2 proceeds through soluble TsF_1 which is presented to the precursors of Ts_2 on I-J^+ factor-presenting cells. This interaction between TsF_1-presenting cells and Ts_2 precursors appears to determine the subsequent H-2-restricted suppressor function. Since the Ts_1 population is also I-J^+ and bears surface TsF_1-like molecules, it is possible that the direct interaction of Ts_1 and precursors of Ts_2 results in the induction of H-2 and allotype-restricted Ts_2 activity. However, at present there is no evidence for this direct Ts_1-precursor-Ts_2 interaction.

3. *Role of Accessory Signal(s)*

A vast majority of TsF_1 studied to date requires antigen as an accessory signal to induce Ts_2 cells irrespective of the mode of induction, varied biochemical nature, and the presence or absence of genetic restrictions imposed on the function of inducer TsF_1.[108,113,114] The requirement for antigen in the induction of Ts_2 was first demonstrated by Germain et al. in the GAT system.[108] Several hypotheses which explain the requirement of antigen have been put forth. These include: (1) interaction of antigen and TsF_1 results in the formation of neodeterminants that favor the activation of Ts_2; (2) presence of antigen may serve as a focusing signal to direct TsF_1 to its appropriate target; and (3) the TsF_1 may represent one of the subunits required for the formation of a biologically active molecule to induce Ts_2, while the other subunit comes from an antigen-stimulated population. In all these cases, TsF_1 plus antigen induce Ts_2 cells with specificity for antigen and not for Id.[108,113]

In the ABA and NP systems where a major dominant CRI is present, antigen is not necessary for the induction of Ts_2 cells by TsF_1. Both the in vivo[65,66] and hybridoma-derived[95,111] TsF_1 induce Ts_2 in the apparent absence of antigen. Since antigen is not present in the case of TsF_1 derived from long-term hybridoma cultures, the argument that trace amounts of antigen are bound to TsF_1 can be ruled out in these systems. Since TsF_1 in these systems bear CRI, it was postulated that the CRI-bearing TsF_1 was sufficient to trigger Id-specific Ts_2, while in systems which lack a major CRI, antigen is also required in the inductive signal.[113] The exception to this rule was observed in the TMA system which is dominated by a major CRI. The induction of Id-specific Ts_2 by TMA-TsF_1 requires the presence of the TMA ligand.[83] Inoculation of TsF_1 alone into naive A/J mice does not generate efferent-acting Ts_2 cell activity as long as 1 month after TsF_1 injection.[96] If, however, TsF_1 is administered along with the TMA ligand, a Ts_2 population appears within 1 week which is indistinguishable from the Ts_2 induced by the tyr (TMA) antigen alone (vide supra). As previously noted, this Ts_2 population binds to the major CRI associated with serum antibodies as well as the m.c. anti-TMA antibody, B-5.4. Manipulation of the second signal (antigen) has yielded some insight into its role in generating Id-binding Ts_2. Normally, we administer soluble TsF_1 i.v. and at the same time the tyr(TMA) antigen is inoculated i.p. in FCA. If, however, we substitute L-tyrosine-*p*-azophenylarsonate (tyr[ABA]) in FCA or give FCA alone along with TsF_1, a Ts population is generated which can suppress DTH responses at the efferent phase. However, this population does not have specificity for the m.c. B-5.4, unlike the TsF_1 + tyr(TMA)-induced Ts_2 population.[96] It is not known whether this population binds Id other than that found on the prototypical B-5.4 m.c. antibody. Two points can be made from these experiments: (1) TsF_1 requires a second signal to generate efferent-phase Ts activity and (2) tyr(TMA) is absolutely required for the generation of Id-specific Ts_2 which bind to the m.c. B-5.4 antibody. Although the mechanisms responsible for the induction of B-5.4-specific Ts_2 are unknown, there are several possibilities which can explain these data. The first involves the interaction of TsF_1 with its specific ligand, the tyr(TMA) antigen. The combination may be necessary either to create or expose Id determinants on TsF_1 which cross react with B-5.4 Id specificities. This complex, perhaps presented by macrophage, then serves to induce the appropriate Ts_2 population to a fully mature efferent-acting cell type. Another possibility involves the direct intervention of B cells which bear surface B-5.4-like receptors. The TsF_1-ligand complex may stimulate these B cells which, in turn, directly or indirectly influence the Ts_2 specificity. There are now several examples of the role of B-cell Ig and its influence on the development of the Ts cell repertoire.[115-121] A variation on this possibility involves the interaction of the tyr(TMA) as a separate antigenic signal with the appropriate B-cell compartment. Although the monovalent antigen tyr(TMA) does not induce anti-TMA antibody formation, it does perturb TMA-specific B cells.[122] Any expansion of the B-5.4-bearing B cells could then influence the TsF_1-induced Id-specific Ts_2 repertoire. Finally, the TsF_1 may combine with a tyr(TMA)-induced T- or B-cell product to form a complete biologically active molecule in order to induce Id-specific Ts_2 precursors. More work is necessary to better understand the mechanisms responsible for Ts_2 induction by TsF_1 and the tyr(TMA) antigen.

As mentioned previously, Id-bearing NP and ABA-TsF_1 induce Ts_2 in the absence of antigen or other signals. Perhaps the difference in the antigen requirement between these and the TMA system lies in the chemical nature of the TsF_1 involved. Whereas the ABA-TsF_1 is made up of two polypeptide chains,[123] TMA-TsF_1 is composed of only a single chain.[83] In the former, one chain bears I-J, while the other contains the antigen binding site(s). The TMA-TsF_1 bears I-J and Id determinants as well as the antigen binding site on a single chain.[83,112] The two-chain structure may contain all the necessary inductive signals, while the single-chain structure lacks a critical signal which is supplied by the antigen.

The structural differences in these inducer molecules would suggest that these TsF_1 originate from different Ts_1 populations. This is somewhat surprising, since the Ts_1 examined in the ABA,[13] NP,[124] and TMA[23] DTH systems appear virtually identical. The Ts_1 populations function only at the induction phase of the response, bind antigen, express the I-J and $Ly1^+2^-$ phenotype, and suppress across H-2 barriers. However, a key difference is the lack of allotype restriction for the function of TMA-TsF_1[83] in contrast to ABA- and NP-TsF_1. It is clear from a variety of antigen systems (both Id and non-Id-defined systems) that a formulation of a consensus pathway at the induction level is not possible at this time.

It is clear that Ts_2 are induced in response to Ts_1/TsF_1 in both Id and non-Id-defined systems. In the former, the Ts_2 population is Id specific[65,69,83] and the latter antigen specific.[108,113,125] The question remains whether Id-specific Ts_2 are utilized in the non-Id-defined systems and vice versa, i.e., do antigen-specific Ts_2 function in the Id-dominated systems? Evidence for Id-specific Ts exists in GT[126] and GAT[127] systems which normally utilize antigen-specific Ts_2.[107,108,125] Functional Id-specific Ts_2 hybridomas have been generated by either in vivo injection of GT-TsF_1[126] or generated in vitro by incubation of spleen cells with GAT-TsF_1[127] and subsequent fusion of the induced population with the BW 5147 thymoma cell line. Thus, Id-specific Ts exist in these systems, but do not appear to function under normal conditions. Regarding the reciprocal situation, we have attempted and failed to detect an antigen-specific Ts_2-like population in the Id-dominated TMA system. To our knowledge, this type of cell has not been detected after Id^+ Ts_1/TsF_1 induction in other Id-dominated systems as well.

There is thought that in the Id-dominated systems, the equivalent of the antigen-specific Ts_2 may be the Id^+ antigen-binding Ts_3 population. However, this cell type, best characterized in the DTH systems, does not appear to be induced by Ts_1/TsF_1, but is coinduced with DTH effector cells after antigen stimulation. The Ts_3 subset remains dormant until acted upon by Id-specific Ts_2/TsF_2. These conditions are clearly different from that of the antigen-specific Ts_2 which is induced by Ts_1/TsF_1 plus antigen and not by antigen alone. At present, the relationship between the suppressor pathways utilized in the Id- and non-Id-dominated systems is not clearly understood. Certainly, more work is needed to determine which cells, if any, are shared between these systems or do these systems represent independent parallel suppressor circuits? Resolution of these questions will depend upon a thorough identification of existing Ts subsets and the elucidation of signals which are required to trigger the various subsets.

C. Mode of Action

In this section we will explore the mechanisms by which Id-specific Ts_2 bring about immune suppression. These cells have been studied at both the cell-mediated (primarily DTH) and humoral immune response levels. We will first review the studies in DTH systems where a great deal of consistent data indicate that the Ts_2 population does not function as the final effector suppressor, i.e., the cell itself or its product(s) is not directly responsible for suppression. Secondly, we will discuss the systems where suppression of antibody responses has been studied. This category is the more controversial in that evidence exists for and against the Ts_2 as a final effector Ts cell type.

1. DTH Regulation

a. Ts_3-Mediated Suppression

Sy et al.[128] first demonstrated that efferent-acting Ts in the 1-fluoro-2,4-dinitrobenzene (DNFB) contact sensitivity system do not function unless a distinct cyclophosphamide (CY)-sensitive, I-J-positive, Ts subset was present along with the target immune T cells. This cell type, called the Ts auxiliary (Ts-aux), was found to be specifically induced by antigen, MHC and Igh restricted, and did not function to suppress unless acted upon by the efferent Ts population.[128,129] These findings led investigators to examine whether Id-specific Ts_2 also depended upon a similar Ts cell type. This was found to be the case in several DTH systems; consistent with previous nomenclature in the Id systems, this cell type was termed Ts_3.[12] This cell possesses I-J in the NP system[82] and Ly 1^-2^+ determinants in the TMA system,[98] binds antigen in the TMA system,[84] and bears surface Id in the ABA[97] and TMA[98] systems. These cells are induced with antigen along with the immune effector T cells, but remain dormant until acted upon by Ts_2/TsF_2. Both MHC and Igh restrictions govern their function.[67,82,130] It was originally suggested that the dual genetic restriction might be the result of combined presentation of the anti-Id receptor along with Ia determinants on Ts_2 to Ts_3.[82] Alternatively, Ts_2 may combine with two distinct Ts_3 populations, one via Ia interaction, the other via an Id-anti-Id interaction. More recent studies in the NP system indicate that these restrictions lie at the level of specialized antigen-presenting cells, the so-called factor-presenting cells.[131] In these studies I-J^b- or I-J^k-restricted hybridoma-derived TsF_2 was pulsed onto Igh-similar B10.A(5R) (I-J^k) or B10.A(3R) (I-J^b) splenic adherent cells which were then injected i.v. into recipients previously primed for NP-specific cutaneous hypersensitivity responses. Although soluble I-J^b TsF_2 failed to function in 5R recipients (I-J^k), when pulsed onto I-J-compatible 3R adherent cells (I-J^b), suppression was observed after inoculation of the pulsed adherent cells into the 5R recipients. However, when the same TsF_2 was added to I-J-incompatible 5R adherent cells and inoculated into 5R recipients, no suppression was produced. These results demonstrate that the I-J restriction of TsF_2 is directed toward determinants on the adherent accessory cell population. Thus, the data suggest that TsF_2 may not directly interact with the Id^+ Ts_3 population, but with an accessory-cell population necessary for presentation of TsF_2 to Ts_3.

The Igh restriction between Ts_2 and Ts_3 appears to be due to the necessity of Id-anti-Id interactions between the interacting cell populations. Insight into these interactions came from the studies of Sy et al.[97] in the ABA system. These authors demonstrated that Id-specific Ts_2 induced with A/J-derived Id^+ antibody coupled to SC failed to function in the Igh disparate BALB/c strain of mouse. However, these cells produced suppression when adoptively transferred into the Igh congenic CAL.20 strain which had the capacity to generate the appropriate Id^+ Ts_3 target. Interaction of the transferred Ts_2 with Id^+ Ts_3 resulted in the suppression of DTH-mediating T cells which lacked surface Id and, thus, was considered Id-nonspecific suppression. Thus, the failure to generate suppression in the Igh disparate strain was attributed to the lack of an Id^+ Ts_3 target and not to failure of these mice to generate Id-specific Ts_2. Furthermore, the results suggested that the Ts_3 was the final effector Ts cell type in this system.

Experiments in the TMA system confirm and extend these observations. Despite the fact that the A/J strain of mice has the ability to produce CRI associated with both anti-ABA[13] and anti-TMA[132] antibodies, immunization with TMA-SC results in the generation of only the TMA-binding,[84] Id^+ Ts_3 subset.[98] The Id binding TMA-TsF_2 can only activate Ts_3-containing lymphocyte populations induced with homologous TMA-SC and not populations induced by ABA-SC or NP-SC, presumably, because heterologous immunogen-induced Ts_3 cells lack appropriate Id structure(s) necessary for interaction.[84] In the same studies, we also showed that a brief in vitro incubation of Ts_3 with TsF_2 was sufficient to trigger Ts_3 to suppress in vivo DTH responses. Furthermore, once the Ts_3 cells were triggered appropriately, they suppressed unrelated ABA- and NP-directed cutaneous hypersensitivity responses in CY-treated recipients. Thus, the TMA-binding, Id^+ Ts_3 cells serve as a final effector Ts population mediating antigen-nonspecific suppression. In the NP system, the m.c. TsF_3, the product of a presumed Ts_3 hybridoma, suppresses immune responses in an antigen-specific fashion in CY-treated mice.[133] Furthermore, the TsF_3 is restricted by both H-2 and allotype-gene products for function. It is not very clear whether the Ts_3 or TsF_3 represents the final effector in the NP system. Nevertheless, the data obtained in all three systems collectively indicate that the anti-Id Ts_2/TsF_2 definitely do not represent the final effector Ts cell population or the effector Ts molecules in cell-mediated immune responses; rather they appear to represent an intermediary transducer cell and/or molecules important for communication between the Id^+ Ts_1 and Ts_3 populations.

b. T Acceptor Subset-Mediated Suppression

Very recent studies in the NP[134] and TMA[85] systems indicate the potential role of yet another terminal-phase Ts subset, the T acceptor (Tacc) cell. Zembala and co-workers[135-138] first described the role of Tacc in mediating suppression of contact sensitivity responses by hapten-specific efferent-acting TsF_2. The Tacc subset does not require specific antigen to be induced and is easily generated by epicutaneous application of irrelevant contact sensitizers. The Tacc does not appear to bear inherent antigen receptors and acquires specificity only after accepting hapten-specific TsF. Thus, ''armed'' Tacc is a CY-sensitive, $Ly\text{-}1^-2^+$, $I\text{-}J^+$, and Fc receptor-positive T cell. Once the binding sites of surface-attached TsF are occupied by the specific hapten and similar I-J products as that of the TsF, the Tacc is then triggered to release nonspecific inhibitor(s). Thus, the Tacc functions as a final effector Ts cell type in several systems which do not possess a dominant CRI.

Although this cell type has not been functionally detected under normal circumstances in the NP or any other Id-dominated antigen system in vitro, incubation of Tacc first with hybridoma-derived NP-TsF_3 and then with NP-SC resulted in the release of nonspecific inhibitor of contact sensitivity.[134] Based on these findings, it was postulated that activation of Ts_3 by Id-specific TsF_2 results in the release of TsF_3 which, in turn, arms the Tacc.[16] Once this cell plus adsorbed TsF_3 encounter the homologous NP ligand plus I-J products. it is activated to release nonspecific inhibitors of contact sensitivity. In this scheme, Ts_2/TsF_2 interacts with only the Ts_3 population which, in turn, activates the Tacc to effect suppression.

In the TMA system, evidence has accumulated to suggest that either the Ts_3[84] or Tacc[85] can alternatively be used as a final effector suppressor after activation by Id-specific TsF_2. The initial observations came from in vivo studies which suggested that the Tacc could substitute for the Ts_3 population.[96,139] Earlier studies in the TMA system demonstrated that under certain conditions, Id-specific Ts_2-bearing mice fail to suppress TMA-specific DTH responses due to a Ts_3 dysfunction.[98] However, we have been able to restore Ts_2-mediated suppressor function by reconstituting the defective mice with not only Ts_3 cells,[98] but also with the Tacc population.[139] Both of these transferred populations depended upon the presence of the Ts_2 cells in these host mice. These experiments suggested the possibility that the Ts_2 population could alternatively utilize either of the populations. We have further tested this possibility by employing transfer protocols in which either of these populations was first incubated in vitro with affinity-purified Id-binding TsF_2 before transfer into normal TMA-DTH-primed recipients.[84,85] Since these recipients were treated with CY to eliminate the Ts_3 and Tacc subsets, any observed suppression was considered to be mediated by the transferred cells. Thus, the donor cells were considered the final effector/suppressor population. The results from these protocols clearly demonstrated that Id-specific TsF_2 could functionally interact with either the Tacc or Ts_3 population. Several control protocols established the absolute requirement for TsF_2 interaction with either of the populations. Furthermore, binding

Table 1
BINDING PROPERTIES OF Ts_3 AND TACC CELLS[84,85]

Type of cell tested	Fractionated cells incubated with TMA-TsF_2	Suppression transferred (%)
Ts_3	TMA-BSA adherent	*73*
	TMA-BSA nonadherent	0
	ABA-BSA adherent	23
	ABA-BSA nonadherent	*102*
Tacc	TMA-BSA adherent	0
	TMA-BSA nonadherent	*58*
	ABA-BSA adherent	15
	ABA-BSA nonadherent	*81*

Note: The Ts_3 was primed by s.c. immunization of A/J mice with TMA-SC and the Tacc by skin painting with 10 m*M* diazonium salt of ABA mixed in dimethylsulfoxide. Five days later, draining lymph nodes and spleens were harvested and T cells were enriched by panning the lymphoid cells on petri dishes coated with affinity-purified rabbit antimouse Ig. The recipient A/J mice were immunized s.c. with TMA-SC 5 days earlier and treated with CY on day 1. Mice were challenged in the footpads with diazotized TMA within 2 hr of cell transfer. The footpad swelling response was measured the following day. Significant suppression is shown in italics.

experiments on antigen-coated petri dishes as well as other functional properties unique to the different cell types indicated that we were not dealing with a mixture of terminal phase populations, i.e., a Tacc population was contaminated with Ts_3 and vice versa. An example of one of these experiments is seen in Table 1. Normal A/J mice were primed subcutaneously with TMA-SC, a procedure known to induce Ts_3 and effector DTH cells.[84,98] Because Tacc are induced in a nonspecific manner,[134-138] it was possible that this population was also coinduced by TMA-SC injection. Since the Ts_3 population possesses hapten-specific receptors[84] while the Tacc bear no known intrinsic receptors,[136] the primed population was first incubated on TMA-protein-coated petri dishes. The cells were subsequently separated into an antigen-adherent and nonadherent population. After a brief incubation with Id-specific TsF_2, these treated populations were then transferred into CY-treated TMA-DTH-primed recipients to assess their suppressor activity. The results show that only the adherent TsF_2-treated population transferred suppression. Had the unseparated population contained Tacc, the nonadherent population, after TsF_2 treatment, would have transferred suppression. It could, however, be argued that prior to separation of the two populations, the Tacc could have passively acquired TsF_3 from the Ts_3 population. If this had been the case, the TMA-SC-primed T-cell population should have transferred suppression without the need for TsF_2 incubation, since Tacc armed with hapten-specific TsF require only the homologous hapten plus self-I-J products to release nonspecific inhibitor.[134-137] Since the purified Ts_3-containing T cells never transferred suppression without in vitro treatment with TsF_2, this possibility was ruled out. Thus, the data argue against the possibility of coinduction of Tacc with Ts_3 cells after TMA-SC immunization.

The contention that the protocols employed for in vivo induction of Ts_3 or Tacc do not result in a mixture of these cells was further supported by a reciprocal experiment performed with Tacc cells. In this case, normal A/J mice were primed by skin painting with the diazonium salt of ABA which induces Tacc as well as effector T cells mediating contact sensitivity.[85] The enriched T-cell populations were incubated on TMA-BSA-coated petri dishes in an identical fashion as described above. After separation of adherent and nonadherent cells, the two populations were separately incubated in vitro with TMA-TsF_2 and and transferred into TMA-DTH-primed CY-treated recipients to assess suppressive activity. The results show that in this case only the nonadherent population transferred suppression (Table 1). The failure of TMA-binding fraction to transfer suppression demonstrated that TMA-binding Ts_3 was not induced by a procedure known to induce Tacc activity. Furthermore, when the ABA-primed population was incubated in petri dishes coated with ABA-BSA, the adherent population also failed to be activated by TMA-TsF_2, indicating that an ABA-binding Ts_3-like population was also not responsible for the observed suppression. Thus, these experiments confirmed that the Tacc population was not contaminated with hapten-binding Ts_3 cells. Host contribution of Ts_3 or other similar Ts cell types has been precluded by CY treatment. Taken together, it appears that the Ts_2 population serves as a bifurcation point in the TMA suppressor pathway and can mediate suppression of DTH through one of two alternate pathways: $Ts_1 \rightarrow Ts_2 \rightarrow Ts_3$ or $Ts_1 \rightarrow Ts_2 \rightarrow$ Tacc.

2. Antibody Regulation

In spite of a large body of evidence for the involvement of Id-specific Ts_2 in B-cell control, it is not clear how the preferential suppression of Id^+ B-cell clones is brought about. In the A-CHO system, it was suggested that Id-bearing T helper cell precursors are the immediate target.[53] The Id^+ B cells themselves are considered to be the target of Id-specific Ts_2 in the ABA system.[56,57,79] In the PC system, it was suggested that either B cells[59] or T-15 Id^+ helper T cells[25] are the target of Ts_2. Evidence has been presented in the NP system for two types of Id-specific Ts_2. One type is induced by i.v. tolerization of mice with NP-SC and depends on the presence of NP-binding, Ly-1^-,2^+, I-J^+, NP^b-Id-bearing Ts_3 cells to suppress antibody responses in vitro.[72] More recently, the same group has described a Ts_2 (T_{sid}) cell which is generated by primary immunization with NP-KLH and appears to be a final effector cell type, since it does not depend on the Ts_3 subset to suppress in vitro anti-NP antibody response.[77]

Along these lines, we have evidence in the TMA system for a Ts_2 cell which functions in a somewhat similar manner to the T_{sid} population. We have shown that a single injection of tyr(TMA) in FCA results in the appearance of distinct Ts subsets in a sequential non-overlapping manner, i.e., 2 weeks after tyr(TMA) injection, we detect only an Id-bearing Ts_1 population[23] and by 6 weeks, only an Id-specific Ts_2 subset.[67] When these mice were immunized with TMA coupled to protein at the 2- or 6-week time period, interesting results were obtained. In the Ts_1-bearing mice, both the Id^+ and Id^- components of the anti-TMA PFC response were suppressed[23] (Table 2). In contrast, the Id^+ PFC were preferentially suppressed in the Ts_2-bearing mice.[21,23] Further analysis revealed that the Ts_2-bearing mice had lost the ability to generate the functional Ts_3 subset and could no longer suppress TMA-specific DTH responses.[98] Despite this loss of Ts_3, the Ts_2-bearing mice maintained the ability to suppress Id^+ PFC. Taken together, the data suggested that under these circumstances the Id^+ B cells were the immediate target of the Id-specific Ts_2 population. On the other hand, the data from the Ts_1-bearing mice left open the possibility that Ts_3 were activated (via induced Ts_2) to release nonspecific inhibitors which accounted for the suppression of both Id^+ and Id^- PFC. Thus, like the NP system, evidence is presented that Id-specific Ts_2 can suppress B-cell responses by several cellular mechanisms.

Although the above systems presented no clear-cut evidence that B cells are the immediate target of Id-specific Ts, the MOPC 315 myeloma system offers a unique opportunity to examine this question. Lynch and colleagues have shown that multiple injections of the MOPC 315 myeloma protein into syngeneic BALB/c mice lead to the appearance of Id-specific Ts cells.[91] The introduction of MOPC 315 myeloma cells into these mice resulted in the suppression of myeloma protein secretion. In these protocols, transplantable myeloma cells were placed inside cell chambers and introduced into the peritoneum of mice. These

Table 2
MODE OF ACTION OF Ts_1 AND Ts_2 ON ANTIBODY PRODUCTION[23]

Group immunized	Suppression of anti-TMA IgG plaque-forming cell response (%)		
	Total	Id^+	Id^-
Ts_1-bearing mice	*73*	*70*	*75*
Ts_2-bearing mice	40	*98*	22

Note: A/J mice which received 100μg of tyr(TMA) in FCA i.p. were immunized i.p. with 100μg of TMA-BSA in FCA either 2 weeks (Ts_1-bearing mice) or 6 weeks (Ts_2-bearing mice) later. These mice were boosted 3 weeks later with 50 μg of soluble TMA-BSA and their spleen cells were plaqued 1 week later. Significant suppression is shown in italics.

chambers were impermeable to cellular movement in and out of the capsule, but allowed the exchange of molecules between the host and the interior of the chamber. Since the chambers precluded direct cell contact between the host Ts cells and the myeloma target cells, suppression appears to have been mediated by factors released from the Ts population. Very similar results have also been generated in vitro[76] and again indicate that a soluble factor derived from Id-specific Ts mediates suppression. Since M315 production by the myeloma cells is independent of T helper activity, it is clear that the immediate target of the Ts was not a T helper population. In addition, the target myeloma cells were apparently cultured free of other T cells and macrophages in the chambers. Thus, it is clear that soluble factors derived from Ts function by direct interaction with the myeloma cells. Although the data strongly argue that the product of an Id-specific Ts is responsible for suppression, the possibility that other Ts, such as the Ts_3 or Tacc, serve as the final effector cannot be completely ruled out.

Abbas et al., in a similar myeloma system, have also presented results which indicate that B cells are the direct target of Ts products. They observed that BALB/c mice injected i.v. with syngeneic SC coupled with the M315 protein developed Id-specific Ts that inhibit in vitro IgA secretion by MOPC 315 cells after 3 to 4 days of coculture.[64] Immunization with M315-coupled SC subcutaneously, followed by administration of a soluble extract of the i.v.-induced Id-specific Ts_1 cell, lead to the generation of an effector Ts_2 population that was also Id specific and inhibits myeloma function within 1 day.[75] The Ts_2 cells are $Ly\text{-}1^-,2^+$ and, unlike the results of Milburn and Lynch,[76] require the presence of an $I\text{-}A^+$ accessory cell population which was required for concentrating and/or presenting soluble TsF_2 to myeloma target cells.[140,141] It was not clear, however, whether the actual suppression was mediated by Id-specific TsF_2 or by another T cell such as Ts_3 or Tacc in the immune cell sample used in these studies.

The MOPC 315 myeloma system has also been utilized to study the molecular mechanisms involved in the selective suppression of myeloma protein secretion by Id-specific Ts. MOPC 315 myeloma cells suppressed by Id-specific Ts were analyzed for mRNA levels using hybridization techniques and cDNA probes specific for α or λ_{II} light chain constant regions.[142] Using this approach it was determined that suppressed MOPC 315 cells contained normal levels of α heavy chain mRNA,[143] whereas little λ_{II} light chain mRNA was detected.[142] Furthermore, these studies also revealed that the Ts simultaneously inhibited the expression of a truncated λ_I mRNA, which has been shown to be the product of an aberrantly rearranged λ gene in MOPC 315 cells. The results implied that λ_I and λ_{II} genes are coordinately regulated despite the fact that the aberrantly rearranged λ_I gene and the productively rearranged λ_{II} gene reside on different copies of chromosome 16.[144] It appears that the events which result in the preferential suppression of λ mRNA are initiated at the cell surface by engagement of the M315 surface receptor by the Ts product. The ensuing suppressive events can be reversed by protease treatment of the MOPC 315 cells and additional culture.[145,146] Studies by Abbas and colleagues[147] suggest that these surface events are highly specific and only that portion of the Ig-producing apparatus of the cell that is linked to the surface Id is affected. In this system, Id-specific Ts were generated against the MPC 11 myeloma protein (IgG_{2b},K) or the MOPC 315 myeloma protein (IgA,λ_2), each of which suppresses myeloma secretion only in their homologous systems. These Ts were cultured independently along with a MOPC 315-MPC 11 hybrid line which secretes both IgG_{2b},k and IgA,λ_2 molecules. In the presence of the M315 Id-specific Ts, only the M315 protein secretion was suppressed and vice versa. These results are consistent with a linked coordinated suppression which initiated at the surface receptor level and is specific for the expressed surface Id.

In summary, from the foregoing discussion of this entire section, it is evident that T and B cells are not necessarily regulated in the same fashion by Id-specific Ts cells. On the one hand, suppression of DTH and other similar cell-mediated responses definitely require one or more terminal-phase Ts subset beyond the Ts_2 population. Controversy still exists whether or not Ts_3 and Tacc interact sequentially or whether they serve as alternative targets of Ts_2 to produce suppression in hypersensitivity responses. On the other hand, it appears that Id-specific Ts_2-mediated antibody suppression does not always depend on other terminal-phase suppressors. It appears, in some cases, additional Ts are required, while in others Ts_2 directly shut down B cells. At present, the significance of these multiple cellular mechanisms are not clearly understood, nor is it precisely known how or what regulatory signals govern which pathway that is to be utilized.

IV. A NOVEL EFFERENT SUPPRESSOR T CELL SPECIFIC FOR T-CELL-ASSOCIATED ID

In this section we will describe a novel Ts cell with specificity for Id which is associated with the TsF_1 molecule and apparently not shared with immunoglobulins. As reported earlier,[83] administration of TMA-TsF_1 alone does not induce detectable efferent-acting Ts activity even as long as 1 month after TsF_1 inoculation.[96] If, however, the TsF_1-primed spleen cells were mixed with similar cells from mice separately primed with the tyr(TMA) antigen in FCA, this combination suppressed DTH responses at the efferent phase.[148] This necessary complementation requires T cells in both populations, and each appears to be functionally distinct. Interestingly, the population originally induced with the tyr(TMA) antigen can be induced either with complete or incomplete Freund's adjuvant alone, suggesting a polyclonal induced cell type with no apparent antigen specificity. However, this nonspecific T-cell population is absolutely required but not sufficient for effector-mediated suppression of the DTH response. There does not appear to be any genetic restriction between the TMA-TsF_1 and the nonspecifically induced complementing cell type. Rather, the non-specific T cells have to be genetically matched (I-J subregion) with that of the DTH-primed recipient mice. Furthermore, no Igh match is required between the nonspecific T cells or the TMA-TsF_1-induced population and the recipients, indicating no apparent role for Igh-determined gene products in this novel suppressor pathway. Thus, the only genetic restriction in this system is imposed by the nonspecific T cell. Furthermore, analysis of this T cell indicates that it has very distinct properties from the previously described final effector Ts_3 and/or Tacc.

In contrast to the nonspecific T cell the complementing TMA-TsF_1-induced cell does not impose any genetic restriction, but appears to contribute to the specificity of immune suppression. Induction of this population is specific in that only TMA-TsF_1 and not control spleen cell lysate-induced cells can complement nonspecific cells to produce suppression. Moreover, such a cell complementation results in suppression of only TMA and not heterologous hapten-specific DTH or cutaneous hypersensitivity responses. These results demonstrate that the specificity of suppression mediated by this cellular complementation is very different from that of the conventional Ts_2-Ts_3 or Ts_2-Tacc interactions described earlier. Furthermore, suppression by the complementing cells does not depend on any additional CY-sensitive cell type provided by DTH-primed recipient mice. Considering the specificity of suppression and the nature of the cells, it appears that the TMA-TsF_1-induced Ts interact in a specific way with TMA-specific DTH-mediating cells.[148]

Since there does not appear to be an Igh restriction between the target DTH and suppressor cells, it is not likely that the suppressor population has specificity for Ig-associated Id. This has been examined, and unlike the conventional tyr(TMA) antigen +TMA-TsF_1-induced Ts_2,[83] the TsF_1 alone induced Ts population does not bind to petri dishes adsorbed with Id-bearing polyclonal anti-TMA antibodies nor to the monoclonal Id+ B-5.4 andibody.[96] Moreover, these cells do not bind to antigen-coated dishes. Further studies revealed that this population has affinity for the inducing agent itself, TMA-TsF_1 (Table 3). Thus, these cells could be absorbed on petri dishes coated with TMA-TsF_1-containing splenic lysate, but not on dishes coated with similar preparations of ABA-specific TsF_1. To verify that the binding was due to the recognition of determinants associated with the TsF_1. molecule and not to other components present in the lysate material, we took advantage of the fact that TsF_1 binds the TMA ligand and bears I J^k determinant to prepare affinity reagents.[83] Either the TMA ligand or the monoclonal KY-76 (anti-I-J^k) antibody was coupled to Sepharose® 4B beads. TsF_1-containing material was then passed through either of these immunoadsorbent columns, washed, and the bound material eluted with 2 *M* KCl. The eluate and flow-through material from these immunoadsorbent columns was then used to coat petri dishes. TsF_1-induced cells were then incubated in these various dishes, and after an appropriate time, both the adherent and nonadherent populations were collected and tested for suppressor activity. Suppressor activity was only found in the adherent populations from dishes coated with eluates from the TMA and anti-I-J^k columns. Suppressor activity was not found in nonadherent populations from the same dishes. These results indicate that the TsF_1-induced T-cell population has specificity for Id associated with the TMA-binding, I-J^+, TMA-TsF_1. Since we cannot detect binding to Id^+ anti-TMA antibodies, we argue that this specificity is directed toward T-cell-associated Id which may not be found on anti-TMA antibodies. Since these TsF_1-induced cells function across H-2 and Igh barriers, the TsF_1-associated Id may, in fact, be conserved and expressed on T-cell structures among many mouse genotypes. Thus, the factor-induced Ts possess specificity and function distinct from the conventional Ts_2 heretofore described. The precise mechanisms by which these cells are preferentially induced over the Ig-Id or antigen-specific Ts_2, as well as their physiological function, are not clear. Nevertheless, the results indicate that the immune system has the potential to employ functionally different Ts subsets which communicate either by shared Ig-Id or T-cell-associated Id. The interrelationship between the two distinct pathways and their independent contribution to suppression in any given immune response is not known and will require a great deal of study before the complexities of these multiple suppressor pathways are understood.

V. PHYSIOLOGICAL SIGNIFICANCE

A. Split Suppression

It is clear from the study of Id-dominated antigen systems that Id-specific Ts_2 serve as

Table 3
TsF_1-INDUCED CELLS SPECIFICALLY BIND TO TMA-TsF_1

Material used for coating petri dishes[a]	Fractionated TsF_1-induced T cells tested	Suppression transferred (%)
Id^+ anti-TMA antibodies	Adherent	0
	Nonadherent	*76*
TMA-BSA	Adherent	14
	Nonadherent	*90*
Splenic lysate containing TMA-TsF_1	Adherent	*81*
	Nonadherent	26
Splenic lysate containing ABA-TsF_1	Adherent	26
	Nonadherent	*81*
TMA-binding TsF_1	Adherent	*90*
	Nonadherent	20
I-J^+ TMA-TsF_1	Adherent	*90*
	Nonadherent	0

Note: Normal A/J mice were injected with TMA-TsF_1 i.v. (2×10^7 cell equivalent splenic lysate per day per mouse) for 3 consecutive days and spleens were harvested on day 7.[148] The T cells were enriched by panning on anti-Ig-coated dishes and further incubated on petri dishes previously coated with indicated material. Adherent and nonadherent cells were collected and transferred i.v. into recipient mice after mixing with the required accessory T-cell population. Recipient A/J mice were primed for TMA-specific DTH responses 4 days earlier. Mice were challenged the day after the cell transfer and footpad swelling response was measured 24 hr later. Significant suppression is shown in italics.

[a] Petri dishes were coated with Id^+ anti-TMA antibodies or with TMA-BSA as described earlier.[67] Splenic cell lysates devoid of debris and membrane fractions were also used to coat the dishes. In some cases, TMA-TsF_1 was passed through either TMA-Sepharose® or m.c. KY-75 (anti-I-J^k) antibody-coupled Sepharose® column and the bound material was eluted and used for coating the dishes.

pivotal cells in suppressor networks connected by Id-anti-Id interactions. Its role in suppression of DTH responses appears to be that of a transducer cell, i.e., it bridges the inducer Ts_1 and effector Ts_3 populations. However, there is suggestive evidence that these cells can suppress Id-bearing T_{DTH} cells in the absence of a Ts_3 or Tacc cell type in an interstitial nephritis experimental model system.[78] In addition, as previously discussed in the myeloma systems, these Ts can suppress Ig production in B cells in the apparent absence of any Ts_3 or T acceptor population which normally serves as the final effector. Thus, the Ts_2 can function as a transducer or final effector cell type depending upon the nature of the target immune effector population (T or B cell) and/or the presence or absence of complementary surface Id on these cells. Furthermore, another degree of flexibility can be seen at this level. For example, in the TMA system we have demonstrated Ts_2-mediated Ab suppression[21,23] without concomitant suppression of DTH responses in mice which were previously immunized (6 weeks prior) with the monovalent antigen tyr(TMA).[98] These mice contain Id-specific Ts_2,[67] but fail to intrinsically suppress TMA-specific DTH responses.[98] These Ts_2 were capable of suppressing TMA-DTH after adoptive transfer into normal syngeneic recipients which were previously primed for TMA-DTH responses.[67] The apparent inability of the Id-specific Ts_2 to function intrinsically was not due to a compensation by Id-negative

T_{DTH}.[98] Rather, the inability of Ts_2 to function was due to the absence or functional loss of the Id-bearing Ts_3 subset in these mice. This defect was rescued by adoptively transferring TMA-binding,[139] Id-bearing, Thy-1$^+$, Lyt 1$^-$2$^+$ Ts_3[98] obtained from normal syngeneic donor mice immunized with TMA-SC. Despite the fact that these mice fail to suppress DTH and lack Ts_3 function, they were capable of inhibiting the Id$^+$ component of an induced anti-TMA antibody response.[21,23] This Id-specific suppression was mediated by the resident Ts_2 population in these mice. This situation serves to illustrate the flexibility built into the TMA-specific suppressor cascade, in that suppression at the Ts_2 level can be split, i.e., an antibody component can be down regulated while the host is still capable of mounting a DTH response.

B. Autoregulation

Since the transducer Ts_2 communicates with both the Ts_1 and Ts_3 populations through Id-anti-Id interactions, there is the potential that the Ts_2 subset plays a key role in the regulation of both Ts_1 and Ts_3. Jerne's network hypothesis[1] implies two kinds of interactions: enhancing and suppressive, as a result of a paratope-idiotope interaction which is vectorial in nature. The interactions with receptors through their paratopes are stimulatory, while interactions through the idiotopes of these same receptors are suppressive. Although there are no direct demonstrations that such stimulatory and suppressive effects occur in any of the suppressor pathways described so far, there is, however, some data to suggest that this may be the case. The fact that Id-bearing Ts_1/TsF_1 with or without antigens induce Id-specific Ts_2 may represent the stimulatory effect of these interactions. In this instance, surface Id on Ts_1 interact with the paratopes of Id-specific surface receptors on Ts_2, which results in activation. On the other hand, do mature Ts_2 down regulate the Ts_1 population through the same paratope-idiotope interaction once sufficient numbers of Ts_2 are generated? Very indirect evidence suggests that this is a possibility. As previously stated, a single inoculation of the tyr(TMA) antigen leads to the sequential appearance of Ts_1 and Ts_2 populations.[23,67] At the time when abundant Ts_2 cells can be detected, we have no evidence for the coexistence of Ts_1, leaving open the possibility that Ts_2 may play an active role in the disappearance of the Ts_1 population. We have tested in vivo whether the presence of dominant Ts_2 populations can influence Ts_1 function. Normally, the transfer of a Ts_1-containing splenic population results in the induction of an Id-specific Ts_2 population 1 week after the cell transfer.[83] However, if Ts_2 cells are first mixed with the Ts_1 population and then transferred, no Ts_2 function can be detected at the 1-week time point in the recipient mice.[96] These results suggest that Ts_1 and Ts_2 functionally neutralize each other, presumably by complementary receptor interactions. The data confirm the neutralization effect previously observed in in vitro antibody[59] and in vivo contact sensitivity systems.[68] We have no further data to explain the possible mechanisms which bring about this neutralization effect. Obviously, much work is needed to interpret this type of experiment.

Suppression of DTH responses mediated by Ts_2 depends upon a functional interaction with the Ts_3 subset. In this case, the anti-Id surface receptor on Ts_2 may serve as the mirror image of antigen[1,149-151] and interact with the paratope of the Ts_3 antigen binding surface receptor. This interaction would normally result in the activation and eventual function of the Ts_3 subset. However, it is also possible under certain conditions that the Ts_2-Ts_3 interaction could result in the down regulation of Ts_3 since the latter also bear surface Id. In this case the Ts_2 surface anti-Id receptor, rather than serve as a mirror image of antigen, interacts through its paratope with Ts_3. This interaction should result in the suppression of Ts_3 function, since the receptor on Ts_3 is stimulated through an idiotope rather than its paratope. As previously described, the Ts_3-defective-tyr(TMA)-primed mice at certain time points possess large numbers of Ts_2, but fail to intrinsically suppress DTH responses.[98] It may be that the Ts_2 are directly responsible for this failure to activate Ts_3 function. This mechanism may also be responsible for the failure to generate Ts_3 activity in these mice even after transfer of normal Ts_3 precursors and subsequent priming with TMA-SC.[139] Further work will be needed to answer whether this unique Ts lesion is directly related to the Id-specific Ts_2 dominance.

C. Other Considerations

Since Id-specific Ts_2 have been shown to suppress some aspects of myeloma function,[64,144] the question was raised whether these cells function in tumor immunity. Kresina et al.[152] have tested this question in mice transplanted with hybridomas producing Id^+ anti-ABA antibodies. The hybridomas were transferred either into normal mice or mice in which Id-specific Ts_2 cells had been generated. Interestingly, resistance to tumor growth was observed in the Ts_2-bearing mice. Although it was not clear whether resistance to the tumors was mediated solely by the Ts_2 population, the results suggest that these cells can potentially contribute to tumor resistance. On the other hand, there is a suggestion that Id-specific T cells play a significant role in tumor growth which may not be beneficial to the tumor-bearing host.[153] These cells are thought to be involved in the selection of Ig-loss variants in myeloma populations. The proliferation of Id-negative variants due to the presence of Id-specific T cells may represent one mechanism by which myelomas escape immune surveillance.

Despite the variety of systems in which Id-specific Is_2/TsF_2 have been described, including an infectious disease model,[93] interstitial nephritis,[78] and tumor systems,[144] their physiological role remains obscure. Their presence suggests an important role, particularly in the context of the Id-network theory. However, to date no definitive evidence has been presented which provides significant insight into the physiological role of these cells. What effect, if any, the absence of these cells would have on the immune system and, more importantly, on the general welfare of the organism is not known. The development of mutant strains of laboratory animals and/or the identification of abnormalities in which Id-specific Ts are absent may provide some insight into the physiological role of these cells.

REFERENCES

1. **Jerne, N. K.,** Towards a network theory of the immune system, *Ann. Immunol. (Inst. Pasteur),* 125C, 373, 1974.
2. **Eichmann, K.,** Expression and function of idiotypes on lymphocytes, *Adv. Immunol.,* 26, 195, 1978.
3. **Janeway, C. A., Sercarz, E. E., and Wigzell, H., Ed.,** *Immunoglobulin Idiotypes,* Academic Press, New York, 1981.
4. **Westen-Schnurr, I., Ed.,** *Idiotypes: Antigens on the Inside,* Editiones Roche, Basel, 1982.
5. **Bona, C. A. and Kohler, H., Eds.,** *Immune Networks, New York Academy of Science, New York,* 418, 1983.
6. **Rajewsky, K. and Takemori, T.,** Genetics, expression, and function of idiotypes, *Annu. Rev. Immunol.,* 1, 569, 1983.
7. **Kohler, H., Urbain, J., and Cazenave, P. A., Eds.,** *Idiotype in Biology and Medicine,* Academic Press, New York, 1984.
8. **Greene, M. I. and Nisonoff, A., Eds.,** *The Biology of Idiotypes,* Plenum Press, New York, 1984.
9. **Moller, G., Ed.,** Idiotypic networks, *Immunol. Rev.,* Vol. 79, 1984.
10. **Gershon, R. K.,** T cell control of antibody production, *Contemp. Top. Immunobiol.,* 3, 1, 1974.
11. **Tada, T. and Okumura, K.,** The role of antigen-specific T cell factors in the immune response, *Adv. Immunol.,* 28, 1, 1979.
12. **Germain, R. N. and Benacerraf, B.,** A single major pathway of T lymphocyte interactions in antigen-specific immune suppression, *Scand. J. Immunol.,* 13, 1, 1981.
13. **Greene, M. I., Nelles, M. J., Sy, M.-S., and Nisonoff, A.,** Regulation of immunity to the azobenzenearsonate hapten, *Adv. Immunol.,* 32, 254, 1982.
14. **Green, D. R., Flood, P. M., and Gershon, R. K.,** Immunoregulatory T-cell pathways, *Annu. Rev. Immunol.,* 1, 439, 1983.

15. **Bellone, C. J. and Jayaraman, S.,** The use of a small synthetic antigen to study immune regulation by way of idiotypes, *Ann. N.Y. Acad. Sci.*, 418, 74, 1983.
16. **Dorf, M. E. and Benacerraf, B.,** Suppressor cells and immunoregulation, *Annu. Rev. Immunol.*, 2, 127, 1984.
17. **Asherson, G. L., Colizzi, V., and Zembala, M.,** An overview of T suppressor cell circuits, *Annu. Rev. Immunol.*, 4, 37, 1986.
18. **Hart, D. A., Wang, A. L., Pawlak, L. L., and Nisonoff, A.,** Suppression of idiotypic specificities in adult mice by administration of antiidiotypic antibody, *J. Exp. Med.*, 135, 1293, 1972.
19. **Cosenza, H. and Kohler, H.,** Specific suppression of the antibody response by antibodies to receptors, *Proc. Natl. Acad. Sci. U.S.A.*, 69, 2701, 1972.
20. **Eichmann, K.,** Idiotype suppression. I. Influence of the dose and of the effector functions of anti-idiotypic antibody on the production of an idiotype, *Eur. J. Immunol.*, 4, 296, 1974.
21. **Alevy, Y. G. and Bellone, C. J.,** Antiphenyltrimethylamino immunity in mice. II. L-tyrosine-p-azophenyltrimethylammonium-induced suppressor T cells selectively inhibit the expression of B-cell clones bearing a cross-reactive idiotype, *J. Exp. Med.*, 151, 528, 1980.
22. **Takemori, T. and Rajewsky, K.,** Specificity, duration and mechanism of idiotype suppression induced by neonatal injection of monoclonal anti-idiotope antibodies into mice, *Eur. J. Immunol.*, 14, 656, 1984.
23. **Jayaraman, S. and Bellone, C. J.,** Hapten-specific responses to the phenyltrimethylamino hapten. IV. Occurrence of mechanistically distinct idiotypic suppressor T cells before the appearance of anti-idiotypic suppressor T cells induced by the monovalent antigen L-tyrosine-p-azophenyltrimethylammonium, *J. Immunol.*, 130, 2519, 1983.
24. **Benjamin, D. C. and Teale, M.,** Tolerance to azobenzenearsonate: preferential loss of the major normal cross-reactive idiotype, *J. Immunol.*, 120, 202, 1978.
25. **Caulfield, M. J., Luce, K. J., Proffitt, M. R., and Cerny, J.,** Induction of idiotype-specific suppressor T cells with antigen/antibody complexes, *J. Exp. Med.*, 157, 1713, 1983.
26. **Kim, B. S.,** Mechanisms of idiotype suppression. I. *In vitro* generation of idiotype-specific suppressor T cells by anti-idiotype antibodies and specific antigen, *J. Exp. Med.*, 149, 1371, 1979.
27. **McKearn, J. P. and Quintans, J.,** Idiotype-specific tolerance: preferential alteration of idiotype expression after neonatal exposure to tolerogen, *J. Immunol.*, 124, 1983, 1980.
28. **Tokuhisa, T. and Rajewsky, K.,** Antigen induces chronic idiotype suppression, *Proc. Natl. Acad. Sci. U.S.A.*, 82, 4217, 1985.
29. **Nakanishi, K., Sugimura, K., Yaunta, Y., Maeda, K., Kashiwamura, S. I., Honjo, T., and Kishimoto, T.,** A T15-idiotype-positive T suppressor hybridoma does not use the T15 V_H gene segment, *Proc. Natl. Acad. Sci. U.S.A.*, 79, 6984, 1982.
30. **Kraig, E., Kronenberg, M., Kapp, J. A., Pierce, C. W., Abruzzini, A. F., Sorensen, G. M., Samelson, L. E., Schwartz, R. H., and Hood, L. E.,** T and B cells that recognize the same antigen do not transcribe similar heavy chain variable region gene segments, *J. Exp. Med.*, 158, 192, 1983.
31. **Binz, H. and Wigzell, H.,** Antigen-binding, idiotypic T-lymphocyte receptors, *Contemp. Top. Immunobiol.*, 7, 113, 1977.
32. **Eichmann, K. and Rajewsky, K.,** Induction of T and B cell immunity by anti-idiotypic antibody, *Eur. J. Immunol.*, 5, 661, 1975.
32. **Julius, M. H., Cosenza, H., and Augustin, A. A.,** Evidence for the endogenous production of T cell receptors bearing idiotypic determinants, *Eur. J. Immunol.*, 8, 484, 1978.
34. **Frischknecht, H., Binz, H., and Wigzell, H.,** Induction of specific transplantation immune reactions using anti-idiotypic antibodies, *J. Exp. Med.*, 147, 506, 1978.
35. **Sy, M.-S., Brown, A. R., Benacerraf, B., and Greene, M. I.,** Antigen- and receptor-driven regulatory mechanisms. III. Induction of delayed-type hypersensitivity to azobenzenearsonate with anti-cross-reactive idiotypic antibodies, *J. Exp. Med.*, 151, 896, 1980.
36. **Strassman, G., Lifshitz, R., and Mozes, E.,** Elicitation of delayed-type hypersensitivity responses to poly (L Tyr, L Glu)-poly (DL Ala)-poly (1 Lys) by anti-idiotypic antibodies, *J. Exp. Med.*, 152, 1448, 1980.
37. **Thomas, W. R., Morahan, A., Walker, I. D., and Miller, J. F. A. P.,** Induction of delayed-type hypersensitivity to azobenzenearsonate by a monoclonal anti-idiotype antibody, *J. Exp. Med.*, 153, 743, 1981.
38. **Jayaraman, S. and Bellone, C. J.,** Hapten-specific responses to the phenyltrimethylamino hapten. I. Evidence for idiotype-anti-idiotype interactions in delayed-type hypersensitivity in mice, *Eur. J. Immunol.*, 12, 272, 1982.
39. **Arnold, B., Wallich, R., and Hammerling, G. J.,** Elicitation of delayed-type hypersensitivity to phosphorylcholine by monoclonal anti-idiotypic antibodies in an allogeneic environment, *J. Exp. Med.*, 156, 670, 1982.
40. **Kohler, H. and Bona, C.,** Idiotype vaccines, *Int. Rev. Immunol.*, Vol. 1, 1986.

41. **Eichmann, K.,** Idiotype suppression. II. Amplification of a suppressor T cell with anti-idiotypic activity, *Eur. J. Immunol.,* 5, 511, 1975.
42. **Boltomly, K., Mathieson, B. J., and Mosier, D. E.,** Anti-idiotype induced regulation of helper cell function for the response to phosphorylcholine in adult BALB/c mice, *J. Exp. Med.,* 148, 1216, 1978.
43. **Yamamoto, H., Nonaka, M., and Katz, D. H.,** Suppression of hapten-specific delayed-type hypersensitivity responses in mice by idiotype-specific suppressor T cells after administration of anti-idiotypic antibodies, *J. Exp. Med.,* 150, 818, 1979.
44. **Sy, M.-S., Bach, B. A., Dohi, Y., Nisonoff, A., Benacerraf, B., and Greene, M. I.,** Antigen and receptor driven regulatory mechanisms. I. Induction of suppressor T cells with anti-idiotypic antibodies, *J. Exp. Med.,* 150, 1216, 1979.
45. **Thomas, W. R., Morahan, G., and Miller, J. F. A. P.,** Induction of suppressor T cells by monoclonal anti-idiotype antibody in strains of mice not expressing the idiotope in hyperimmune serum, *J. Immunol.,* 130, 2079, 1983.
46. **Cerny, J., Cronkhite, R., and Heusser, C.,** Antibody response of mice following neonatal treatment with a monoclonal anti-receptor antibody. Evidence for B cell tolerance and T suppressor cells specific for different idiotopic determinants, *Eur. J. Immunol.,* 13, 244, 1983.
47. **Bona, C., Lieberman, R., House, S., Green, I., and Paul, W. E.,** Immune response to leven. II. T independence of suppression of cross-reactive idiotypes by anti-idiotype antibodies, *J. Immunol.,* 122, 1614, 1979.
48. **Heusser, C. H., Etlinger, H. M., and Julius, M. H.,** Thymus-independent induction and antigen-dependent recovery of idiotype-specific suppression, *Cell. Immunol.,* 76, 148, 1983.
49. **Rothstein, T. L., Miller, R. A., Parker, D. J., Kelly, E., Vastola, A. P., and Marshak-Rothstein, A.,** Induction of idiotype suppression in the anti-azophenylarsonate response of T-depleted A/J mice, *J. Exp. Med.,* 159, 1283, 1984.
50. **Bangassar, S. A., Kapasalis, A. A., Frake, P. J., and Nisonoff, A.,** Competition for antigen by cell populations having receptors with the same specificity but of different idiotype, *J. Immunol.,* 114, 610, 1975.
51. **Eig, B., Ju, S. T., and Nisonoff, A.,** Complete inhibition of the expression of an idiotype by a mechanism of B cell dominance, *J. Exp. Med.,* 145, 1574, 1977.
52. **Ward, K., Cantor, H., and Nisonoff, A.,** Analysis of the cellular basis of idiotype-specific suppression, *J. Immunol.,* 120, 2016, 1978.
53. **Hetzelberger, D. and Eichmann, K.,** Idiotype suppression. III. Induction of unresponsiveness to sensitization with anti-idiotypic antibody: identification of the cell types tolerized in high zone and in low zone, suppressor cell-mediated, idiotype suppression, *Eur. J. Immunol.,* 8, 839, 1978.
54. **Woodland, R. and Cantor, H.,** Idiotype-specific T helper cells are required to induce idiotype-positive B memory cells to secrete antibody, *Eur. J. Immunol.,* 8, 600, 1978.
55. **Owen, F. L., Ju, S. T., and Nisonoff, A.,** Binding to idiotypic determinants of large proportions of thymus-derived lymphocytes in idiotypically suppressed mice, *Proc. Natl. Acad. Sci. U.S.A.,* 74, 2084, 1977.
56. **Owen, F. L., Ju, S. T., and Nisonoff, A.,** Presence of idiotype-specific suppressor T cells of receptors that interact with molecules bearing the idiotype, *J. Exp. Med.,* 145, 1559, 1977.
57. **Owen, F. L. and Nisonoff, A.,** Effect of idiotype specific suppressor T cells on primary and secondary responses, *J. Exp. Med.,* 148, 182, 1978.
58. **Hammerling, G. J. and Eichmann, K.,** Expression of Ia determinants on immunocompetent cells, *Eur. J. Immunol.,* 6, 565, 1976.
59. **Kim, B. S. and Greenberg, J. A.,** Mechanisms of idiotype suppression. IV. Functional neutralization in mixtures of idiotype-specific suppressor and hapten-specific suppressor T cells, *J. Exp. Med.,* 154, 809, 1981.
60. **Kim, B. S. and Massey, P. B.,** Induction of T15-specific suppressor T cells in mice with the CBA/N defect by neonatal injection with anti-T15 idiotype antibody, *J. Immunol.,* 128, 1145, 1982.
61. **Bona, C. and Paul, W. E.,** Cellular basis of regulation of expression of idiotype. I. T-suppressor cells specific for MOPC 460 idiotype regulate the expression of cells secreting anti-TNP antibodies bearing 460 idiotype, *J. Exp. Med.,* 149, 592, 1979.
62. **Sy, M.-S., Bach, B. A., Brown, A., Nisonoff, A., Benacerraf, B., and Greene, M. I.,** Antigen- and receptor-driven regulatory mechanisms. II. Induction of suppressor T cells with idiotype-coupled syngeneic spleen cells, *J. Exp. Med.,* 150, 1229, 1979.
63. **Dohi, Y. and Nisonoff, A.,** Suppression of idiotype and generation of suppressor T cells with idiotype-conjugated thymocytes, *J. Exp. Med.,* 150, 909, 1979.
64. **Abbas, A. K., Perry, L. L., Bach, B. A., and Greene, M. I.,** Idiotype-specific T cell immunity. I. Generation of effector and suppressor T lymphocytes reactive with myeloma idiotypic determinants, *J. Immunol.,* 124, 1160, 1980.

65. **Sy, M.-S., Dietz, M. H., Germain, R. N., Benacerraf, B., and Greene, M. I.,** Antigen- and receptor-driven regulatory mechanisms. IV. Idiotype-bearing I-J$^+$ suppressor T cell factors induce second-order suppressor T cells which express anti-idiotypic receptors, *J. Exp. Med.*, 151, 1183, 1980.
66. **Deitz, M. H., Sy, M.-S., Benacerraf, B., Nisonoff, A., Greene, M. I., and Germain, R. N.,** Antigen- and receptor-driven regulatory mechanisms. VII. H-2-restricted anti-idiotypic suppressor factor from efferent suppressor T cells, *J. Exp. Med.*, 153, 450, 1981.
67. **Jayaraman, S. and Bellone, C. J.,** Hapten-specific responses to the phenyltrimethylamino hapten. II. Regulation of delayed-type hypersensitivity by genetically restricted, anti-idiotypic suppressor T cells induced by the monovalent antigen L-tyrosine-p-azophenyltrimethylammonium, *Eur. J. Immunol.*, 12, 278, 1982.
68. **Miller, S. D., Butler, L. D., and Claman, H. N.,** Suppressor T cell circuits in contact sensitivity. I. Two mechanistically distinct waves of suppressor T cells occur in mice tolerized with syngeneic DNP-modified lymphoid cells, *J. Immunol.*, 129, 461, 1982.
69. **Weinberger, J. Z., Germain, R. N., Benacerraf, B., and Dorf, M. E.,** Hapten-specific T cell responses to 4-hydroxy-3-nitrophenyl acetyl. V. Role of idiotypes in the suppressor pathway, *J. Exp. Med.*, 152, 161, 1980.
70. **Sherr, D. H. and Dorf, M. E.,** Hapten-specific T cell responses to 4-hydroxy-3-nitrophenyl acetyl. IX. Characterization of idiotype-specific effector-phase suppressor cells on plaque-forming cell responses *in vitro*, *J. Exp. Med.*, 153, 1445, 1981.
71. **Sherr, D. H., Ju, S.-T., and Dorf, M. E.,** Hapten-specific T cell responses to 4-hydroxy-3-nitrophenyl acetyl. XII. Fine specificity of anti-idiotypic suppressor T cells (Ts_2), *J. Exp. Med.*, 154, 1382, 1981.
72. **Sherr, D. H. and Dorf, M. E.,** Hapten-specific T cell responses to 4-hydroxy-3-nitrophenyl acetyl. XIII. Characterizaton of a third T cell population involved in suppression of *in vitro* PFC responses, *J. Immunol.*, 128, 1261, 1982.
73. **Taniguchi, N., Usui, M., Okuda, K., and Matuhasi, T.,** Hapten-pullulan conjugate-induced CMI suppression: demonstration of a common pathway of suppressor cells involving idiotypic interactions, *J. Immunol.*, 129, 1816, 1982.
74. **Flood, P. M., Philipps, C., Taupier, M. A., and Schreiber, H.,** Regulation of myeloma growth *in vitro* by idiotype-specific T lymphocytes, *J. Immunol.*, 124, 424, 1980.
75. **Abbas, A. K., Takaoki, M., and Greene, M. I.,** T lymphocyte-mediated suppression of myeloma function *in vitro*. IV. Generation of effector suppressor cells specific for myeloma idiotypes, *J. Exp. Med.*, 155, 1216, 1982.
76. **Milburn, G. L. and Lynch, R. G.,** Immunoregulation of murine myeloma *in vitro*. II. Suppression of MOPC-315 immunoglobulin secretion and synthesis of idiotype-specific suppressor T cells, *J. Exp. Med.*, 155, 852, 1982.
77. **Sherr, D. H. and Dorf, M. E.,** Characterization of anti-idiotypic suppressor T cells (Tsid) induced after antigen priming, *J. Immunol.*, 133, 1142, 1984.
78. **Neilson, E. A., McCafferty, E., Mann, R., Michaud, L., and Clayman, M.,** Tubular antigen-derivatized cells induce a disease-protective, antigen-specific, and idiotype-specific suppressor T cell network restricted by I-J and Igh-V in mice with experimental interstitial nephritis, *J. Exp. Med.*, 162, 215, 1985.
79. **Hirai, Y. and Nisonoff, A.,** Selective suppression of the major idiotypic component of an antihapten response by soluble T cell-derived factors with idiotypic or anti-idiotypic receptors, *J. Exp. Med.*, 151, 1213, 1980.
80. **Minami, M., Okuda, K., Furusawa, S., Benacerraf, B., and Dorf, M. E.,** Analysis of T cell hybridomas. I. Characterization of H-2- and Igh-restricted monoclonal suppressor factors, *J. Exp. Med.*, 154, 1390, 1981.
81. **Sherr, D. H., Ju, S. T., Weinberger, J. Z., Benacerraf, B., and Dorf, M. E.,** Hapten-specific T cell responses to 4-hydroxy-3-nitrophenyl acetyl. VII. Idiotype-specific suppression of plaque-forming cell responses, *J. Exp. Med.*, 153, 640, 1981.
82. **Sunday, M. E., Benacerraf, B., and Dorf, M. E.,** Hapten-specific T cell responses to 4-hydroxy-3-nitrophenyl acetyl. VIII. Suppressor cell pathways in cutaneous sensitivity responses, *J. Exp. Med.*, 153, 811, 1981.
83. **Jayaraman, S. and Bellone, C. J.,** Hapten-specific responses to the phenyltrimethylamino hapten. V. A single chain antigen-binding I-J$^+$ first-order T suppressor factor requires antigen to induce anti-idiotypic second-order suppressor T cells, *J. Immunol.*, 134, 1010, 1985.
84. **Jayaraman, S. and Bellone, C. J.,** Interaction of idiotype-specific third-order T suppressor subset results in antigen-nonspecific suppression, *Cell Immunol.*, 101, 72, 1986.
85. **Jayaraman, S. and Bellone, C. J.,** Idiotype-specific T suppressor factor alternatively interacts with a nonspecific T acceptor-like cell to mediate immune suppression, *Cell. Immunol.*, 101, 363, 1986.

86. **Gorczynski, R. M., Kennedy, M., Khomasurya, B., MacRae, S., and Cunningham., A. J.,** Individual-specific (idiotypic) T-B cell interactions regulating the production of anti-2,4,6-trinitrophenyl antibody. I. Generation of suppressor T cells and antibody directed against immunocompetent cells, *Eur. J. Immunol.*, 10, 781, 1980.
87. **Gorczynski, R. M., Khomasurya, B., Kennedy, M., MacRae, S., and Cunningham, A. J.,** Individual-specific (idiotypic) T-B cell interactions regulating the production of anti-2,4,6-trinitrophenyl antibody. II. Developement of idiotype-specific helper and suppressor T cells within mice making an immune response, *Eur. J. Immunol.*, 10, 788, 1980.
88. **Braley-Mullen, H.,** Activation of distinct subsets of T suppressor cells with type III pneumococcal polysaccharide coupled to syngeneic spleen cells, *Ann. N.Y. Acad. Sci.*, 392, 165, 1982.
89. **Malley, A. and Dresser, D. W.,** Regulation of timothy grass pollen IgE antibody formation. I. In-vitro induction of suppressor T cells by soulble T suppressor factors, *Immunology*, 49, 463, 1983.
90. **Sakato, N., Semma, M., Eisen, H. N., and Azuma, T.,** A small hypervariable segment in the variable domain of an immunoglobulin light chain stimulates formation of anti-idiotypic suppressor T cells, *Proc. Natl. Acad. Sci. U.S.A.*, 79, 5396, 1982.
91. **Rohrer, J. W., Odermatt, B., and Lynch, R. G.,** Immunoregulation of murine myeloma: isologous immunization with M315 induces idiotype-specific T cells that suppress IgA secretion by MOPC-315 cells *in vivo, J. Immunol.*, 122, 2011, 1979.
92. **Grouix, B. and Scott, D. W.,** Role of self carriers in the immune response and tolerance. VIII. Suppression of the MOPC-104E idiotypic response by idiotype-modified self, but not by dextran-modified self, *J. Immunol.*, 130, 86, 1983.
93. **Abe, T. and Colley, D. G.,** Modulation of *Schistosoma mansoni* egg-induced granuloma formation. III. Evidence for an anti-idiotypic, I-J-positive, I-J-restricted, soluble T suppressor factor, *J. Immunol.*, 132, 2084, 1984.
94. **Okuda, K., Minami, M., Sherr, D. H., and Dorf, M. E.,** Hapten-specific T cell responses to 4-hydroxy-3-nitrophenyl acetyl. XI. Pseudogenetic restrictions of hybridoma suppressor factors, *J. Exp. Med.*, 154, 468, 1981.
95. **Aoki, I., Minami, M., and Dorf, M. E.,** A mechanism responsible for the induction of H-2 restricted second order suppressor T cells, *J. Exp. Med.*, 157, 1726, 1983.
96. **Jayaraman, S. and Bellone, C. J.,** unpublished data, 1986.
97. **Sy, M.-S., Nisonoff, A., Germain, R. N., Benacerraf, B., and Greene, M. I.,** Antigen- and receptor-driven regulatory mechanisms. VIII. Suppression of idiotype-negative p-azobenzenearsonate-specific T cells results from the interaction of an anti-idiotype second-order T suppressor cell with a cross-reactive-idiotype-positive, p-azobenzenearsonate-primed T cell target, *J. Exp. Med.*, 153, 1415, 1981.
98. **Jayaraman, S. and Bellone, C. J.,** Hapten-specific responses to the phenyltrimethylamino hapten. III. Mice whose delayed-type hypersensitivity responses cannot be abrogated by the presence of anti-idiotypic suppressor T cells lack a critical modulatory T cell function, *J. Exp. Med.*, 155, 1810, 1982.
99. **Takaoki, M., Sy, M.-S., Tominaga, A., Lowy, A., Tsurufuji, M., Finberg, R., Benacerraf, B., and Greene, M. I.,** I-J-restricted interactions in the generation of azobenzenearsonate-specific suppressor T cells, *J. Exp. Med.*, 156, 1325, 1982.
100. **Minami, M., Honji, N., and Dorf, M. E.,** Mechanism responsible for the induction of I-J restrictions on Ts_3 suppressor cells, *J. Exp. Med.*, 156, 1502, 1982.
101. **Minami, M., Furusawa, S., and Dorf, M. E.,** I-J restrictions on the activation and interaction of parental and F_1-derived Ts_3 suppressor cells, *J. Exp. Med.*, 156, 465, 1982.
102. **Sherr, D. H., Minami, M., Okuda, K., and Dorf, M. E.,** Analysis of T cell hybridomas. III. Distinctions between two types of hapten-specific suppressor factors that affect plaque-forming cell responses, *J. Exp. Med.*, 157, 515, 1983.
103. **Sy, M.-S., Dietz, M. H., Nisonoff, A., Germain, R. N., Benacerraf, B., and Greene, M. I.,** Antigen- and receptor-driven regulatory mechanisms. V. The failure of idiotype-coupled spleen cells to induce unresponsiveness in animals lacking the appropriate V_H genes is caused by the lack of idiotype-match targets, *J. Exp. Med.*, 152, 1226, 1980.
104. **Hirai, Y., Lamoyi, E., Dohi, Y., and Nisonoff, A.,** Regulation of expression of a family of cross-reactive idiotypes, *J. Immunol.*, 126, 71, 1981.
105. **Hirai, Y., Sy, M.-S., Grene, M. I., and Nisonoff, A.,** Suppressor T cells induced by idiotype-coupled cells function across an allotype barrier, *J. Immunol.*, 126, 2064, 1981.
106. **Tada, T.,** Regulation of the antibody response by T cell products determined by different I subregions, in *The Immune System: Genetics and Regulation,* Sercarz, E. E., Herzenberg, L. A., and Fox, C. G., Eds., Academic Press, New York, 1977, 345.
107. **Waltenbaugh, C., Theze, J., Kapp, J. A., and Benacerraf, B.,** Immunosuppressive factor(s) specific for L-glutamic acid^{50}-L-tyrosine^{50} (GT). III. Generation of suppressor T cells by a suppressive extract derived from GT-primed lymphoid cells, *J. Exp. Med.*, 146, 970, 1977.

108. **Germain, R. N., Theze, J., Kapp, J. A., and Benacerraf, B.,** Antigen-specific T-cell-mediated suppression. I. Induction of L-glutamic acid^{60}-L-alanine^{30}-L-tyrosine^{10} specific suppressor T cells in vitro requires both antigen-specific T-cell-suppressor factor and antigen, *J. Exp. Med.*, 147, 123, 1978.
109. **Cantor, H. and Gershon, R. K.,** Immunological circuits: cellular composition, *Fed. Proc. Fed. Am. Soc. Exp. Biol.*, 38, 2058, 1979.
110. **Alevy, Y. G., Witherspoon, C., and Bellone, C. J.,** Anti-TMA immunity in mice. III. Induction of L-tyrosine-p-azophenyltrimethylammonium [tyr(TMA)]-specific helper T cells by the monovalent antigen or idiotypic antisera, *J. Immunol.*, 126, 2390, 1981.
111. **Takaoki, M., Sy, M.-S., Whitaker, B., Nepom, J., Finberg, R., Germain, R. N., Nisonoff, A., Benacerraf, B., and Greene, M. I.,** Biologic activity of an idiotype-bearing suppressor T cell factor produced by a long-term T cell hybridoma, *J. Immunol.*, 128, 49, 1982.
112. **Jayaraman, S. and Bellone, C. J.,** The role of idiotypic determinants in syngeneic and allogeneic immune suppression, *Fed. Proc. Fed. Am. Soc. Exp. Biol. Abstr.*, 43, 1799, 1984.
113. **Tsurufuji, M., Benacerraf, B., and Sy, M.-S.,** An antigen-specific signal is required for the activation of second-order suppressor T cells in the regulation of delayed-type hypersensitivity to 2,4,6-trinitrobenzene sulfonic acid, *J. Exp. Med.*, 158, 932, 1983.
114. **Adorini, L., Colizzi, V., Doria, G., and Ricciardi-Castagnoli, P.,** Immunoregulation of lysozyme-specific suppression. II. Hen egg-white lysozyme-specific monoclonal suppressor T cell factor suppresses the afferent phase of delayed-type hypersensitivity and induces second-order suppressor T cells, *Eur. J. Immunol.*, 14, 826, 1984.
115. **L'age-Stehr, J., Teichmann, H., Gershon, R. K., and Cantor, H.,** Stimulation of regulatory T cell circuits by immunoglobulin-dependent structures on activated B cells, *Eur. J. Immunol.*, 10, 21, 1980.
116. **Calkins, C. E.,** Interactions between primed and unprimed cells in the regulation of *in vitro* antibody responses. I. Role of "plasma cells" as inducers of suppression, *Eur. J. Immunol.*, 12, 70, 1982.
117. **Shimamma, T., Hashimoto, K., and Sasaki, S.,** Feedback suppression of the immune response *in vivo*. I. Immune B cells induce antigen-specific suppressor T cells, *Cell. Immunol.*, 68, 104, 1982.
118. **Taylor, C. E., Stashak, P. W., Caldes, G., Prescott, B., Chused, T. E., Brooks, A., and Baker, P. J.,** Activation of antigen-specific suppressor T cells by B cells from mice immunized with type III pneumococcal polysaccharide, *J. Exp. Med.*, 158, 703, 1983.
119. **Sy, M.-S., Lowy, A., HayGlass, K., Janeway, C. A., Jr., Gurish, M., Greene, M. I., and Benacerraf, B.,** Chronic treatment with rabbit anti-mouse μ-chain antibody alters the characteristic immunoglobulin heavy-chain restriction of murine suppressor T-cell factors, *Proc. Natl. Acad. Sci.*, 81, 3846, 1984.
120. **Usui, M., Ju, S.-T., and Dorf, M. E.,** The expression of idiotypic determinants on suppressor T cells is independent of T cell Igh phenotype, *J. Mol. Cell. Immunol.*, 1, 293, 1984.
121. **Flood, P. M., Janeway, C. A., Jr., and Gershon, R. K.,** B cell-deprived mice lack functional expression of certain T suppressor cell subsets, *J. Mol. Cell. Immunol.*, 1, 167, 1984.
122. **Prange, C. A., Green, C., Nitecki, D. E., and Bellone, C. J.,** Antigen-binding lymphocytes in guinea pigs. I. B cell expansion to the monovalent antigen L-tyrosine-p-azophenyltrimethylammonium (tyr(TMA)) in the absence of antibody production, *J. Immunol.*, 118, 1311, 1977.
123. **Lowy, A., Flood, P. M., Tominaga, A., Drebin, J. A., Dambrauskas, J., Gershon, R. K., and Greene, M. I.,** Analysis of hapten-specific T suppressor factors: genetic restriction of TsF_1 activity analyzed with synthetic hybrid suppressor molecules, *J. Immunol.*, 132, 640, 1984.
124. **Weinberger, J. Z., Germain, R. N., Ju, S. T., Greene, M. I., Benacerraf, B., and Dorf, M. E.,** Hapten-specific T-cell responses to 4-hydroxy-3-nitrophenyl acetyl. II. Demonstration of idiotypic determinants on suppressor T cells, *J. Exp. Med.*, 150, 761, 1979.
125. **Kapp, J. A. and Araneo, B.,** Antigen-specific suppressor T cell interaction. I. Induction of an MHC-restricted suppressor factor specific for L-glutamic acid^{50}-L-tyrosine^{50}, *J. Immunol.*, 128, 2447, 1982.
126. **Lei, H-Y. and Waltenbaugh, C.,** Regulation of immune responses by I-J gene products. IV. Distinct suppressor factors derived from "nonresponder" A strain mice, *J. Immunol.*, 133, 1723, 1984.
127. **Poon, R. Y. M., Kapp, J. A., Pierce, C. W., and Sorensen, C. M.,** Characterization of two monoclonal idiotype-binding suppressor T cell factors specific for the antibody response to L-glutamic acid^{60}-L-alanine^{30}-L-tyrosine^{10} (GAT). *J. Immunol.*, 137, 3709, 1986.
128. **Sy, M.-S., Miller, S. D., Moorhead, J. W., and Claman, H. N.,** Active suppression of 1-fluro-2,4-dinitrobenzene-immune T cells. Requirement of an auxiliary T cell induced by antigen, *J. Exp. Med.*, 149, 1197, 1979.
129. **Miller, S. D., Butler, L. D., and Claman, H. N.,** The role of suppressor T cell networks in the regulation of DNFB contact sensitivity. Receptor-anti-receptor interactions in efferent suppression, *Ann. N.Y. Acad. Sci.*, 392, 122, 1982.
130. **Weinberger, J. Z., Benacerraf, B., and Dorf, M. E.,** Hapten-specific T cell responses to 4-hydroxy-3-nitrophenyl acetyl. IV. Interaction of effector suppressor T cells is restricted by H-2 and Igh-V genes, *J. Exp. Med.*, 151, 1413, 1980.

131. **Usui, M., Aoki, I., Sunshine, G. H., and Dorf, M. E.,** Requirements for suppressor T cell activation, *J. Immunol.,* 133, 1137, 1984.
132. **Alevy, Y. G., Witherspoon, C. D., Prange, C. A., and Bellone, C. J.,** Anti-TMA immunity in mice. I. The appearance of cross-reactive idiotype(s) to the trimethylammonium (TMA) hapten in A/J mice, *J. Immunol.,* 124, 215, 1980.
133. **Okuda, K., Minami, M., Furusawa, S., and Dorf, M. E.,** Analysis of T cell hybridomas. II. Comparisons among three distinct types of monoclonal suppressor factors, *J. Exp. Med.,* 154, 1838, 1981.
134. **Asherson, G. L., Dorf, M. E., Colizzi, V., Zembala, M., and James, B. M. B.,** Equivalence of conventional anti-picryl T suppressor factor in the contact sensitivity system and monoclonal anti-NP TsF_3: their final nonspecific effect via the T acceptor cell, *Immunology,* 53, 491, 1984.
135. **Zembala, M., Asherson, G. L., and Colizzi, V.,** Hapten-specific T suppressor factor recognizes both hapten and I-J region products on haptenized spleen cells, *Nature (London),* 297, 411, 1982.
136. **Zembala, M., Asherson, G. L., James, B. M. B., Stein, V. E., and Watkins, M. C.,** Anti-haptene T suppressor factor acts through an $I\text{-}J^+$, $Ly1^-2^+$, T acceptor cell that releases a nonspecific inhibitor of the transfer of contact sensitivity when exposed to antigen, *J. Immunol.,* 129, 1823, 1982.
137. **Asherson, G. L., Colizzi, V., Zembala, M., James, B. B. M., and Watkins, M. C.,** Nonspecific inhibitor of contact sensitivity made by T-acceptor cells: triggering of T cells armed with antigen-specific T-suppressor factor (TsF) requires both occupancy of the major histocompatibility complex recognition site by soluble I-J product and cross-linking of the antigen recognition sites of the TsF, *Cell. Immunol.,* 83, 389, 1984.
138. **Zembala, M., Colizzi, V., Asherson, G. L., and Watkins, M. C.,** Non-specific inhibitor made by T acceptor cells inhibits both the afferent and efferent stage of the contact sensitivity reaction, *Immunology,* 52, 599, 1984.
139. **Jayaraman, S. and Bellone, C. J.,** The use of nonspecific T acceptor cells to overcome the aberrant function of antigen-specific third-order T suppressor cells, *Cell. Immunol.,* 107, 326, 1977.
140. **Moser, A., Tominaga, A., Greene, M. I., and Abbas, A. K.,** Accessory cells in immune suppression. I. Role of $I\text{-}A^+$ accessory cells in effector phase idiotype-specific suppression of myeloma function, *J. Immunol.,* 131, 1728, 1983.
141. **Moser, G., Kauffman, M. G., and Abbas, A. K.,** Accessory cells in immune suppression. II. Evidence for presentation of idiotype-specific suppressor factors to B cell targets by $I\text{-}A^+$ accessory cells, *J. Immunol.,* 134, 2867, 1985.
142. **Parslow, T. G., Milburn, G. L., Lynch, R. G., and Granner, D. K.,** Suppressor T cell action inhibits the expression of an excluded immunoglobulin gene, *Science,* 220, 1389, 1983.
143. **Milburn, G. L., Parslow, T. G., Goldenberg, C., Granner, D. K., and Lynch, R. G.,** Idiotype-specific T cell suppression of light chain mRNA expression in MOPC-315 cells is accompanied by a posttranscriptional inhibition of heavy chain expression, *J. Mol. Cell. Immunol.,* 1, 115, 1984.
144. **Lynch, R. G. and Milburn, G. L.,** The use of myeloma cells to study immunoregulatory mechanisms, *Immunol. Today,* 4, 326, 1983.
145. **Rohrer, J. W., Odermatt, B., and Lynch, R. G.,** Idiotype-specific suppression of MOPC-315 IgA secretion *in vivo:* reversible blockade of secretory myeloma cells by soluble mediators, *J. Immunol.,* 121, 1799, 1978.
146. **Milburn, G. L. and Lynch, R. G.,** Anti-idiotypic regulation of IgA expression in myeloma cells, *Mol. Immunol.,* 20, 931, 1983.
147. **Abbas, A. K., Burakoff, S. J., Gefter, M. L., and Greene, M. I.,** T lymphcyte-mediated suppression of myeloma function *in vitro.* III. Regulation of antibody production in hybrid myeloma cells by lymphocytes, *J. Exp. Med.,* 152, 969, 1980.
148. **Jayaraman, S. and Bellone, C. J.,** A novel suppressive activity: complementation between a T cell induced with first-order T suppressor factor and an I-J restricted antigen-nonspecific T cell, *Cell. Immunol.,* 101, 351, 1986.
149. **Lindenmann, J.,** Speculations on idiotypes and homobodies, *Ann. Immunol. (Inst. Pasteur),* 124C, 171, 1973.
150. **Lindenmann, J.,** Homobodies: do they exist?, *Ann. Immunol. (Inst. Pasteur),* 130C, 311, 1979.
151. **Jerne, N. K., Roland, J., and Cazenave, P.-A.,** Recurrent idiotopes and internal images, *EMBO J.,* 1, 243, 1982.
152. **Kresina, T., Baine, Y., and Nisonoff, A.,** Adoptive transfer of resistance to growth of an idiotype-secreting hybridoma by T cells from idiotypically suppressed mice, *J. Immunol.,* 130, 1478, 1983.
153. **Ghosh, S. K. and Bankert, R. B.,** Generation of heavy chain-loss mutants in a B cell hybrid mediated by syngeneic idiotype-specific spleen cells, *J. Immunol.,* 133, 1677, 1984.

INDEX

A

B

C

D

E

F

J

K

L